HIKE LIST

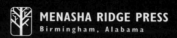

MENASHA RIDGE PRESS
Birmingham, Alabama

60 HIKES
WITHIN 60 MILES

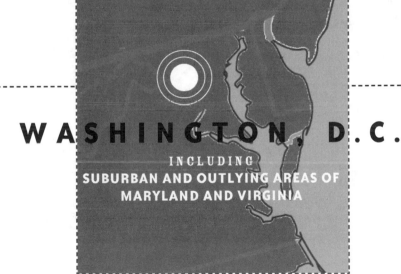

WASHINGTON, D.C.

INCLUDING
SUBURBAN AND OUTLYING AREAS OF
MARYLAND AND VIRGINIA

SECOND EDITION

PAUL ELLIOTT

DISCLAIMER

This book is meant only as a guide to select trails in the Washington, D.C., area and does not guarantee hiker safety in any way—you hike at your own risk. Neither Menasha Ridge Press nor Paul Elliott is liable for property loss or damage, personal injury, or death that result in any way from accessing or hiking the trails described in the following pages. Please be aware that hikers have been injured in the Washington area. Be especially cautious when walking on or near boulders, steep inclines, and drop-offs, and do not attempt to explore terrain that may be beyond your abilities. To help ensure an uneventful hike, please read carefully the introduction to this book, and perhaps get further safety information and guidance from other sources. Familiarize yourself thoroughly with the areas you intend to visit before venturing out. Ask questions, and prepare for the unforeseen. Familiarize yourself with current weather reports, maps of the area you intend to visit, and any relevant park regulations.

Copyright © 2007 Paul Elliott
All rights reserved
Printed in the United States of America
Published by Menasha Ridge Press
Distributed by Publishers Group West
Second edition, fourth printing 2010

Library of Congress Cataloging-in-Publication Data

Elliott, Paul, 1955–
    60 hikes within 60 miles, Washington, D.C.: including suburban and outlying areas
of Maryland and Virginia/by Paul Elliott.—2nd ed.
        p. cm.
    ISBN 13: 978-0-89732-555-4
    ISBN 10: 0-89732-555-9
        1. Hiking—Washington Region—Guidebooks. 2. Washington Region—
    Guidebooks. I. Title: Sixty hikes within sixty miles, Washington, D.C. II. Title.

GV199.42.W17 E44 2005
917.5304'42—dc22

                                                                            2005056160

On the cover: Weverton Cliffs, overlooking the Potomac River. Photo by Paul Elliott
Cover and text design by Stephen Sullivan
Maps by Steve Jones and Paul Elliott
Photos on pages x, 107, 157, and 188 by Patrick Wamsley; photos on pages 59 and 74 by Randy Bowman; photo on page 150 by Carol Wolter; photo on page 164 by Karen Jones; photos on pages 172 and 180 by Frank Wodarczyk; photos on pages 229, 236, and 245 by GB Ludwig
All other photos by Paul Elliott

Menasha Ridge Press
P.O. Box 43673
Birmingham, AL 35243
www.menasharidge.com

FOR ALL OF THE CHILDREN AND SOME OF THE ADULTS NAMED ON PAGES vii–viii, AND IN REMEMBRANCE OF DAVID, MARGOT, TILLI, MAURICE, SALLY ANNE, JACOB, AND ALEXA EDELMAN; SOPHIA WYATT; JACK EDDLEMAN; ARTHUR BARTSCH; JENELLE McCARN; HILDE LION, FRANCESKA RAPKIN; ROBERTO REYES; AND PAUL EDELMAN. — PAUL ELLIOTT

TABLE OF CONTENTS

ACKNOWLEDGMENTS

I am grateful to the 1.3 gazillion people who have contributed directly and indirectly to this book over exactly the same number of years. Among them have been the landscape shapers and environmental stewards, park makers and rangers, trail builders and maintainers, historians and visionaries, hikers and other trail users, and bards and other writers whose paths I have used or crossed on my way here—plus Mother Nature and Lady Luck. Nearly all are unknown to me, but all have my collective thanks.

I'm also beholden to people whose names and generosity I know well. The book's first edition came about because, a decade after Ellen Kohn first took me hiking, Janis Knorr took me to Menasha Ridge Press (MRP) editor Bud Zehmer. For that edition, Bud, Scott Wilson, and Ray Abercrombie re-scouted several hikes; Carol Ivory helped me subject groups to test outings; Dick Terwilliger lent me his measuring wheel; Cliff Noyes gave me his hike-and-paddle outing (now Hike 58); hike evaluators Brigitte Savage, Annie Glenn, and Carol, Claire, and Isabelle Wolter helped keep me on track; and editors Bud Zehmer and Russell Helms and cartographer Steve Jones saw the book into print.

For the second edition, with its many new hikes and revised old ones, it's been my lucky lot to also have had help from the hiking community's David Bailey, Henri Comeau, Mike Darzi, Helen Epps, Jim Finucane, Paul Fofonoff, Ric Francke, Glenn Gillis, Bruce Glendening, Dick Hillman, Rhonda Krafchin, Gary Kosciusko, Mark Nelson, Bill Niedringhaus, Mary Ann Ray, Paul Ray, Paul Rowe, Patrick Wamsley, and Frank Wodarczyk; trail tester Lut Van Damme, gimlet-eyed Brian Kulak; role models Sheila Bach, Maggie Chan, and David Rumon; and especially naturalist-photographer GB Ludwig. I also acknowledge having been graciously spoiled by MRP president Molly Merkle, editors Russell Helms and Ritchey Halphen, and map whiz Steve Jones.

Lastly, my thanks in advance go to each of the following children on the chance that they will come to know, value, and protect our hiking venues and the rest of the environment—and also help do away with the concrete clover leaf as our national flower: Adrian Kamel, Aidan Mantho, Alissa Rumon, Alyssa Marie Prete, Arthur Ostrega, Austin Grant, Becca Estes, Ben Riber, Brent Vanderheyden, Bridget Holt, Cailin Lechner, Cameron Poole, Cate Perakslis, Cecilia Sherland, Claire Roberts, Claire Wolter, Chloe Perakslis, Christopher Seyfried, Cloé Berge, Cody Perakslis, Dana Randall, Daniel Edelman, Danny Johnston, Derek Vanderheyden, Dillon Ramsey, Ellie Raynor, Emma Estes, Erik McIntosh, Evan Lechner, Francie Zehmer, Gabriel Mouellem, Gregory Kline, Hannah Edelman, Hillary Lynch, Imogen Poole, Isabelle Wolter, Jack Holt, Jamie Zehmer, JD Corrales, Jonathan Edelman, Johnny Estes, Joshua Rose Schmidt, Kai Knorr, Kasper Rapkin, Kate Randall, Katelyn Johnston, Katie Clark, Katie McIntosh, Klara Drees-Gross, Lauren Grant, Lauren Horowitz, Lauren Ramsey, Leah Rumon, Lucas Farr, Lucas Horowitz, Luciano Mantho, Lucy Frost-Helms, Lyndon Wolf, Madelyn Wolf, Mariah Johnston, Max Strackbein, Maximilian Mueller, Monica Moore, Morgan Ipsale, Narcisa Medgidia, Natalie Drees-Gross, Nicholas Grillias, Peter Manthos, Philip Hepworth, Philip Manthos, Rigel Farr, Sandra Kohn, Sean Edelman, Shane Strackbein, Sophie Hepworth, Spenser J. Wyatt, Tanya Whisnant, Timothy Grillias, Toma Meyer, Trey Anthony Ipsale, William Bancroft, William Sherland, Wyatt Moore, Zachary Poole, and Zoe Roberts.

—PAUL ELLIOTT

FOREWORD

Welcome to Menasha Ridge Press's *60 Hikes within 60 Miles,* a series designed to provide hikers with information needed to find and hike the very best trails and other hiking routes in and around cities usually underserved by good guidebooks.

Our strategy is simple: First, find a hiker who knows the area and loves to hike. And second, ask that person to spend a year hiking, mapping, photographing, and describing the very best hiking routes around in terms of difficulty, scenery, condition, elevation change, and all other categories of information that are important to hikers. "On each hike, pretend you are a new hiker to the area and think about what any hiker would want to know," we tell each author. "Imagine their questions; be clear in your answers."

An experienced hiker and professional writer, Paul Elliott has come up with 60 of the best hikes in the Washington, D.C., metropolitan area. From urban hikes that make use of parklands and streets to flora-and-fauna-rich treks along the Potomac to aerobic outings in the mountains, Elliott provides hikers (and walkers) with a great variety of hikes—and all within roughly 60 miles of D.C.

You'll get more out of this book if you take a moment to read the Introduction, which explains how to read the hike profiles and listings. The Maps section will help you understand how useful topos can be on a hike, and Appendix B will tell you where to get them. And though this is a "where-to," not a "how-to," guide, those of you who have not hiked extensively will find the Introduction of particular value.

As much for the opportunity to free the mind as to free the body, let Paul Elliott's hikes elevate you above the urban hurry.

All the best,
The Editors at Menasha Ridge Press

ABOUT THE AUTHOR

I am a writer and editor by longtime trade. I stumbled into the profession in Chicago and liked it enough to then jump into the Manhattan publishing world, first as a house editor and then as a self-employed book writer and freelance editor. Moving to the Washington, D.C., area, I continued to freelance and write books, and also put in a couple of extended employee stints, first with a federal contractor and then at a science institute. I opted for self-employment again in 2000, when I was asked to write more books—one of which became the first edition of this hiking guide.

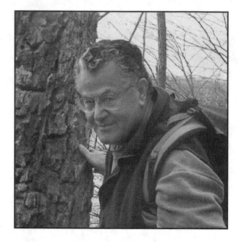

By then, I had become a recreational hiker with a growing enthusiasm for hiking's wonderful mix of exercise possibilities, vista visions, floral and faunal sightings, seasonal change, chanced-upon historic sites, social and cultural opportunities, personal challenges, and assorted surprises. With the help of kindred spirits, I had learned a lot firsthand about the D.C. area's richly diversified landscape, with its long-range mountains and beaches, and everything in between—and all lying within easy driving range. And I was already leading hikes for both the Sierra Club and Appalachian Mountain Club.

So off I went, with notebook and pen in hand, to devise and describe 60 hikes. It was the first writing project I had ever tackled that required almost all of the research to be done outdoors and on foot—and that provided me with lots of exercise as well. It also took me two years and roughly 2,000 miles of legwork to complete ("2,000" because I did each hike at least three times, and also explored variants; "legwork" because I did some of those miles by bike to save time). Oddly, though, it was only later that I made the connection between this project and my early training as a geographer.

With the book's publication in 2002, I finally had an answer to the question, What does it take to write such a book? And now, four-plus years later, I can also answer the question, What's so special about the second edition?

To find out, read the Preface.

PREFACE

"I like walking because it is slow, and I suspect that the mind, like the feet, works at about three miles an hour. If this is so, then modern life is moving faster than the speed of thought, or thoughtfulness."
—Rebecca Solnit,
Wanderlust: A History of Walking, page 10

In researching and writing the first edition of this book, I had two basic objectives in mind. One was to tell or remind both local residents and visitors about the exceptional hiking opportunities available in the Washington, D.C., metropolitan area—and not just in exurbia and suburbia, but also in the city itself. The metro area has something to offer to just about anyone with an interest in hiking. Taken together, these many somethings reflect the area's rich diversity of landscape, parklands, trails, wildlife, city life, historical heritage, cultural resources, and recreational opportunity, as well as its modest tradition of preservation and conservation. What's more, hiking in the metro area is very much a rewarding four-season enterprise.

My other objective in writing the book was—and remains—to provide residents and visitors with a reliable means of exploring the local world of hiking on their own—and without relying on organized group outings. My intent was to present them with tempting choices, tell them what to expect, motivate them to get out there, and enable them to experience on-course, safe, and enjoyable outings. I urged them to select their hikes wisely, appropriately; read my words and maps attentively; and take along a compass and at least one companion (and a cell phone, too). And I warned them that trail signage and landmarks sometimes disappear and guidebooks tend to get out-of-date.

For that first edition, I created an eclectic mix of 60 hikes that ranged in location from the central city to and through the suburbs and beyond to the foothills and mountains in the west and the

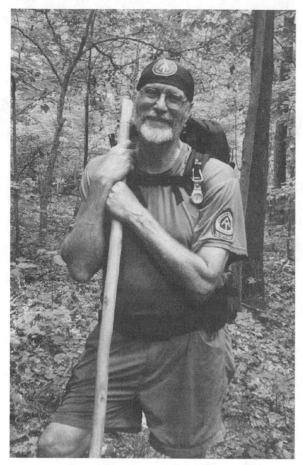

> In summer, on Hikes 46, 47, 53, 54, 59, or 60, say hello to the Potomac Appalachian Trail Club's Ridgerunners on patrol.

lowlands in the east. The hikes fell into three categories: variants on traditional hikes in already popular hiking locales, new hikes in such locales, and new hikes in underused areas. All in all, I think that I met my objectives and that the first edition turned out quite well. However, I had wildly underestimated the amount of time it would take me to complete the book, with so much time being taken up by my having to rehike some trail segments and test-hike my drafted directions. So I now know what it takes to write such a book: mostly time, plus good descriptive skills, good legs, good luck, and persistence in using what I think of as the "trail and error" method.

It was the passage of yet more time after publication that spurred my ambition to update the book by continuing to monitor the existing hikes and find new ones (and check them out by leading group hikes), and by becoming more involved with—and educated by—local hiking, environmental, and conservation organizations. I also came to understand the importance of both preserving public space and supporting the acquisition of more of it, as well as of extending access to private land through the use of trail easements. And I came to appreciate the vital role played by the various federal, state, and local agencies and especially by such local nonprofits as the Potomac Appalachian Trail Club (the area's chief trail builder and maintainer), the Appalachian Trail Conservancy, the Potomac Conservancy, the Piedmont Environmental Council, the C&O Canal Association, and the Potomac Heritage Trail Association, plus the organizations listed in Appendix A.

The result is this second edition, which is certainly bigger (more pages, more words, more photos—and one more hike, as I'll explain), and possibly better than the first one. The book has been redesigned, and the formerly alphabetized hikes have been reorganized into five major locational categories. And the 60 hikes in this second edition include 13 new hikes (Hikes 17, 20, 22, 24, 33, 38, 41, 45, 48, 52, 56, 57, and 60). Nearly all of these new ones involve rarely-if-ever-used or newly created hiking locales (Hike 41, for example, uses a park that, in 2006, was still be to officially opened). The book also includes 9 significantly revised ones (Hikes 3, 5, 25, 26, 29, 35, 36, 53, and 59), along with updates in all of the other 38 hikes. And I have had to drop only 12 hikes, the 13th being covered by combining two hikes (now Hike 35).

In addition, working closely with me, the editors have revamped the Introduction, and I strongly encourage you to read it, especially if you're a beginning or rusty hiker, because it explains the internal organization of the hike listings. We also have devised new categories for the section on Hiking Recommendations (in that section, by the way, "little elevation change" means less than 1,000 feet of change, and "lots of elevation change" means more than 3,000 feet of change).

Also, to give you a sense of each hike's difficulty level, I have applied a rating scale based on a simple formula that combines horizontal distance and elevation change (up or down). On this scale, each mile of distance counts for 1 point and every 400 feet of elevation change also count for 1 point. You'll find each hike's difficulty rating in its Key-at-a-Glance Information box. Here are the rating categories (essentially the same ones I used in the book's first edition):

Very easy	**under 5 points**
Easy	5–7.9
Easy–moderate	8–10.9
Moderate	11–13.9
Moderate–hard	14–16.9
Hard	17–19.9
Quite hard	20–22.9
Very hard	23–25.9
Extremely hard	26 or more

In this second edition, I again have indulged myself by incorporating into the text various unidentified quotes and paraphrases from sayings, poems, and other writings on the chance that some readers like literary puzzles (example: the Thoreau-ly lyric line "The bluebird carries the sky on his back"). These passages are buried in Hikes 10, 14, 15, 18, 23, 26, 27, 31, 32, 34, 35, 36, 39, 44, 53, and 55, and in the Acknowledgments and this Preface. See if you can find them, and then tell me who said or wrote what. If you're right, I'll feature you in the third edition of the book and also send you a copy of it.

To supplement the information sources cited in almost every hike listing, here is a short and idiosyncratic reading list in which I skip over the standard reference tomes and Web sites and encourage you to read or at least sample certain publications that have enriched this book and my life. The first among these is a Rebecca Solnit's enlightening and provocative *Wanderlust: A History of Walking*, which takes the form of a wonderfully multifaceted, quirky, and quotation-rich rumination on bipedalism.

To learn more about the metro area's abundant plant and animal life, dip into Richard L. Berman and Deborah McBride's *Natural Washington* (which covers much of the metro area); Cristol Fleming, Marion Blois Lobstein, and Barbara Tufty's *Finding Wildflowers in the Washington–Baltimore Area;* Barbara Medina and Victor Medina's *Central Appalachian Wildflowers* and Leonard M. Adkins's *Wildflowers of the Appalachian Trail* (both of which have clear and useful color photos and succinct text passages); Louis J. Halle's *Spring in Washington* (an elegant, now-60-year-old essay on the city and nearby areas, with emphasis on birdlife); Melanie Choukas-Bradley and Polly Alexander's *City of Trees* (a lovely guide to where they are and what they are); and the various plant, bird, butterfly, and other checklists available at area parks and preserves. Also look for *A Birder's Guide to Montgomery County,* a book from the Maryland Ornithological Society's Montgomery County Chapter that also identifies some little-known hiking venues. And for a one-of-a-kind illustrated ground-level guide that's not region specific but still the best there is after six decades, consult Olaus J. Murie's classic *Animal Tracks.* I also recommend visiting Bob Pickett's Trail and Field Notes Web site (**www.patc.net/hiking/pickett**), where you'll find the observations and musings of an ardent and prolific local naturalist.

From time to time, though, consider ignoring me and taking Walt Whitman's advice: "You must not know too much, or be too precise or scientific about birds and trees and flowers and watercraft; a certain free margin, and even vagueness—perhaps ignorance, credulity—helps your enjoyment of these things."

For detailed information on the manmade C&O Canal, delve into Thomas F. Hahn's *Towpath Guide to the C & O Canal*; Mike High's *C&O Canal Companion*; and "*184 Miles of Adventure: Hiker's Guide to the C&O Canal,*" a map-based booklet put out by the Mason-Dixon Council of the Boy Scouts of America.

Useful books on Washington itself include the justifiably still revered, monumental, and bracingly opinionated *Washington: City and Capital,* prepared in 1937 by the Federal Writers' Project; Candace H. Stapen's scholarly, tightly packed, and anecdote-laced *Washington D.C.;* E. J. Applewhite's *Washington Itself* (with eccentric emphasis on matters architectural); Dex Nilsson's *The Names of Washington, D.C.* (what's named for whom, etc.); Douglas E. Evelyn and Paul Dickson's richly illustrated *On This Spot: Pinpointing the Past in Washington, D.C.;* Gail Spilsbury's homage to the Olmsteds, *Rock Creek Park;* and Benjamin Franklin Cooling III and Walton H. Owen II's definitive *Mr. Lincoln's Forts: A Guide to the Civil War Defenses of Washington.*

In winding up this second edition, I find myself empathizing with a British encyclopedist who, after putting his tome to bed, would sit back, he said, and pick slivers of information out of his brain, and with a French poet of the same era who believed that one does not finish a poem—one simply abandons it. But I am comforting myself by making notes for the third edition. So, if you have any comments or corrections—or a puzzle solution, please contact me. Try reaching me through Menasha Ridge Press, or write to me directly at P.O. Box 9781, Alexandria, VA 22304, or **metrohiker@yahoo.com** (and put my first name on the subject line to help keep me safe from spam).

—PAUL ELLIOTT

HIKING RECOMMENDATIONS

HIKES WITHIN CAPITAL BELTWAY

HIKES WITH LITTLE ELEVATION CHANGE

HIKES WITH LITTLE ELEVATION CHANGE (CONTINUED)

HIKES WITH LOTS OF ELEVATION CHANGE

HIKES GOOD FOR VIEWING FLORA OR FAUNA

HIKES FEATURING SCENIC BODIES OF WATER

HIKES WITH VISTA-RICH OVERLOOKS

HIKES RICH IN HISTORIC SITES

SECLUDED HIKES

HIKES FROM 5 TO 10 MILES (CONTINUED)

HIKES FROM 10 TO 15 MILES

HIKES FROM 15 TO 20 MILES

HIKES MORE THAN 60 MILES

60 HIKES
WITHIN 60 MILES

WASHINGTON, D.C.
INCLUDING
SUBURBAN AND OUTLYING AREAS OF MARYLAND AND VIRGINIA

SECOND EDITION

INTRODUCTION

Welcome to *60 Hikes within 60 Miles: Washington, D.C.* If you're new to hiking or even if you're a seasoned trailsmith, take a few minutes to read the following introduction. We explain how this book is organized and how to use it.

WHAT'S IN EACH HIKE LISTING

Each listing contains seven key items: a locator map, an "In Brief" hike summary, a "Key At-a-Glance Information" box, directions to the trailhead, a trail map, a detailed hike description, and a note about nearby and related activities. Together, these items provide you with a means of assessing each hike in advance.

LOCATOR MAP

After narrowing down the general area of the hike on the overview map (on the book's inside front cover), use the locator map, along with the directions also given in the listing, to find the trailhead.

IN BRIEF

This synopsis offers a snapshot of what to expect along the way, mostly in general terms of the hike's location and its chief attractions for hikers.

KEY AT-A-GLANCE INFORMATION

This box gives you a quick idea of the hike's specifics. It covers 13 or 14 basic elements.

LENGTH Specifies the hike's length from start to finish. For many hikes, author Paul Elliott notes that there are shorter options. They're explained in the hike description, and you can use them—together with the hike's difficulty rating (see next page)—to customize the hike to match your ability, inclination, or time constraint.

CONFIGURATION Characterizes the hiking route's overall shape if it could be seen from overhead. Most of the hikes are loops, out-and-backs, or modifications of these two types. There are also a few figure eights, one-ways, and more-exotic configurations.

DIFFICULTY Indicates the degree of effort an average hiker is likely to need to make on the hike. Using a simple formula of distance and elevation change, Paul applies a scale ranging from "Very Easy" to "Extremely Hard," as he explains in the Preface.

SCENERY Summarizes what you can expect in general terms of terrain, vegetation, land use, water bodies, and views.

EXPOSURE Reveals how much sunshine will land on your shoulders on a clear day. Paul's exposure scale uses "open" and "shady" proportionately, and makes allowance for the effects of trees, cliffs, buildings, and the changing seasons.

TRAFFIC Indicates how busy the trail might be on an average day. Trail traffic, of course, will vary from day to day and season to season.

TRAIL SURFACE Notes how crowded or uncrowded the hiking route is likely to be, allowing for the time of day, week, and season.

HIKING TIME Provides a practical range based on Paul's own experience and his perception of the average hiker.

SEASON Names the best season for doing the hike, in Paul's opinion.

ACCESS Reveals the days and the times of day when the hiking route is officially open, and whether hikers must pay usage fees or obtain permission to hike.

MAPS Identifies United States Geological Survey and other maps that usefully supplement the trail map in each hike listing, and also identifies some map sources (others are given in Appendix B).

FACILITIES Tells of toilets, public phones, and water sources available along or near the hiking route—or simply specifies "None."

FOR MORE INFORMATION Explains where to get more.

SPECIAL COMMENTS Reminds you about such matters as park or gate closings, trails susceptible to flooding or freezing, and hunting seasons that could affect your plans.

DIRECTIONS

Follow these driving directions carefully, with the locator map in hand, to get to the trailhead and park legally. Some hikes include public-transportation options.

DESCRIPTION

The description is the heart of each hike listing. Here, Paul presents what is essentially a combination of essay and hiking guide in which he creates a vivid and concise picture of the venue's natural and human history and provides easy-to-follow instructions and a map to keep you on course. Ultimately, the description is your chief tool in deciding what hikes to try—and to repeat.

NEARBY/RELATED ACTIVITIES

Each hike listing includes suggestions for other things to do. Paul's novel suggestions include places to detour privately, swim, picnic, bird, row, take a ranger-led tour or sunset boat ride, dine indoors, pick fruit, attend an outdoor play or concert, sample a festival, dig into history, explore an oddball museum, hike by moonlight, stargaze, find Alpenglow, ride a horse (on a trail or antique carousel), make ice cream by hand, browse for books, and meditate in a peace park.

BE SENSIBLE ABOUT THE WEATHER

The Washington, D.C., metropolitan area has a generally temperate climate that favors year-round hiking, although deep freezes and major storms occur from time to time in the winter and the often hot and humid summers take some getting used to. If you make prudent decisions about which of these 60 hikes to try, what to take with you, and what the weather is likely to be, you can count on being able to hike enjoyably and safely on most days of the year.

During the winter, early-morning temperatures are usually near the freezing mark, and frosts are not uncommon throughout much of the area. Remember that winter weather in the mountains tends to be more severe than elsewhere, so pay attention to mountain-weather forecasts. Some winters bring little or no snow—and some bring warm spells. Even a mild winter tends to be a gray season of short days, but (Paul tells us) winter hiking in the area has its devotees, who enjoy the absence of leaves, insects, and crowds and who delight in the opened-up vistas.

Average daily temperatures by month in Washington, D.C. (degrees Fahrenheit)

	Jan	Feb	Mar	Apr	May	Jun
High	43	47	55	66	76	84
Low	24	26	33	42	52	62

	Jul	Aug	Sep	Oct	Nov	Dec
High	89	87	80	69	58	48
Low	60	59	52	41	34	25

On the hottest days of summer, from late July to early September, try to go hiking first thing in the morning and look for hikes that have heavy shade—or for trails in the mountains, where temperatures are routinely lower (generally, one degree lower for every 1,000 feet of elevation gain). Keep in mind that even late in the day, the temperature and humidity won't have dropped enough to be really comfortable. Also be wary of thunderstorms, which are the area's most common weather hazard in summer.

All in all, the best hiking weather in the Washington area occurs in the fall and spring. Autumn can be glorious, especially from September to early December, during Indian summer. With the return of spring, between about mid-March and mid-May, comes balmy weather, the reawakening of the plant world, and the reappearance of songbirds and lots of hikers.

LEARN ABOUT USING MAPS

The maps in this book have been produced with great care and, when used with the hike descriptions, will direct you to the trailhead and keep you on course during the hike. However, for superior detail and other valuable information about the terrain you'll be traversing, you should also use the United States Geological Survey's 7.5-minute series topographic maps (Paul identifies the ones that cover most of his hikes).

If you're new to hiking, you might be wondering, "What's a topographic map?" In short, a topo indicates not only linear distance but elevation as well, using contour lines. Contour lines spread across the map like dozens of intricate spiderwebs. Each line represents a particular elevation, and at the base of each topo, a contour's interval designation is given. If the contour interval is 200 feet, then the height difference between each contour line is 200 feet. Follow five contour lines up on the same map, and the elevation has increased by 1,000 feet.

You can find topo maps at local outdoor stores and some bike shops, as well as online at many Web sites. For the 7.5-minute USGS maps, visit the USGS Web site, **topomaps.usgs.gov**. These and other topo maps—and aerial photographs—also can be found at **terraserver.microsoft.com** and **www.topozone.com**. Another valuable map resource in Washington is the Library of Congress, which has a treasure trove of maps that the public can use and photocopy.

PRACTICE TRAIL ETIQUETTE

Whether you're on a city walk or on a long hike, remember that great care and resources (from nature as well as from tax dollars) have gone into creating the trails and paths. Taking care of them begins with you, the hiker. Treat the trail, wildlife, flora, and your fellow hikers with respect. Here are a few general ideas to keep in mind while hiking:

1. **Hike on open trails only. Respect trail and road closures (ask if you're not sure), avoid trespassing on private land, and obtain any required permits or authorization. Leave gates as you found them or as marked.**

2. **Leave no trace of your visit other than footprints. Be sensitive to the land beneath your feet. This also means staying on the existing trails and not creating any new ones. Be sure to pack out what you pack in. No one likes to see trash someone else has left behind. Also, consider packing out at**

least some of the trash you find along the trail (Paul tells us that, in the D.C. area, many parks no longer provide trash receptacles).

3. **Never spook animals.** Give animals extra room and time to adjust to you.

4. **Plan ahead.** Know your equipment, your ability, and the area in which you are hiking—and prepare accordingly. Be self-sufficient at all times; carry necessary supplies for changes in weather or other conditions. A well-executed trip is a satisfaction to you and not a burden or offense to others.

5. **Be respectful of and courteous to everyone you meet while hiking.**

BE SURE YOU HAVE AND DRINK ENOUGH WATER

One of the keys to hiking both enjoyably and safely in the Washington area is keeping well hydrated. So be sure to take along enough water. How much is enough? The answer depends chiefly on the length and duration of the hike and the ambient temperature. One year-round standard recommended by some local hiking clubs is to carry at least one quart for every five miles to be covered. During the summer, Paul tells us, it's not uncommon for hikers doing, say, 10 to 12 miles with even modest elevation change to carry three or four quarts.

Try to start any hike with potable water. Many—but not all—of the hikes in this book have drinking water available at the trailhead or along the way. But if you must use water that's not from a reliable tap, make sure you purify it; otherwise, you run the risk of infection. That's because waterways throughout the area—including high-mountain streams and springs—can be sources of unwelcome bacteria (such as *Giardia intestinalis*, *Cryptosporidium,* and *Escherichia coli*), as well as viruses and other pollutants.

Accordingly, some hikers purify suspect water with very effective and only slightly distasteful tetraglycine-hydroperiodide tablets (sold under such names as Potable Aqua, Globaline, and Coughlan's), or they employ portable, lightweight filters. Unfortunately, even the best filters can't remove everything, but they can reduce the infection risk to a very low level.

All in all, the two best ways of being safe are to take potable water with you or boil untreated water for five or more minutes (if that's practical). The pleasures of hiking—and the displeasure of getting sick—make such relatively minor efforts worth every one of the minutes involved.

USEFUL THINGS TO TAKE ON THE HIKE

Choose sensibly from the following list (prepared by Paul):

Bandana

Companion or companions

Cell phone

Cold-weather clothing (e.g., hat, gloves, extra layers, dry socks)

Compass

Duct tape

Emergency blanket or poncho lightweight)

Emergency fire starter (e.g., household dryer lint) in waterproof container (e.g., film canister)

First-aid kit

Flashlight (plus extra batteries)

Food

Insect repellent

Maps or trail guides

Medications (just your own, if any)

Pocketknife

Raingear

Safety pins

Sunblock

Sunglasses

Toilet paper

Twine and fishing line (for repairs)

Water

Waterproof matches or pocket lighter

Water-purification tablets or water filter (on longer hikes)

Whistle

YOUR FIRST-AID KIT

Be sure to carry a kit. The following are the basics:

Ace bandages or Spenco joint wraps

Antibiotic ointment (Neosporin or the generic equivalent)

Aspirin or acetaminophen

Band-Aids

Benadryl or the generic equivalent— diphenhydramine (an antihistamine, in case of allergic reactions)

Butterfly-closure bandages

Gauze (one roll)

Gauze compress pads (a half-dozen 4 in. x 4 in.)

Hydrogen peroxide or iodine

Matches or pocket lighter

Moleskin/Spenco "Second Skin"

A prefilled syringe of epinephrine (for those known to have severe allergic reactions to such things as bee stings)

Snakebite kit

Sunscreen

Water-purification tablets or water filter (see note above)

Whistle (more effective in signaling rescuers than your voice)

Pack these items in a waterproof bag or bags. Also, between hikes, remember to check expiration dates periodically. If you hike a lot, also think about taking a first-aid class.

HOW TO DEAL WITH POTENTIAL TRAIL HAZARDS

It's easy to get into trouble when hiking. Here are some tips about taking care of yourself on the trail—in addition to making it a point to hike with at least one companion:

KNOW WHERE YOU ARE

Guard against getting lost on the hike. Have a map and trail guide with you, along with a compass—and know how to use all three. Try to keep track of where you are at all times. If you lose your way, the safest thing to do is retrace your steps. If backtracking gets you further lost, stop and seek help. Watch for other hikers or call for help on a cell phone or by using your whistle (three short blasts is the universal distress signal)—or by yelling collectively with your companions. In general, you should stay put if it's getting dark.

WATCH YOUR STEP

A common hiking hazard is tripping and falling down, thanks to rocks, tree roots, or uneven or slippery surfaces. Injury, especially to a lower limb, can take the fun out of any hike. So pay attention to Paul's comments about trail surfaces, and be smart, when on tricky trails, about when to admire the view and when to watch where you put your feet.

GET OFF THE TRAIL BY DUSK

Hiking after dark can be hazardous, so make sure you finish while there's still daylight. Take note of Paul's time estimates for each hike, and leave room for a margin of error (his or yours). Keep a working flashlight in your pack.

AVOID POISON IVY AND STINGING NETTLES

Poison ivy thrives throughout the area, in both the city and countryside. It's a climbing vine and also a shrubby form of groundcover, identified by its telltale three leaflets to a leaf (hence the old adage "Leaves of three, let it be"). Recognizing and avoiding contact with it is the most effective way to prevent the painful, oozing, and itchy rashes caused by urushiol, the oil in the plant's sap. Urushiol occurs in all parts of the plant (including

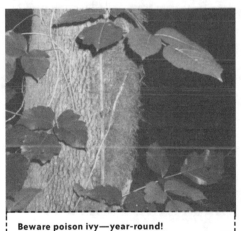

Beware poison ivy—year-round!

the hairy vines that climb trees) and is active year-round. Within 48 hours of skin's exposure to the oil, raised lines and/or blisters may appear, accompanied by itching.

On exposure, sluice the skin with water (also rub the area with wet mud and then rinse). Then, when you can, wash the area with soap, dry it thoroughly, and, if a rash eventually appears, apply calamine lotion repeatedly to help dry it out. If itching or blistering is severe, seek medical attention. Also wash any urushiol-contaminated clothes or hiking gear. Remember that sensitivity to urushiol varies greatly from one person to the next, and that it tends to increase over time with repeated rash outbreaks.

Stinging nettles, with their typical sawtooth-edged leaves, are a perennial that line some trails during warm-weather months. You'll remember them if your bare skin brushes against them, but the stinging doesn't last long for most people (minutes or hours, depending on individual sensitivity). The best prevention method is wearing long pants.

PROTECT YOURSELF AGAINST BITING AND STINGING INSECTS

During the warm-weather months in the Washington area, hikers are likely to be bugged mostly by mosquitoes, bees and wasps, ticks, and biting flies. There are also no-see-ums, chiggers, and even poisonous spiders, but Paul claims that they're rarely encountered. In all cases, though, practice prevention by using effective insect repellents and also wearing long-armed and long-legged clothing with a tight weave.

Mosquitoes are the most common irritant, especially in the city itself and close-in urban areas, where the Asian tiger mosquito (*Aedes albopictus*)—an aggressive daytime biter—has become established over the past decade. Over the same period, local health authorities have also become concerned about the possible spread of West Nile virus (WNV) by infected native Culex mosquitoes. However, as of late 2006, there have been very few cases of WNV virus in this area. Nevertheless, health authorities recommend that people going outdoors take active measures to prevent getting bitten.

Bees and wasps (including hornets and yellowjackets) are occasionally aggressive, especially in the fall. Most people get stung when they venture too close to the underground lairs of yellowjackets. Be vigilant, and if you're highly allergic to bee or wasp stings (which can be fatal), be sure to carry an epinephrine-loaded syringe.

Ticks are also common and troublesome. They attach themselves to hikers walking through long grass, brushing past trailside bushes, or sitting on dead tree trunks. You won't feel them land on you or bite you, but it takes them a while to get settled on you and start feeding. In this area, the species of medical concern are the deer tick (about the size of the period at the end of this sentence), which may be infected with Lyme disease, and the dog tick (up to a half inch long), which may carry Rocky Mountain spotted fever. Insect repellents containing DEET are known to be effective deterrents. Most importantly, though, be sure to inspect yourself visually at the end of the hike, and then later, while taking a shower, do a complete body check. For ticks that are already embedded, removal with tweezers is best. (To learn more about dealing with ticks, visit **www.emedicinehealth.com/ticks/article_em.htm.**)

STEER CLEAR OF ALL ANIMALS—AND HUNTERS

The Washington area has a rich variety of animals, large and small, and hikers are usually thrilled to see most of them. However, you need to give all animals you encounter a wide berth, both for their sake and yours. Although rarely dangerous, they can be a threat under certain circumstances, as when surprised or cornered by humans. So be watchful, and do not, for example, get between a female bear and her cubs, try to pet a coyote, feed a deer, or approach a lethargic fox during the daytime (it could be rabid).

Also stay away from all snakes. There are only two poisonous ones—the timber rattlesnake and the copperhead—and neither is aggressive if left alone. Be careful where you put your hands and feet when crossing rocks or downed tree trunks, especially in the late summer and early fall, when snakes seek out the sun. Also carry a snakebite kit.

During the hunting season, wear orange, be noisy, and avoid hunters in areas where hunting is allowed. Remember that Maryland, Virginia, and West Virginia are among the few states that ban hunting on Sundays on both public and private lands. Take note of Paul's warnings about certain hikes. If you feel uneasy, stay away altogether.

HIKING WITH CHILDREN

No one is too young for a nice hike in the woods or through a city park. Parents can carry infants and toddlers in special carriers. Older children, of course, can follow along with adults. Use common sense to judge a child's capability, endurance, and boredom factor. When packing for the hike, remember the children's needs as well as your own. Make sure children are adequately clothed and shod for the weather, and remember that they dehydrate quickly. Most children should be able to do at least segments of some of the shorter hikes in this book—as well as the three short and easy hikes that Paul specifically recommends for them (see page xix).

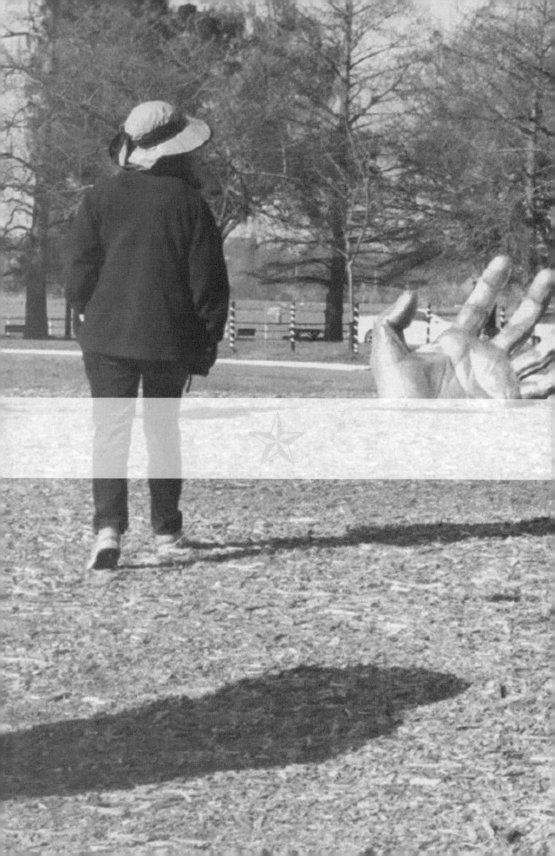

WASHINGTON, D.C.

01 LINCOLN MEMORIAL TO LINCOLN PARK

KEY AT-A-GLANCE INFORMATION

LENGTH: 8.6 miles (with shorter options)

CONFIGURATION: Loop

DIFFICULTY: Easy–moderate

SCENERY: Parklands, public buildings

EXPOSURE: Mostly open

TRAFFIC: Light–moderate; heavier in tourist season, weekends, holidays

TRAIL SURFACE: Mostly pavement

HIKING TIME: 4–5 hours

SEASON: Year-round

ACCESS: Lincoln Memorial closes at midnight; no other restrictions

MAPS: USGS Washington West; ADC Metro Washington; posted map on display boards on and near Mall

FACILITIES: None at trailhead; toilets, water, phones in museums and other public buildings on or near Mall; toilets in ranger station on Independence Avenue near 17th Street; stand-alone toilets on Mall

FOR MORE INFORMATION: Contact National Capital Parks, (202) 619-7222 or www.nps.gov/nacc

SPECIAL COMMENTS: Mall and Capitol Hill are high-security areas; obey signs; don't trespass; be prepared to modify your route if necessary; finish hike by dusk

IN BRIEF

Roaming the Mall and Capitol Hill on foot serves as a wonderful introduction to hiking in the nation's capital—and to learning firsthand about the city's heritage and treasures.

DESCRIPTION

Each Fourth of July, half a million folks crowd onto Washington's Mall for a special birthday celebration. Between one Fourth and the next, they and others frequent the Mall's museums, monuments, and memorials and gather to play, picnic, stroll, jog, bike, relax, protest, march, and sightsee. The Mall, in effect, serves as the nation's front yard, town square, commons, pulpit, soapbox, park, and memorial garden. It's also a great hiking venue where one can take self-propelled voyages of discovery and rediscovery. And it's small enough to cover on foot, but large enough for a hiker to get some exercise—and avoid the crowds.

This 8.6-mile, clockwise loop ranges across the Mall and beyond to Capitol Hill, and it features sites of historic and cultural interest, with emphasis on both Abe Lincoln and, inevitably, war. But it's planned as a daytime

----

Directions ───────────────→

Head for Washington's Mall area. Park near the trailhead—the Smithsonian Metro station entrance within the Mall (near Independence Avenue and 12th Street SW). Arrive early on crowded warm-weather weekends and holidays; beware local parking regulations. Or use the Metro: Smithsonian station is on Orange, Blue lines; Metrobuses operate on nearby streets. Contact Metro, (202) 637-7000 or www.wmata.com.

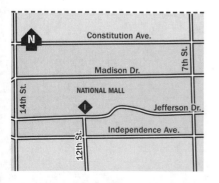

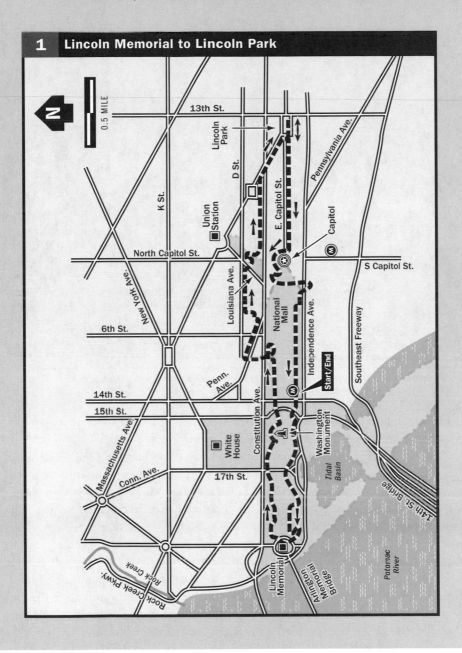

1 Lincoln Memorial to Lincoln Park

and outdoor hike (except for one indoor peek at the biggest Lincoln). Detour indoors if you want to, but do maintain a good pace between stops, be careful crossing streets, and use the paths and sidewalks. And for a shorter hike, just make free use of a street map. Note that "the Mall" is usually taken to be the grand 2.2-mile stretch of open space between the Lincoln Memorial and the U.S. Capitol. Officially, though, the Mall—or National Mall—is only the part east of

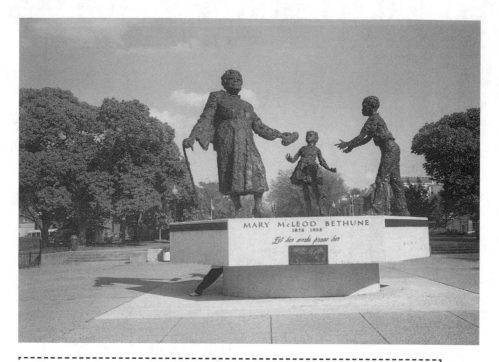

This monument in Lincoln Park was the city's first to honor an African American. (FYI: those trees in back bear chestnuts.)

14th Street, and the memorial itself lies in West Potomac Park. But worry not. The entire area is under National Park Service jurisdiction.

To get started from the Smithsonian Metro station on the Mall, head south (toward Independence Avenue) for about 20 yards. Turn right onto a broad paved path alongside Jefferson Drive. Follow the path across 14th and 15th streets NW, then turn left and almost immediately turn right onto a short, narrow, paved, downhill path. At the bottom, turn left onto another paved path. Follow it west along Independence Avenue and past the Sylvan Theater and an information-equipped ranger station. At 17th Street, cross at the traffic light. Look or veer left to see the hike's first war-related memorial, on a traffic island. Erected in 1912, it depicts American Revolution naval hero (and later Russian admiral) John Paul Jones ("I have not yet begun to fight"), but supplies no details.

On the other side of 17th Street, proceed straight through the possibly grandiose National World War II Memorial, opened in 2004. Then continue westward on a paved path, but detour to the left to visit a circular bandstand, built in 1931 as Washington's World War I memorial. Then return to the paved path and proceed past some yellow-topped bollards (security structures that have proliferated on the Mall, each costing $7,500) to a four-way intersection. There, turn left and tour the Korean War Veterans Memorial. Dedicated in 1995, it depicts soldiers in winter. Made of stainless steel, the grim figures are reflected in a polished black granite wall on which many faces are faintly etched.

Return to the intersection, head for the nearby Lincoln Memorial, and climb the 56 steps (Lincoln died at age 56). Enter the great chamber to face the seated marble figure that's four-and-a-half times life-size. Notice Lincoln's fingers, bent to form "A" and "L" in sign language (Lincoln supported education for the deaf; sculptor Daniel French had a deaf son). An inscription above Lincoln's head celebrates his having saved the Union, but ignores his role in ending slavery. As the writer later explained, the memorial—opened in 1922—was meant to help heal the North–South rift, so it was best to "avoid the rubbing of old sores." But architect Henry Bacon had the chamber walls inscribed with the Gettysburg Address and the second inaugural address, which make clear Lincoln's views. Before leaving, look for the inscription marking the spot where Martin Luther King delivered his now-memorable "I Have a Dream" speech in 1963.

Then descend the steps, swing left, and head for the Vietnam Veterans Memorial. After passing an information kiosk, stop near a flagpole to see a three-guys-with-guns sculpture. Then take the paved path along the base of a sunken black granite wall carrying the names of the Vietnam War dead and missing. When dedicated in 1982, the memorial designed by Maya Lin consisted solely of the engraved wall. As she later wrote, "I did not want to civilize war by glorifying it or by forgetting the sacrifices involved." But her design provoked controversy. That led to *Three Servicemen* being added in 1984. The nearby Vietnam Women's Memorial, showing three nurses aiding a fallen soldier, was added in 1993.

From there, retrace your steps to the last junction and walk straight (east) on a paved path through Constitution Gardens. At a small lake, swing left and follow the paved waterside path to an elevated plaza. Cross it, staying left, and swing left onto a diagonal paved path leading to 17th Street. Circle the nearby boarded-up stone house. An 1835 lock house, it is both the Mall's oldest building and a reminder that a canal once ran along what are now Constitution Avenue and 17th Street. The canal was paved over in the 1870s, but the area west of 17th was a mosquito-infested marsh until the 1920s. Cross 17th, turn right, and proceed to the first paved path leading uphill to the left. Take it to reach the sublimely abstract Washington Monument. When finished in 1884, the shaft topped out at about 555.5 feet. It's still the city's tallest masonry structure. But it's sinking at a rate of 5.64 inches a century and will disappear by the year 118,900.

Circle to the left around the monument and take the paved path leading down to the ticket kiosk on 15th Street. Cross that street and 14th Street, and head east along Madison Drive for five blocks, past the American history and natural history museums. Then turn left to walk through a butterfly garden that's colorful in the spring and summer, but consistently butterfly-less. At Constitution Avenue, turn right to cross 9th Street. Then turn right to circle through the six-acre National Sculpture Garden. Opened in 1999, it's part of the nearby National Gallery of Art (the Mall's only non-Smithsonian museum). It features serious and whimsical modern sculptures set around what doubles as a summer fountain and winter ice-skating rink.

From there, cross Constitution and walk north on 9th Street. At Pennsylvania Avenue, turn right onto the avenue. On that corner, next to the National Archives, note the memorial to Franklin D. Roosevelt that FDR himself requested; it's desk-sized, unlike the 1997 FDR memorial at the Tidal Basin. Continue along the avenue, cross to the other side at 6th Street, turn right, pass the relocated Newseum (to open in 2007), and head for the Embassy of Canada. Walk up the steps, stand in the small rotunda, sing, and listen to the acoustic effects incorporated into the striking 1989 building. Roam the open courtyard, with its hanging garden and Bill Reid's beguiling bronze sculpture, *The Spirit of Haida Gwaii.* Then cross a brick driveway to enter John Marshall Park. Cross to the far side to check on a playful 1988 chess game between two men seated on a low wall.

Head uphill through the park, past a statue of Marshall (the country's fourth chief justice, who lived in a 4th Street rooming house) and across two streets, to view a thin and austere Lincoln, at the hike's halfway point. Carved by Lot Flannery, who had known his subject, the 1868 granite statue was funded by citizen donations as the first public monument to Lincoln. Turn right to head east on D Street. Pause to inspect *Guns into Plowshares,* an arresting 1997 sculpture by Esther and Michael Augsburger. Continue for four blocks. Then cross and turn right alongside New Jersey Avenue. At the next corner, turn left onto Louisiana Avenue and then left again into the Japanese American Memorial to Patriotism during World War II.

Opened in 2001, the memorial, or Mahnmal, recognizes the unjust wartime internment of over 120,000 Japanese Americans. It's the only memorial I know that's an apology, as affirmed by Ronald Reagan's inscribed words: "Here we admit a wrong." It also honors the Japanese Americans who served in the armed forces. Designed by Davis Buckley, it includes powerful symbols; a sculpture of two cranes ensnared in barbed wire, a reflecting pool resembling a Zen garden, and a remarkable metal tube that, when sounded, emits a vibrant, templelike bell tone. Leaving the memorial, turn left, walk to the corner of D Street, and cross Louisiana Avenue. Then take a paved path on the right to head south past a pool and a fountain and onto Union Station Plaza, atop a huge government garage. Continue walking through the lovely parklike area toward the Capitol. At Constitution Avenue, turn left and follow the avenue eastward.

At the corner of 2nd Street NE, take a look at the Sewall-Belmont House and its historical plaques. Since 1929, it's been the Women's National Party headquarters. During the War of 1812, it was the only private building torched by the British invaders—after snipers in the house annoyed the British general by hitting his horse. After crossing 2nd Street and Maryland Avenue to stay on Constitution, you'll be in a Capitol Hill area of tree-lined streets and well-kept row houses. Proceed for about five blocks and then swing right onto Massachusetts Avenue and follow it to 11th Street. Then turn right, walk one short block to East Capitol Street, and turn left to enter Lincoln Park.

Follow a paved path to *Emancipation,* a bronze monument paid for by emancipated blacks but designed by whites that depicts a magisterial Lincoln standing next to a crouching African American man. At the 1876 dedication, the keynote speaker, abolitionist and local resident Frederick Douglass, chided sculptor Thomas Ball for the croucher's subservient posture—but his remarks went unreported by local newspapers.

Continue along the path to see the Mary McLeod Bethune Monument and what difference a century can make. Created by Robert Berks in 1974, almost two decades after Bethune's death, the monument shows the educator, civil-rights leader, and National Council of Negro Women founder handing a young boy and girl a rolled document. Composed the year she died and as inscribed on the pedestal, the document is her 68-word "Legacy": "I leave you love. I leave you hope. I leave you the challenge of developing confidence in one another. I leave you a thirst for education. I leave you a respect for the use of power. I leave you faith. I leave you racial dignity. I leave you also a desire to live harmoniously with your fellow man. I leave you finally a responsibility to our young people." When the monument was finished, *Emancipation* was turned to face it. In recent years, Emancipation Day has been revived as an official Washington holiday.

Walk back through the park and head west for ten blocks on boulevard-like East Capitol Street. As the Capitol looms ahead, you'll pass such landmarks as the Folger Shakespeare Library, main Library of Congress building, and Supreme Court building. At 1st Street NE, pause to admire the Capitol and its distinctive cast-iron dome topped by Freedom, a huge bronze statue of a woman that is 19.5 feet high, weighs 7.5 tons, and was installed during the Civil War. Also, check on the Capitol's huge, much-delayed, and overbudget underground visitor center (the largest addition since Lincoln pushed wartime completion of the remodeled building), and mourn the fact that its vista-rich terrace on the west front is now permanently off-limits for post-9/11 security reasons. Then turn right, walk a block north on 1st Street, and turn left onto Constitution Avenue. Cross the well-guarded entrance road, and then swing left onto a walkway that curves downhill to reach a roofless brick structure half-hidden in a small grove. It was designed as a summer retreat for members of Congress by Frederick Law Olmsted when he landscaped the Capitol grounds in the 1870s. Pause to peer into its tiny and charming grotto.

Continuing, turn right at a fork at a nearby stumpy tower (a Capitol ventilation shaft) and follow a curving path (Olmsted didn't like straight lines) to 1st Street NW. Crossing it, note the Peace Monument, which honors the Union seamen who died in the Civil War. Head for the nearby reflecting pool, and then turn left onto a promenade between the pool and a huge memorial to Ulysses S. Grant. Finished in 1922, the memorial depicts soldiers caught up in the frenzy of war, as well as a brooding Grant on horseback. It's realistic without glorifying war. Note the fallen trooper. His face is that of sculptor Henry Merwin Shrady, who labored on the memorial for more than 21 years and died just before it was dedicated. This memorial is the most tersely labeled one I know. It bears just one word: GRANT.

Return to 1st Street and proceed southward, passing an 1887 statue of President James Garfield and then the U.S. Botanic Garden's renovated and dazzling conservatory. At Independence Avenue, cross to explore a small garden packed with assorted and labeled plants set around the large and historic Bartholdi Fountain. Recross Independence, turn left, and head west, past the conservatory and the future National Garden. Turn right onto 3rd Street, cross Maryland Avenue, and turn left onto Jefferson Drive, across from the distinctive National Museum of the American Indian, opened in 2004. Continue westward on Jefferson, past the Air and Space Museum, and across 7th Street. Abreast of the doughnutlike Hirshhorn Museum, swing right to wander through its sunken and well-filled sculpture garden. Emerging on the inner Mall, follow a broad gravel path west to the trailhead. Along the way, you'll pass the Smithsonian Castle and more museums, as well as a working antique carousel.

NEARBY/RELATED ACTIVITIES

During or after the hike, explore the museums and other buildings along the hike route. If you don't mind crowds, repeat the hike during the Mall's annual Smithsonian Folklife Festival or Fourth of July festivities—and allow yourself extra time.

COLUMBIA ISLAND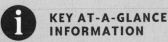

IN BRIEF

Columbia Island is one of Washington's best-kept secrets. Hidden in plain sight, it lies in the Potomac River across from the Lincoln Memorial. Often mistaken for part of Virginia, it serves as a novel and view-rich hiking locale.

Directions ────────────────────➤

From Washington's Mall area, use Constitution Avenue heading west to cross Theodore Roosevelt Memorial Bridge, staying to right. Take first exit to right and then another right onto northbound George Washington Memorial Parkway. Take first exit (within 300 yards) into Theodore Roosevelt Island parking lot on right. To get there from parkway's southbound lanes, cross into Washington, turn around, and follow directions given above. Note: To return to Washington or southbound lanes after hike, drive north on parkway for 0.7 miles and take first exit on left onto Spout Run Parkway; then either take first exit on left to get onto southbound parkway, or continue to Lee Highway, which connects to local streets and Interstate 66.

Or use Metro and your feet to get to trailhead. Take Orange Line or Blue Line train to Rosslyn Metro station and then walk 0.8 miles to trailhead: From main entrance, turn left and walk north (downhill) on North Moore Street, cross North 19th Street, turn right alongside Lee Highway, cross North Lynn Street, turn left and walk north on North Lynn, and cross Lee Highway; at far corner, turn right onto sign-posted Mount Vernon Trail, and follow it to trailhead. Contact Metro, (202) 637-7000 or www.wmata.com.

Another Metro option: Take Blue Line train to Arlington Cemetery station, and then walk 0.2 miles east on Memorial Drive sidewalk to tap into hike route at Seabees Memorial.

(i) KEY AT-A-GLANCE INFORMATION

LENGTH: 5.7 miles

CONFIGURATION: Modified loop

DIFFICULTY: Easy

SCENERY: Waterside parklands, cross-Potomac views of mainland Washington, Metro tracks close-up

EXPOSURE: Mostly open

TRAFFIC: Generally light; moderate on Mount Vernon Trail on warm-weather evenings, weekends, holidays

TRAIL SURFACE: Mostly pavement; some grass, dirt

HIKING TIME: 2.5–3.5 hours

SEASON: Year-round

ACCESS: Mount Vernon Trail closes at dark; Columbia Island closed, midnight–6 a.m.; no other restrictions

MAPS: USGS Washington West

FACILITIES: Toilet at trailhead; toilets, water, phones, cafe at marina; water at LBJ grove

FOR MORE INFORMATION: Contact George Washington Memorial Parkway, (703) 289-2500 or www.nps.gov/gwmp

SPECIAL COMMENTS: Be very careful when crossing roads; best and safest time to do this hike is on weekend mornings or (even better) holiday mornings

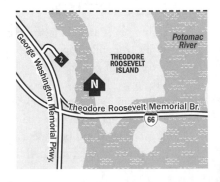

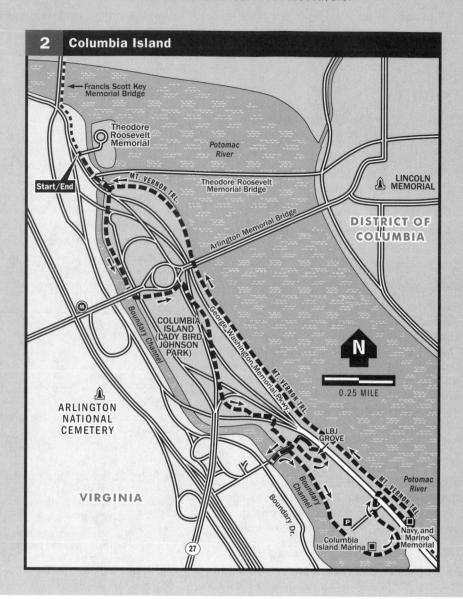

DESCRIPTION

Columbia Island came to be in 1916, when the Potomac River was dredged and the spoils were piled up on the Virginia shore. Because the new land formed an island, it automatically became part of Washington, D.C., thanks to an ancient law denying Virginia even part-ownership of the Potomac. But that didn't prevent Virginia from protesting. The matter was settled in the 1930s, when the District received the island and Virginia received reclaimed land later developed as National Airport. That same decade the island became a key link in the metro area's growing road network. The island was also landscaped, but its primary purpose was to carry motor traffic.

In 1968 the National Park Service designated the 121-acre island as Lady Bird Johnson Park to honor the then–First Lady's efforts to beautify the country. The Lyndon Baines Johnson Memorial Grove was added in 1974, the year after the ex-president died. The island now has many dogwoods, pines, and flowering bushes, as well as myriad daffodils and fine views of mainland Washington and the river.

This hike (a revised and expanded version of my initial island outing) is a 5.7-mile counterclockwise loop that follows much of the perimeter of the mostly flat island. It crosses heavily traveled and high-speed roadways, so be vigilant.

To get started from the parking-lot trailhead (legally in Virginia), march to the lot's south end and proceed on the mostly paved Mount Vernon Trail. At the first T-junction, turn left to stay close to the river. Continuing, you'll get to a concrete bridge with gray metal railings (at the 0.5-mile mark) at the mouth of Boundary Channel, which makes the island an island and legally part of Washington. Beyond the bridge, swing right and climb the slope to reach the northbound parkway lanes (eyes left to watch for traffic). Cross carefully and proceed across a grassy vale to the southbound parkway lanes (eyes right). Cross just as carefully and swing right onto a grassy landscaped area and proceed alongside the channel.

About 50 yards before reaching the arches that support Memorial Drive, turn left and cross the parkway (eyes left). Then climb the grassy slope and, at the top, head for the paved path around the traffic circle at the western end of Arlington Memorial Bridge. Turn right onto that path and walk across the Boundary Channel Bridge (and off the island) to the Seabees Memorial (almost 1 mile into the hike). Completed in 1974, the black granite monument is one of those rare Washington-area memorials that explain their subjects' significance. Walk behind the memorial to get onto a dirt trail that crosses an open grassy area. Follow it, staying left, for about 0.3 miles to a huge sunken sycamore whose lower branches start at ground level.

Then return to the Seabees Memorial and cross Memorial Drive with due diligence to visit the rifle-toting *Hiker* (formally, the United Spanish War Veterans Memorial). Erected in 1965, the statue is said to depict an American soldier—not a hiker. Then take the sidewalk back across the bridge and onto the island again. Continue on the paved path around the traffic circle to reach the parkway (2 miles into the hike). Cross defensively (eyes right) to enter Lady Bird Johnson Park. Then, at a T-junction a few feet ahead, detour a few yards to the left to read the plaque. Then reverse course and head generally southward on the paved path.

Cross the next roadway perceptively (eyes right) and continue. At the next fork, turn right and head gently uphill. On reaching the next roadway, cross with great care (eyes right) and keep going, slightly uphill and across a bridge. On reaching the roadway after that, cross the same way and descend a grassy slope. Then head across the grass toward a large roadside sign and cross the roadway alertly (eyes right). On the other side, swing left onto a dirt trail and stay with it as it swings right through open woodlands close to Boundary Channel.

On reaching a gravel path and fork, stay to the right, and then turn right at the next T-junction to take a wooden bridge across the channel to visit Virginia in sight

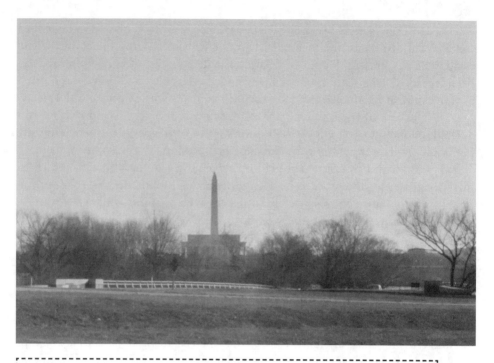

Seen from Columbia Island, the city seems to have sprouted a new edifice; it could be the Washington-Lincoln Memorial.

of the looming Pentagon (at the hike's 2.8-mile and almost-halfway mark). There, push Lady Bird Johnson's labeled button and listen closely. Then go back over the bridge to continue on a broad flagstone path that swings right and then left to reach the center of the 15-acre LBJ Memorial Grove. There, set on a circular paving-stone plaza rimmed with white pines, is a rough-hewn 19-foot-high slab of Texas granite.

Retrace your steps on the flagstone path to the first junction. There, turn left onto a gravel path; then go right at the next fork and walk through Columbia Island marina's parking lot to the cafe's patio. Then take the access road to the parkway, where green signs mark a pedestrian crossing (3.5 miles into hike). Cross vigilantly, turn right, and take a narrow paved path alongside the parkway to get to seven aluminum seagulls skimming the crest of a large aluminum wave breaking across a granite base. That's the Navy and Marine Memorial, created by Ernest Bagni del Piatti and erected in 1934. Read the eloquent inscription. Then head for the river, but pause to read a large sign. Dated 1990, it's the memorial's inscription translated into bureaucratese. Then get onto the paved riverside path (Mount Vernon Trail), turn left, and hike 2 miles back to trailhead, staying to the right at each intersection.

NEARBY/RELATED ACTIVITIES

For a glorious postscript, do the 2-mile circuit around Roosevelt Island (see Hike 4, page 27, for details and a map).

POTOMAC PARK AND SOUTHWEST WASHINGTON

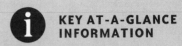

IN BRIEF

Extending south from the Mall, Washington's Potomac Park is just the place for a hike that features waterfront views, the Tidal Basin, memorials, paved paths, and much open space, especially when combined with the history-rich streets of Southwest Washington.

DESCRIPTION

Potomac Park is one of the youngest parks of Washington, dating literally from the 1880s. And Southwest Washington is one of the oldest parts of the city, dating from the 1790s. Together, these two parts make up a one-of-a-kind venue where adventuresome hikers can combine vigorous outdoor exercise with exposure to history and the outdoors—and a colorful fish market. My 9.2-mile circuit hike stays close to the water in going around Potomac Park and the Washington Channel, and then zigzags through the neighborhood streets.

   To get started from the Smithsonian Metro station on the Mall, head south (toward Independence Avenue) for about 20 yards. Turn right onto the paved path along Jefferson Drive. Follow it across 14th and 15th streets NW; then turn left and follow 15th Street to

KEY AT-A-GLANCE INFORMATION

LENGTH: 9.2 miles (with shorter option)

CONFIGURATION: Modified loop

DIFFICULTY: Easy–moderate

SCENERY: Parklands, waterfront views, street scenes

EXPOSURE: Mostly open

TRAFFIC: In Tidal Basin area, moderate–heavy in cherry-blossom season especially on weekends, holidays; lighter at other times; elsewhere, light year-round

TRAIL SURFACE: Pavement

HIKING TIME: 4–5 hours (including refueling shop at wharf)

SEASON: Year-round, but best in nonhot weather

ACCESS: No restrictions

MAPS: USGS Washington West; ADC Metro Washington

FACILITIES: None at trailhead; toilets, water, phones at Tidal Basin memorials, elsewhere in park, in Mall museums

FOR MORE INFORMATION: Contact National Capital Parks—Central, (202) 619-7222 or www.nps.gov/nacc; Cultural Tourism D.C., www.culturaltourismdc.org

SPECIAL COMMENTS: Finish hike by dusk

Directions

Head for Washington D.C.'s Mall area. Park near trailhead—Smithsonian Metro station entrance within Mall (near Independence Avenue and 12th Street SW). Arrive early on crowded warm-weather weekends and holidays; beware local parking regulations (read signs carefully). Or use Metro: Smithsonian station is on Orange, Blue lines; Metrobuses operate on nearby streets. Contact Metro, (202) 637-7000 or www.wmata.com.

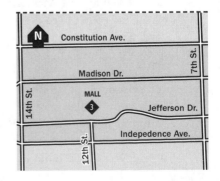

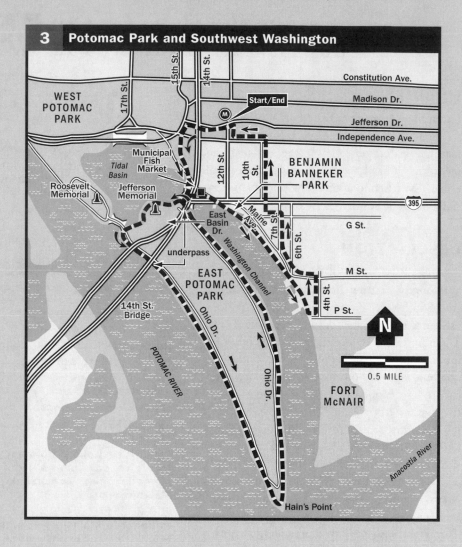

3 **Potomac Park and Southwest Washington**

Independence. Cross to continue on Raoul Wallenberg Place (appropriately close to the U.S. Holocaust Memorial Museum). Then cross Maine Avenue, walk a few yards, and go left onto the paved path that flanks the Tidal Basin and then becomes a sidewalk that bumps over the basin's hidden outlet. Next, turn right to leave the sidewalk and walk along the Tidal Basin to John Russell Pope's Jefferson Memorial.

You'll be walking through a man-made landscape. In fact, the land itself did not exist until the 1880s. Back then, the area consisted of often-flooded swamplands and mudflats along the silted-up Potomac River. Then along came a man with a plan. He was Peter Hains, an army officer who happened to be between wars (a Civil War veteran, he later served in both the Spanish-American War and World War I). To build up the mudflats and make the river more navigable, he

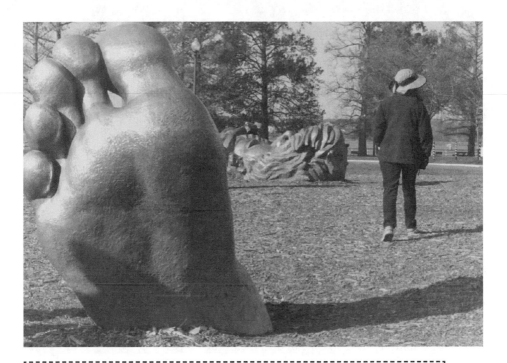

The aluminum giant on Hains Point has been struggling to get up—while being walked across by visitors—since 1980.

ordered the dredging of the river's main channel and Washington Channel, with the spoils to be piled between them, and also on the mudflats.

Held in place by a seawall, the spoils formed a long, uvula-like peninsula. The Tidal Basin was created in the following decade. It was built to collect river water for releasing into the pier-lined Washington Channel when water levels got too low. Subsequently, the new lands were landscaped. In 1912, 3,000 flowering cherry trees—a gift from Japan to the United States—were planted around the Tidal Basin (today, only about a hundred survive; the rest are replacements). Starting in the 1920s the basin also served as a whites-only public swimming pool, complete with a sandy beach, and the federal government operated a 60-acre tourist camp for visiting motorists on the peninsula. The resort disappeared with the construction of the Jefferson Memorial, opened in 1943. Today, the Tidal Basin and the adjoining areas that make up West Potomac Park are a world-famous tourist attraction, and in spring the basin's walkways are wreathed in cherry blossoms and upturned faces.

At the classical-style Jefferson Memorial, pause to take in fine views across the city and of the nearby Roosevelt Memorial (see Hike 4, page 27). Also take a look at the rather uninspired statue of Jefferson (the emphasis seems to be on the great man's great coat). And read the wall panels of Jefferson quotes and speculate why the first panel slightly mangles the Declaration of Independence. Then resume walking west to the junction of East Basin Drive and Ohio Drive, near the basin's inlet. There, turn left and cross East Basin Drive to visit a jolly Virginia statesman in bronze, George Mason, sitting casually on a stone bench. Meander around his colorful-in-spring garden, and then cross Ohio Drive carefully, cross the grass to the seawall, and turn left onto the paved perimeter path that will be your route for the next 4 miles around the peninsula, which is coextensive with East Potomac Park.

This park section remains a recreational area but is dominated by a golf course and playing fields. Continuing, you'll reach Hain's Point (named for the dredger), a windy but bird-rich open spot where the Anacostia River joins the Potomac. After the point, detour to visit *The Awakening*, a huge and literally disjointed aluminum statue created by J. Seward Johnson Jr. in 1980. Then keep going, along the Washington Channel (you'll see Fort McNair on the far side), and follow the path as it cuts left to become a sidewalk that passes under Francis Case Memorial Bridge. Stay on the sidewalk as it swings right and then turns right again alongside Maine Avenue. Pass the Washington Marina, and swing right to get to the Municipal Fish Market—commonly called the Wharf—where cooked food will be waiting.

From the Wharf, get onto the waterfront promenade and keep going. Stop to read the first of several Cultural Tourism D.C. information boards you'll pass on this route—and also consult the boards to get a sense of the neighborhood's long and rich, but troubled, history. It's poignant to realize that so much of the original community has disappeared as a chilling consequence of massive federal experiments in urban renewal starting in the 1950s. Not only were huge tracts simply cleared and rebuilt, but some 20,000 African Americans were displaced.

Follow the promenade to the end, at the Women's *Titanic* Memorial, which, like the Maine-lobsterman statue you'll pass earlier, has no apparent connection to Southwest Washington. Then swing inland on a broad walkway leading to 4th Street SW. Turn left and head north along 4th Street, pausing to take stock on the left of Washington's oldest surviving row houses (street numbers 1315–21), dating from 1794. On reaching M Street, turn left, go two blocks, and then cross M Street and proceed up 6th Street far enough to swing left through the famed Arena Stage theater complex. Emerging on Maine Avenue, continue to 7th Street. Turn right, walk north for three blocks, and turn left onto G Street. Take G to 6th Street, cross at the light, and follow the ramp up to Benjamin Banneker Park.

The park is intended to honor the self-taught African American astronomer, mathematician, and almanac writer who helped survey the site that would become Washington. However, as you'll see, it's in an almost-invisible, noise-polluted location and is badly neglected. Now head north again, along 10th Street and through L'Enfant Plaza (and the Forrestal Building). Cross Independence Avenue, turn left, and walk to 12th Street. There, turn right and return to the trailhead.

For a shorter hike of 6.3 miles, skip Southwest and go directly back to the trailhead from Potomac Park by way of the sidewalk at the Tidal Basin's outlet.

NEARBY/RELATED ACTIVITIES

Given that there are so many—or too many—things to see and do in the Mall area, try something new to you.

ROOSEVELT ISLAND TO ROOSEVELT MEMORIAL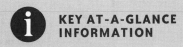

IN BRIEF

The close-in Potomac River parklands are rich in views and include two Roosevelt memorials and a nature preserve. Two memorial bridges enable hikers to some stimulating connections.

DESCRIPTION

Metro-area hikers owe Theodore Roosevelt and his distant relative Franklin Delano Roosevelt at least a grateful nod. During TR's 1901–09 presidency, the country got a forest service and wildlife-refuge system, and the

---

Directions

From Washington's Mall area, use Constitution Avenue heading west to cross Theodore Roosevelt Memorial Bridge, staying to right. Then take first exit to right and then another right onto northbound George Washington Memorial Parkway. Take first exit (within 300 yards) into Theodore Roosevelt Island parking lot on right. To get there from parkway's southbound lanes, cross into Washington, turn around, and follow above directions. *Note:* To return to Washington or southbound lanes after hike, drive 0.7 miles north on parkway and take first left exit onto Spout Run Parkway; then either take first left exit onto southbound parkway or continue to Lee Highway, which connects to local roads and Interstate 66.

Or use Metro and feet to get to trailhead. Take Orange Line or Blue Line train to Rosslyn Metro station and then walk 0.8 miles to trailhead: From main entrance, turn left and walk north (downhill) on North Moore Street, cross North 19th Street, turn right alongside Lee Highway, cross North Lynn Street, turn left and walk north on North Lynn, and cross Lee Highway; at far corner, turn right onto signposted Mount Vernon Trail and follow it to trailhead. Contact Metro, (202) 637-7000 or www.wmata.com.

KEY AT-A-GLANCE INFORMATION

LENGTH: 9.2 miles (with shorter options)

CONFIGURATION: Modified loop

DIFFICULTY: Easy–moderate

SCENERY: River and canal views, street scenes, parklands, woodlands

EXPOSURE: Mostly open; more so in winter

TRAFFIC: Usually light; moderate–heavy on warm-weather evenings, weekends, holidays—more so at FDR Memorial

TRAIL SURFACE: Pavement, dirt, boardwalk, brick

HIKING TIME: 5–6 hours

SEASON: Year-round

ACCESS: TR island open daily, 8 a.m.–dark; Mount Vernon Trail, C&O Canal towpath open until dark; no restrictions elsewhere

MAPS: USGS Washington West; ADC Metro Washington, Northern Virginia; sketch map in free brochure and on bulletin board (both on TR island)

FACILITIES: Toilets, water on TR island; toilets, water, phones at boat center (warm season), FDR memorial, near towpath; toilet, water at volleyball courts; water along Ohio Drive

FOR MORE INFORMATION: See details at end of Description

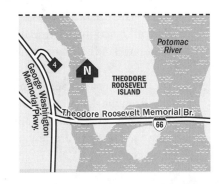

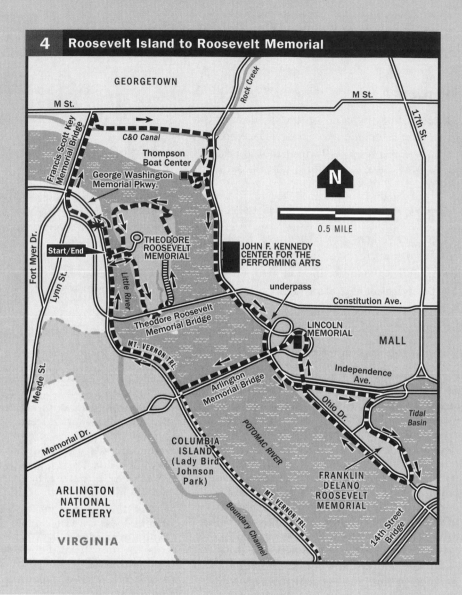

metro area had a hiker in the White House. During FDR's 1933–1945 presidency, the country got many new and improved national parks, including metro-area parklands along both banks of the Potomac.

This 9.2-mile, hill-less, and history- and culture-infused hike loops through these scenic parklands. Managed by the National Park Service (NPS), they include the Franklin Delano Roosevelt Memorial at the Tidal Basin and the Theodore Roosevelt Memorial and nature preserve on Theodore Roosevelt Island. The hike route's trail signs are few, so follow my directions closely. Also be careful about road traffic.

The hike begins with a mini-loop around TR Island, which is part of Washington, not Virginia (see Hike 2, page 19). Long known as Analostan Island, it was a plantation until the Civil War and later a recreation area. Neglected for decades, it was bought by the Theodore Roosevelt Memorial Association in 1931 and given to the NPS. Taken on as a Civilian Conservation Corps project, the island was renamed, stripped of everything man-made, planted with 30,000 trees, and allowed to evolve as a nature preserve. The TR memorial was added in 1967.

To get started, take the footbridge to the heavily wooded island, which is a great place for watching birds, trees, and wildflowers. At a map-equipped bulletin board, turn right and head south on a broad dirt path for 50 yards. At a fork, turn right onto a narrow dirt trail. Then continue, staying to the right at the next junction. After passing under the Theodore Roosevelt Memorial Bridge, turn right again at the next fork. Then follow the trail back under the bridge, and, at a T-junction, turn right and head for the nearby boardwalk.

Where the boardwalk ends, head for the nearby T-junction, turn right, and take the dirt trail leading to the riverbank. There, scan the formerly industrial Georgetown waterfront. Compare what you see with the grimy 1863 view reproduced on a nearby plaque. Also check the writing on the wall—on the bulkheads near a row of high-school and college boathouses. The painters identify their teams and colorfully express their opinions. Heading back, take the first side trail on the right, along the island's northern shore. At a junction, go straight onto a trail heading south. Pass the footbridge and bulletin board, and swing left to follow the curving main path to the TR memorial. That's a large open plaza dominated by a 17-foot-high statue of TR and flanked by large stone tablets inscribed with TR quotations. It seems odd to find such an edifice in a nature preserve.

Then return to the parking-lot trailhead, having hiked almost 2.5 miles. Next, head upriver on the paved Mount Vernon Trail, which crosses the George Washington Memorial Parkway on a footbridge and winds to the foot of the Francis Scott Key Memorial Bridge. Cross the bridge to Georgetown, turn sharply right, and walk through Francis Scott Key Park, with its colorful plantings and plaques that provide the Key facts. Key, who once lived nearby, left because of the C&O Canal construction noise. His bridge was opened in 1924. A poem of his became the official national anthem in 1931. His house was dismantled in 1949.

From the park, descend by steps and ramp to the restored canal. Head east through Georgetown on the dirt—later, brick—towpath, keeping the canal on your right. After passing several locks and basins, the NPS visitor center, and a bust of canal saver William O. Douglas (see Hike 15, page 81), turn right onto the paved Rock Creek Trail and head south along Rock Creek Parkway. At the Thompson Boat Center, detour to cross the parking lot and Rock Creek and reach the waterfront. Walk to the left past the boat center, and take the nearby footbridge to find the concrete post inscribed with "Mile 0" (a towpath marker)—and great views.

Return to the Rock Creek Trail and continue south along the waterfront. Pass the infamous Watergate complex, developed in the 1960s on the site of a former gasworks. Then pass the famous John F. Kennedy Center for the Performing Arts, developed in the same decade on the site of a former brewery. Continuing, you'll go under Roosevelt Bridge at the hike's halfway point (about 4.6 miles) and reach a large flowerbed. Turn left there, cross a side road, and get onto a paved path alongside some volleyball courts. Follow it back to the riverbank and parkway at the foot of the Watergate Steps; then pass under Arlington Memorial Bridge and follow the parkway to where it merges into Independence Avenue at Ohio Drive. There, cross Ohio and continue east on the paved path alongside Independence Avenue.

On reaching a side road (West Basin Drive), cross it, turn right onto a walkway, and proceed across a spur road to the Tidal Basin. Note the plaque marking the site of a future memorial to Martin Luther King Jr. Swing right onto the basinside path and proceed amid the cherry trees. Then turn right to enter the FDR memorial. Completed in 1997, the 7.5-acre memorial is laid out as four walled outdoor enclosures, called "rooms," each devoted to one of FDR's terms of office. Stonework, waterfalls, pools, landscaping, sculptures, and FDR quotations illustrate the years covered, literally and symbolically. Controversy about FDR's concealment of his polio-induced paralysis led to the addition in 2001 of a bronze FDR sitting jauntily in his wheelchair—but minus his customary cigarette holder.

Next, head for the Tidal Basin, turn right onto the perimeter path, and follow it to Ohio Drive. Cross the drive, turn right, and walk north on the paved and scenic riverbank path for 0.75 miles. At Independence Avenue, recross Ohio Drive, cross Independence, and head up the sidewalk. Then cross the Lincoln Memorial's large plaza to reach Henry Bacon Drive (the memorial itself is covered in Hike 1, page 12). Carefully cross Henry Bacon Drive, turn left, and follow the sidewalk leading to Arlington Memorial Bridge (crossing 23rd Street NW and other roadways most carefully en route). Cross the bridge and stay on the sidewalk as it swings right. Then turn sharply right to descend the grassy slope to the riverbank. Turn left onto the Mount Vernon Trail, and head north for about a mile, half of it on boardwalk, to get back to the trailhead.

To shorten the hike to 6.7 miles, just skip the island circuit. For a 5-mile outing, start by going directly to the TR memorial and then use the Mount Vernon Trail and Memorial Bridge to visit the FDR memorial and return.

For more information, contact the NPS's George Washington Memorial Parkway, (703) 289-2500 or www.nps.gov/gwmp, regarding TR Island and the Mount Vernon Trail; the NPS visitor center in Georgetown, (202) 653-5190, regarding the canal and towpath; and the NPS's National Capital Parks–Central, (202) 619-7222 or www.nps.gov/nacc, regarding the FDR memorial.

NEARBY/RELATED ACTIVITIES

Go birding on Theodore Roosevelt Island. Circle the island again—by boat (rent one at Thompson's or at Jack's Boats, under Key Bridge). Study the presidents Roosevelt and revisit both memorials.

U.S. NATIONAL ARBORETUM `05`

IN BRIEF

Tucked away in gritty eastern Washington, the U.S. National Arboretum ranks among the city's finest outdoor treasures and is this book's most botanically diverse hiking venue.

DESCRIPTION

Wedged between New York Avenue and the Anacostia River, the 446-acre arboretum serves primarily as a U.S. Department of Agriculture horticultural research center of global renown. However, for those of us who know, it's also a spacious and exotic recreational area that can dazzle the senses, intrigue the mind, restore the spirit, and exercise the body of the receptive hiker.

Directions

From downtown Washington, D.C., take New York Avenue NE (US 50) heading out of town. Turn right onto Bladensburg Road. Drive about 0.4 miles and turn left onto R Street, which ends in 0.2 miles at the arboretum's main entrance. Drive through gates to parking lot. Or, while on New York Avenue, cross Bladensburg Road to swing right onto service road leading to other gated entrance; once inside, bear right and follow Hickey Lane to R Street parking lot. *Note:* To access westbound New York Avenue after hike, get back on R Street, turn right onto Bladensburg Road, and then take first left, onto Montana Avenue, which runs into New York Avenue.

Or travel by Metro. Take Orange Line or Blue Line train to Stadium Armory Metro station, transfer to Metrobus B2, leave bus at Bladensburg Road and R Street, and walk 0.2 miles along R Street. On weekends and holidays, use Metrobus X6, which runs from Union Station (on Red Line) to arboretum's R Street parking lot. Contact Metro, (202) 637-7000 or www.wmata.com.

KEY AT-A-GLANCE INFORMATION

LENGTH: 7.3 miles (with shorter options)

CONFIGURATION: Modified loop

DIFFICULTY: Moderate

SCENERY: Woodlands, open spaces, exotic plants, odd structures

EXPOSURE: Mostly open

TRAFFIC: Generally very light to light; much heavier on spring weekends

TRAIL SURFACE: Mostly paved; some dirt, gravel, concrete, grass, mulch

HIKING TIME: 4–6 hours (allowing for lingering to take in the sights)

ACCESS: Open daily, 8 a.m.–5 p.m., but 8 a.m.–7 p.m. in June–July (closed on December 25)

MAPS: USGS Washington East; sketch map in free arboretum brochure

FACILITIES: Toilets, water at administration building; toilets at Arbor House and (warm-weather months only) near National Grove of State Trees and in Asian collections

FOR MORE INFORMATION: Call (202) 245-2726 or visit www.usna.usda.gov

SPECIAL COMMENTS: Remember that museum closes at 3:30 p.m., gates leading to riverbank close at 4:30 p.m., and arboretum's entrance gates clang shut at 5 p.m.

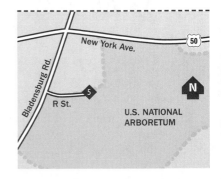

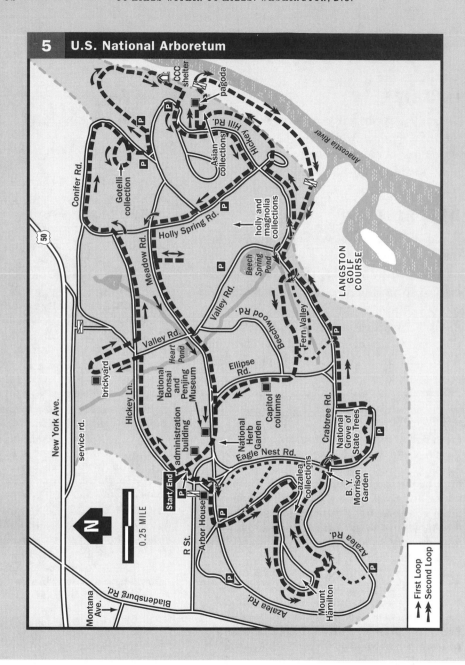

5   U.S. National Arboretum

Although the gently rolling woodlands and grassy open spaces seem serenely naturalistic, the landscape is thoroughly man-made. It represents the transformation of a tract of traditional American farmland into a thriving, one-of-a-kind botanical community consisting of many kinds of plants from around the world. Having led many hikes there for almost a decade, I know that the scenery changes

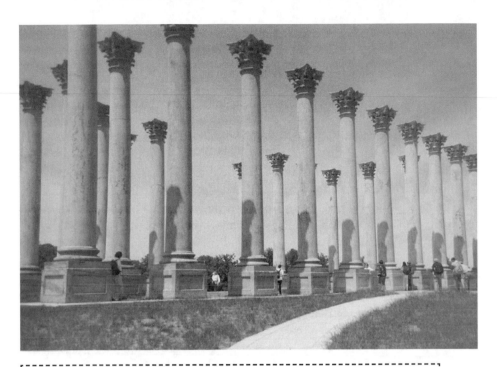

Once part of the Capitol, these columns are now firmly planted at the arboretum, where they may well confound future archaeologists.

with each passing season—and also that blooming plants are to be found in all 12 months. Accordingly, I rank the arboretum as both an educationally and aesthetically rewarding hiking venue at any time of year.

The hike I have devised consists of two wiggly loops totaling 7.3 miles and 1,600 feet of elevation change. Both start at the R Street parking lot and mostly follow clearly signposted paved roads usually used only by a few strollers, joggers, bikers, and car-enclosed sightseers, as well as security patrols. You can shorten or otherwise modify the hike by using my map, the signposts, and the "Hort Hot Spots" and other brochures available at the administration building (visitor center). Also keep in mind that the plants are catalogued, that many of them are labeled, and that the staffers are helpful to visitors.

I suggest starting with the slightly longer (3.7 miles) and flatter of my two loops. Take Hickey Lane heading away from the R Street entrance. At the first intersection, detour to the left to cross a large parking lot to look at the fenced-off beehive kilns that were part of a major brickyard that operated from 1909 to 1972 and used local clay. Then continue on Hickey. Admire the bordering maples, turn left at the next junction, and proceed on Conifer Road. Watch on your right for the Gotelli collection, a five-acre Lilliputian forest of dwarf conifers donated by ardent collector William Gotelli in 1962 and worth a detour. Let yourself be amazed by the single-trunk weeping blue Atlas cedar and other beauties. Also meander through a lovely azalea grove.

Continuing on Conifer, pause to inspect some dawn redwoods. As a plaque explains, the species was classified as extinct when discovered in fossil form in the 1930s, but living specimens were found in China in the 1940s, and some reached the arboretum in 1948. Next, turn left onto Hickey Hill Road and walk gently uphill, swing left through a parking lot, and take a paved path to a circle. There, head gently downhill on the grass to reach and turn right onto a woodland trail overlooking the Anacostia River. Stop at a renovated shelter, originally built in the 1930s by the Civilian Conservation Corps as part of its project to develop the arboretum, which had been authorized by Congress in 1927 (but was not opened to the public until 1949).

After the shelter, walk gently uphill on the grass for 80 yards, and turn left onto a woodland dirt trail and into the impressive Asian collections. Proceed, ignoring all side trails and admiring the cold-hardy camellia bushes. Next, swing left at a fork marked by two huge tulip trees, go through the next two intersections, and pause at a bench-equipped overlook. Then turn right and proceed, watching for a spectacular late-blooming Lu Shan snow camellia the size of a tree. Keep going, up some steps, and turn right onto a short gravel path, along which you'll see three unusual Asian trees: a dove tree, with white leaves that flutter in a breeze; an *Idesia polycarpa* tree, with its heart-shaped leaves and drooping orange-red berries; and a ginkgo tree, with fan-shaped leaves that turn brilliant yellow.

Then turn left onto Hickey Hill Road, follow it downhill for 0.3 miles, and turn right onto Holly Spring Road. Follow that road uphill to a parking area on the left. Pause there to sample the arboretum's hollies and magnolias, on the left. Then continue along the road for 0.3 miles, and then turn left and westward onto aptly named Meadow Road. After about 180 yards, detour left off that road to visit a two-centuries-old willow oak—the arboretum's largest tree. Then follow Meadow Road for 0.5 miles back to the trailhead.

Before doing the hike's second loop, explore the exquisite National Bonsai and Penjing Museum (which closes at 3:30 p.m.). Also roam through the nearby National Herb Garden, where there's much to both smell and see, including old varieties of roses and 800 kinds of herbs. And in summer, look for water lilies and flashy carp in the administration building's patio ponds.

To do the 3.6-mile second loop, leave the parking lot, cross the entrance road, pass the Arbor House gift shop, and head west on Azalea Road. Go 200 yards; then turn left at a small parking lot and head uphill on a paved road leading to the summit of well-wooded Mount Hamilton, one of the city's highest points (240 feet above sea level). There, peer through the trimmed trees to see the distant U.S. Capitol and perhaps puzzle (as I do) over why the nearby clearing contains two broken columns that once graced that building.

Cross the clearing and head downhill on a dirt trail. Take the first left turn, and follow another dirt trail eastward for 0.3 miles across a hillside covered by mature azalea bushes, the legacy of the arboretum's first director, Benjamin Y. Morrison, who personally planted some 15,000 of them in 1946–47. Go through the next intersection and descend to reach the azalea-filled B. Y. Morrison Garden, guarded by a colorful and rare lace-bark pine. Next, descend to Azalea Road, and bear right to follow Eagle Nest Road to the National Grove of State Trees, where all of them are named (including D.C.'s) and some of them have been planted.

Then continue east and north to reach and turn right onto Crabtree Road. Keep going for 0.5 miles, first on Crabtree and then (after turning right) on Hickey Hill Road. At the next intersection, turn right onto a short and uphill dead-end road; stay to the left and watch for a dirt woodland trail going off to the left. Follow that trail for 0.2 miles until you emerge at Hickey Hill Road. Next, step onto an ugly-yellow concrete walkway, follow it for 100 yards, turn left onto another one, and go 30 yards to turn right onto a dirt path leading down into the Asian collections, where you'll reach a pagoda.

From there, take a stepping-stone path downhill and turn left to continue on the yellow walkway. At the bottom, pass through the perimeter fence (the gates are locked at 4:30 p.m.) and onto federal parkland, and then follow a dirt-and-gravel path along the Anacostia for 0.3 miles to return to the arboretum grounds (through another gate) and swing left onto Hickey Hill Road. Then walk to and turn left onto Crabtree Road, and follow it for 200 yards to the first side trail on the right, across from two longleaf pines. Peer past the pines to get a glimpse of historic Langston Golf Course, opened in 1939 as the segregated city's first full course open to African Americans.

Then take the side trail through Fern Valley, a wooded stream valley filled with informatively labeled native-American plants. Cross a stream, turn left, and follow the trail uphill, staying to the right. After passing a beautiful and comfortable wooden bench, watch for and take a dirt trail on the right that leads out of the woods and reaches Ellipse Road. From there, head for an amazing site: 22 capital-topped sandstone columns arranged in austere, Acropolis-like splendor on a low knoll. The columns were installed there in 1990, three decades after completing their first assignment—supporting the Capitol's east portico for 130 years—and after being stored, allegedly in Kenilworth Marsh. Finally, take the nearby concrete walkway lined with saplings—and prematurely labeled the Flowering Tree Walk—back to the administration building area and trailhead.

NEARBY/RELATED ACTIVITIES

Visit the Arbor House gift shop (open from March to mid-December, 10 a.m. to 3 p.m.). Combine this hike with the following one in Kenilworth Aquatic Gardens and Kenilworth Marsh. Heading back downtown on New York Avenue, turn left onto Penn Street (about 1.5 miles from Bladensburg Road) to splurge at the richly stocked, inexpensive, and multiethnic Capital City Market and the D.C. Farmers Market (try to get there before 3 p.m.). Contact the arboretum (see page 31) to learn about its volunteer opportunities and its many program offerings, especially the 5-mile full-moon hikes.

06 KENILWORTH AQUATIC GARDENS AND KENILWORTH MARSH

KEY AT-A-GLANCE INFORMATION

LENGTH: 2.5 miles

CONFIGURATION: Two out-and-backs separated by figure-eight loop

DIFFICULTY: Very easy

SCENERY: Water-lily ponds, marshlands, woodlands

EXPOSURE: Two-thirds shady; less when leaves are down

TRAFFIC: Very light; heavy only during Waterlily Festival (fourth Saturday in July)

TRAIL SURFACE: Mostly hard-packed, pebbly dirt; some gravel, grass, boardwalk

HIKING TIME: 2–2.5 hours (allowing for birding, butterflying, etc.)

SEASON: Year-round

ACCESS: Open daily, 7 a.m.–4 p.m. (but closed on Thanksgiving Day, December 25, January 1)

MAPS: USGS Washington East; sketch map in free gardens pamphlet

FACILITIES: Toilets, water, phones at visitor center; water at parking lot

FOR MORE INFORMATION: Contact National Capital Parks–East, (202) 426-6905, or www.nps.gov/nace/keaq

SPECIAL COMMENTS: Be sure to leave park by 4 p.m., when outer entrance gate is closed

IN BRIEF

The Kenilworth Aquatic Gardens and Kenilworth Marsh, in Washington's gritty eastern section, constitute an alluring botanical gem, a too-well-kept city secret, and a hiking locale worth visiting in any season.

DESCRIPTION

For a short and exotic urban hike that's wonderfully nonurban, visit the Kenilworth Aquatic Gardens and adjoining 77-acre Kenilworth Marsh, located on the east bank of the Anacostia River. There you'll find a combination of tidy garden landscape and mini-wilderness in the collective form of gorgeous water-lily ponds (also a summertime butterfly

Directions

From downtown Washington, take New York Avenue NE (US 50) heading out of town (northeastward). After passing Bladensburg Road intersection and U.S. National Arboretum, go about 2 miles and turn right onto Kenilworth Avenue (DC 201). Head south for 0.4 miles toward Interstate 295 and then take first right (watch for sign for Addison Road and Eastern Avenue) onto Kenilworth Avenue frontage road. Follow large brown "Aquatic Gardens" signs. Go straight at Eastern Avenue T-junction, proceed for two blocks, and turn right onto Douglas Street. Go 0.3 miles to end of Douglas and turn right onto Anacostia Avenue. Then turn left through gate into visitor parking lot—the trailhead. *Note*: Leaving gardens can be tricky because of one-way streets; one option is to return to Kenilworth Avenue frontage road and Douglas Street, turn right onto one-way frontage road, go 1.5 miles, turn right onto Benning Road, go right onto 17th Street, and then, at Bladensburg Road, go either right toward New York Avenue or left toward Capitol Hill area.

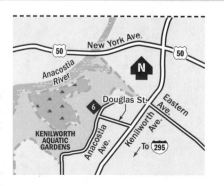

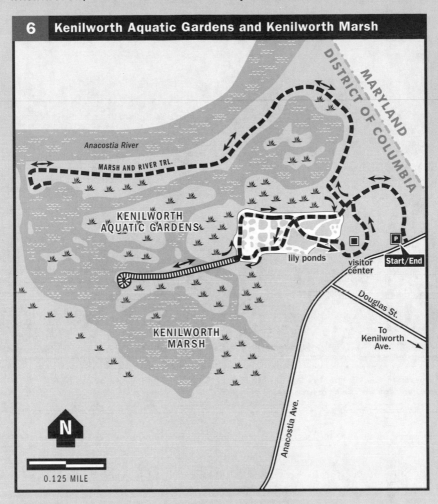

6   Kenilworth Aquatic Gardens and Kenilworth Marsh

hot spot), wildflower-infested woodlands, a plant-and-wildlife-rich tidal marsh, and a lovely air of serenity. I have used these ingredients to devise a 2.5-mile, four-leg excursion. The first leg is an out-and-back 1.5-mile trek on a woodland trail. The second is a stroll through half of the 12-acre lily-pond area. The third is an out-and-back trip on a boardwalk that penetrates the marsh. The fourth covers the pond area's other half.

In planning a Kenilworth visit, remember that the water-lily blooming season lasts from May until September, with color lingering into November. The hardy lilies, which stay outside year-round, have blooms that open during the day and are at their peak in June and July. The lotuses and other tropical lilies, which winter in greenhouses, are at their flowering best in July and August. They include both day bloomers and night bloomers. On a morning visit, you'll see—and smell—the day bloomers as they open and the night bloomers before they

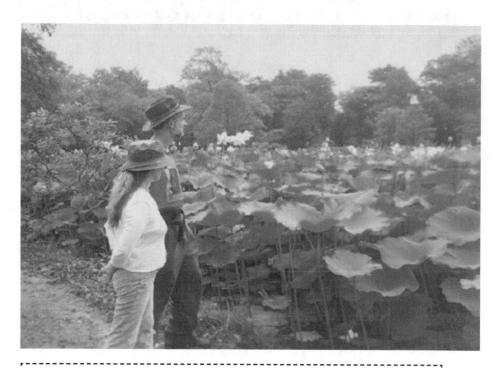

Lotuses, with their fragrant yellow flowers, thrive in summer at Kenilworth, as do hikers who can cope with being in the open.

close. Remember, too, that the park can be glorious at just about any time of year. Winter, for instance, can be a lovely time to watch the sun rise over the marsh.

To get started from the visitor parking lot, head catty-corner from the entrance gate onto an unpaved service road. It follows the perimeter fence and curves left. The greenhouses beyond the fence produce fresh flowers for the White House. After about 300 yards, turn right onto the signposted Marsh & River Trail. A large information board tells about the marsh, including its 1930s decline and 1990s restoration. Both processes involved the U.S. Army Corps of Engineers, although the board mentions only its 1990s role.

The dirt-surfaced Marsh & River Trail follows a man-made spit rimming the Anacostia River (to your right, although summer foliage hides it). Winding through young and mostly deciduous woods for three-quarters of a mile, the trail is thickly flanked by wildflowers, shrubs, and poison ivy. You'll also get glimpses of the marsh and waterfowl, and perhaps a muskrat or otter. The trail ends by hooking to the left along a narrow channel linking the Anacostia River proper to the marsh, and then it peters out at the water's edge. Check out the view, note the distant boardwalk, and then return to the information board. From there, swing right at a bamboo clump and enter the pond area, where grass-topped dikes separate the ponds. (Although I have plotted a figure-eight route through the area, you may want to just wander around freely.)

The ponds date from the late 19th century, when a government clerk named Walter Shaw planted a dozen lilies from his native Maine in an old farm pond. His hobby soon became a business. New ponds were dug, exotic species were imported and cultivated, and Shaw's water gardens became both a thriving enterprise and tourist attraction. In the late 1930s, though, the gardens seemed doomed when the U.S. Army Corps of Engineers embarked on dredging the Anacostia and draining the marsh. But the Department of the Interior stepped in and bought the gardens—for $15,000—and made them the core of a new National Park Service unit. (Administratively, the gardens and marsh now form part of Kenilworth Park, which is part of Anacostia Park.)

Proceed along the broad gravel perimeter path, passing hardy water lilies and other aquatic plants on your left. Then take the first left (where a white ash holds a large branch over the path) onto one of the dikes. Go right at the Y-intersection, pass lotuses on your left and hardy lilies on your right, stay left at the next intersection, and walk straight through the one after that. Then turn right to rejoin the perimeter path. Next, turn left across a small bridge and circle clockwise around a cluster of lotus ponds to reach the boardwalk.

Extending almost a quarter of a mile into the marsh, the boardwalk—and its information boards—introduce visitors to the ecology of a freshwater tidal marsh. You'll see such native plants as cattails, sedges, American lotus, and wild rice, as well as purple loosestrife and other invasive or alien species—and much sky. Where the boardwalk ends, it's possible to see herons and egrets fishing, ducks bobbing, or an osprey or bald eagle flapping by. Contemplate, or even marvel at, the existence of such a place within the city limits. Then retrace your steps to dry land.

Leaving the boardwalk, continue straight on a gravel path and return to the figure-eight pattern by swinging left onto the perimeter path past hardy lilies on your right. The marshlands on the left are a last remnant of the area's original wetlands. Next are the ponds' spectacular South American tropical lilies called *Victoria amazonica,* with their huge floating pads and night-blooming, football-sized flowers. Gawk for a moment, and then continue on the perimeter path as it curves to the right, past more hardy lilies. In this area, watch for smooth wet trails left on the path by beavers that slip into the ponds at night to feast on water-lily roots.

Turn right at the overhanging white-ash branch (oddly, this seems to be the only labeled tree in the gardens and marsh). Swing left at the Y-junction, and head for the rear of the visitor center. There, you'll see specimens of East Indian lotus descended from a couple of centuries-old and remarkably still-viable seeds discovered in Manchuria in 1951. Finally, head for and pass a large conifer, cross a small parking lot, and then turn right onto a narrow gravel trail that leads through a gate and out to the visitor parking lot.

NEARBY/RELATED ACTIVITIES

There's much to do at Kenilworth. Tour the exhibit-packed visitor center. Talk to the rangers. Take a ranger-guided morning tour of the ponds (call for details). Arrange to take a canoe trip through the marshes with the Anacostia Watershed Society, (301) 699-6204 or **www.anacostiaws.org.** (The AWS is devoted to restoring what, alas, was named in 2006 as one of the country's most polluted waterways.) On the fourth Saturday in July, enjoy the Waterlily Festival, which features tours, entertainment, food, and the educational presence of the AWS and other environmental and community groups.

Try combining this hike with part or all of the outing I have devised for the nearby U.S. National Arboretum. The two locales complement one another. Kenilworth provides exotic aquatic gardens and an all-American marsh (allowing for the alien plants) with its avian residents and visitors. The arboretum offers a rich sampling of plants from several continents. And both locales have views to be found nowhere else in the city.

BROOKLAND 07

IN BRIEF

Brookland, in Northeast Washington, is an unusual community of religious and educational institutions, residential areas, and cemeteries. It's a rewarding hiking locale for those who like to use their powers of locomotion, observation, and reflection.

DESCRIPTION

Brookland is a distinctive area that feels more like a separate community than an outlying part of the nation's capital. It's an intriguing, multiethnic expanse of campuses, religious institutions, nonpalatial but mostly stable residential neighborhoods, and historic cemeteries, with only a marginal federal presence. It has a palpable sense of community and friendliness, and, I suggest, ranks as one of the city's best and best-kept secrets.

This hike traces an 8.6-mile figure eight through the community. It's fairly flat, but

---

Directions

From downtown Washington, take New York Avenue (US 50) heading out of town. Soon after passing New Jersey Avenue NW, turn right onto M Street. Go 0.3 miles and turn left onto North Capitol Street. Go about 1.4 miles and turn right onto Michigan Avenue. Go 0.6 miles and then turn left onto Harewood Road and left again into the basilica parking lot (open 8:30 a.m. to 6:30 p.m.). To use Metro, take Red Line train to Brookland-CUA Metro station. Start hike there (see text). Or walk 0.5 miles to trailhead: Leave station through university-side exit on John McCormack Road, and walk across CUA campus to basilica parking lot. Contact Metro, (202) 637-7000 or www.wmata.com.

KEY AT-A-GLANCE INFORMATION

LENGTH: 8.6 miles (with shorter options)

CONFIGURATION: Figure 8

DIFFICULTY: Easy–moderate

SCENERY: Edifices, campus areas, local streets, cemeteries

EXPOSURE: Mostly open

TRAFFIC: Usually very light–light

TRAIL SURFACE: Nearly all pavement

HIKING TIME: 4.5–5.5 hours (assuming minimal time indoors)

SEASON: Year-round

ACCESS: Monastery grounds open daily, 9 a.m.–5 p.m. (except for January 1, Easter Sunday, Thanksgiving Day, Christmas Day); Rock Creek Cemetery open daily, dawn–dusk; National Cemetery open daily, 8 a.m.–5 p.m. (7 p.m. on Memorial Day); no other daytime restrictions

MAPS: USGS Washington East, ADC Metro Washington

FACILITIES: Toilets, water, phones, cafeteria near trailhead (in basilica basement); toilets at Rock Creek Cemetery parish hall; toilets, water, phones elsewhere en route, including monastery and cultural center

SPECIAL COMMENTS: Be sure to finish hike by dusk; CUA campus roadways are not named or signposted

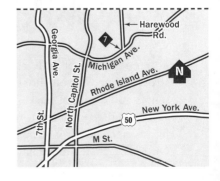

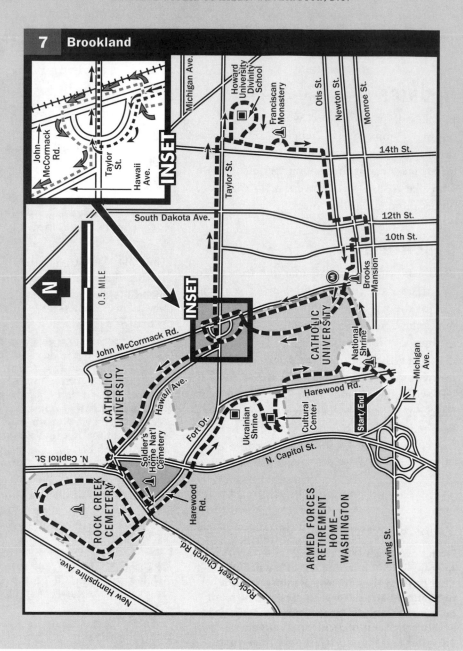

hilly enough to provide about 800 feet of elevation change. And it's mostly a street outing, so you should make wise use of sidewalks, traffic lights, and your senses and common sense. En route, savor the architecturally striking exteriors— and consider returning to explore the interiors. Brookland's street grid and my figure-eight hike route make it easy for you to shorten the basic 8.6-mile hike. Options include shortening the national cemetery loop (deduct up to 0.4 miles)

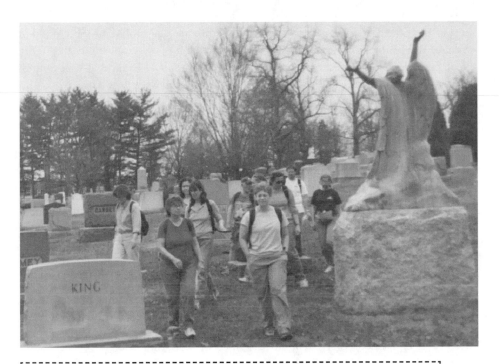

In Rock Creek Cemetery, get an annotated map at the office and then roam in search of
many links to national and local history.
----

or the Rock Creek Cemetery loop (deduct up to 1.5 miles), or doing only the first part (4 miles) or second part (4.6 miles) of the figure eight.

The hike starts at the Basilica of the National Shrine of the Immaculate Conception. (Alternatively, start elsewhere around the figure eight, such as at the Metro station.) The colorfully domed, Byzantine-style basilica is the world's eighth largest church and the largest Catholic church in the Americas. Built between 1920 and 1960, it ranks second only to the Washington Monument among the city's tallest masonry structures, thanks to its 329-foot-high bell tower, which is often loudly appealing.

From the basilica parking lot, cross Harewood Road and take a nearby ramp up to the basilica. Go past the entrance and head east across the mostly Gothic-style Catholic University of America campus. Pass Gibbons Hall, and then swing right onto a descending roadway. At John McCormack Road, cross the road (next to the Brookland-CUA Metro station) and turn left onto the sidewalk, which doubles as part of the Metropolitan Branch Trail (a bike route).

Head north, paralleling the Metro tracks. Just before an overpass, turn left to cross the street and go uphill on a ramp to Taylor Street. There, turn right, and head east on Taylor through a residential area. Then, turn right onto 14th Street and walk uphill and south. Turn left at the first driveway on the left and take a 0.3-mile loop through the spacious grounds of Howard University Divinity School, using the roadways and lawn areas. Then continue up 14th Street. Near the top, turn left to tour the Franciscan Monastery Memorial Church of the Holy Land. Founded in the late 1890s, the complex is the U.S. headquarters for Franciscan activities in the Near East, chiefly the preservation of Christian shrines. The Byzantine-style church and its grounds include copies of these shrines, as well as of the famed Lourdes grotto and Roman catacombs.

Entering at the main gates, turn left to walk along the Rosary Portico. Follow the portico as far as you can, then step into the flower-filled courtyard. Swing left to go around the front of the church, then pass through the portico on the far side to descend to the lower garden. Circle it, then head uphill on a paved path and turn right at a junction to return to the portico. Go through to the courtyard, turn left, and return to the main gates.

Leaving, turn left and continue along 14th Street, which heads downhill. Turn right and west onto Otis Street, and then left and south onto shop-lined 12th Street (pause at the corner to experience the Java Head Café), and then right and west onto Monroe Street. Going right and north at 10th Street, veer left to see one of Brookland's oldest surviving buildings—the now-restored Brooks Mansion. A War of 1812 veteran, Jehiel Brooks, built it in the 1840s on what was then his country property. It remained the family home until Brooks died in the 1880s, when the estate was replaced by subdivisions. The mansion became a Catholic school in the 1890s, when CUA was being developed, and later served as a convent. It then lay derelict for decades until community action saved it from the wreckers.

On 10th Street, turn left onto Newton Street and head for the nearby Metro station. Cross the bus area to the station's east entrance and disappear underground (at the hike's 3.5-mile mark). Emerge at the west entrance and again cross John McCormack Road to get back on the CUA campus. Head uphill and west on the same roadway you used earlier. If you want to do only the hike's first, 4-mile loop, return straight to the trailhead. But to do the full hike, swing right around the end of Pangborn Hall, and follow a walkway north. Then turn right and go down a few steps onto another walkway leading to a grassy circle. There, turn left and head north on a walkway bordering the law school (but pause to circle the school's small courtyard and read the detailed wall plaque).

Continuing north, turn left along a roadway, walk 20 yards, and turn right onto another roadway heading uphill. At the top, turn right onto a brown walkway and go down some steps to a diagonal concrete path that eases downhill. At the bottom, swing left and proceed on a concrete path alongside Ryan Hall and Regan Hall. Turn right onto a sidewalk leading out to John McCormack Road. Turn left and follow that road north. But this time, go under the overpass and turn left onto a ramp leading to the far side of Taylor Street (roughly the hike's halfway mark). Turn right onto Taylor, and then right again onto Hawaii Avenue, which borders CUA's athletic center. Walk uphill to Hawaii's intersection with Alison Street and Clermont Drive.

Cross Clermont and follow Alison uphill to where it joins Rock Creek Church Road. Veer left there to follow that road uphill to its junction with Harewood

Road. There, cross Rock Creek Church Road, turn left, and proceed to Rock Creek Cemetery.

Technically, it's the city's oldest burial ground (1719), but actually predates the city by seven decades. It's also a nonsectarian cemetery that surrounds St. Paul's Episcopal Church, similarly the city's oldest church (although the present building is a 1921 reconstruction of the 1712 original). As you'll discover, the cemetery is an intriguing, 100-acre area enveloped in history. Get a map from the cemetery office and roam (you'll cover up to about 1.5 miles). Count on being surprised by both who is buried there and the fascinating variety of grave markers.

Don't miss the memorial to Marian "Clover" Adams (section E), marked by a now-famous statue created by Augustus Saint-Gaudens. As decreed by her grieving husband, writer and diplomat Henry Adams (later buried alongside her), the memorial has no inscription and the statue is nameless. But the hooded figure is often referred to as Grief, allegedly because Mark Twain said it embodies all human grief. But when Twain asked Adams about the statue's significance, Adams replied that any 12-year-old would know.

On leaving the cemetery, turn left and return to the corner of Rock Creek Church Road and Harewood Road. Cross to get onto Harewood. Head downhill and turn left to enter the U.S. Soldiers' Home National Cemetery. The nation's oldest national cemetery, it dates from 1861, when the Soldiers' Home set aside nine acres as a burial ground for Civil War soldiers. Its filling up so quickly led the government to start Arlington National Cemetery. Although expanded to 16 acres in the 1880s, it's now almost full again, as you'll see when you take a 0.4-mile roadway loop clockwise through the regimented rows of white marble markers. Near the end of the half-mile loop, detour left across the grass to see the oldest graves (the original wooden markers were replaced with marble ones in the 1870s).

On leaving the cemetery, turn left to continue along Harewood Road, with the Soldiers' Home (now officially the Armed Forces Retirement Home—Washington) on your right. Cross North Capitol Street and proceed on Fort Drive, passing Archbishop Carroll High School, named for John Carroll (the country's first Catholic bishop and the founder of Georgetown University).

At a road fork, swing right onto another length of Harewood Road, which marks CUA's western boundary. Continuing, note the imposing Ukrainian Catholic National Shrine of the Holy Family, with its gold domes and open bell tower. It's best viewed from the sidewalk. Next, leave the sidewalk to circle the ultramodern Pope John Paul II Cultural Center, opened in 2001 as a museum and research center. Take the long driveway to the rear and climb a grassy slope to savor the view. Then descend, swing right onto the grass, and walk past the center to follow the edge of the woods to reach Harewood Road again. Cross the road, turn right, and continue downhill and past the Gilbert V. Hartke Theatre, named for the remarkable priest who ran CUA's celebrated drama program. At the bottom of the hill, recross the road to reach the parking-lot trailhead.

For more information about places along the hike route, contact the basilica, (202) 526-8300 or **www.nationalshrine.com;** the university, (202) 319-5000 or **www.cua.edu;** the monastery, (202) 526-6800 or **www.myfranciscan.com;** Rock Creek Cemetery, (202) 829-0585; the national cemetery (202) 829-1829; the Ukrainian shrine, (202) 526-3737 or **www.ucns-holyfamily.org;** and the cultural center, (202) 635-5400 or **www.jp2cc.org.**

NEARBY/RELATED ACTIVITIES

Sample Brookland's other temptations, all on or near the hike route: The insides of the places you pass; the large and tasty crab cakes at the Hitching Post, (202) 726-1511; the ambience at Colonel Brooks' Tavern, (202) 529-4002 and (in summer) neighboring Island Jim's Crab House and Tiki Bar, (202) 529-4002; a play or summer opera at the Hartke Theatre, (202) 319-5367; or an avant-garde dance performance at Dance Place, (202) 269-1600. Also explore nearby and nicely landscaped Trinity University, (202) 884-9700 or **www.trinitydc.edu.**

UPPER NORTHWEST WASHINGTON MILITARY SIGHTS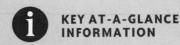

IN BRIEF

March across northern Rock Creek Park and through streets. Check fort attacked in only Confederate raid on Washington. Pay respects at Union cemetery. Retreat through woods. Regroup at civilian cabin. Reconnoiter second fort. Disband.

DESCRIPTION

Hiking not only meshes well with other interests but also can lead to new discoveries. That's how I discovered Fort Stevens and Fort DeRussy in upper Northwest Washington and learned about the only Civil War attack on the city. Later, after finding other historic sites in the vicinity, I devised this hike. The 7.3-mile hike is a counterclockwise loop with about 1,100 feet of elevation change. It starts and ends in the rolling woodlands of northern Rock Creek Park. In between, it pops eastward

----

Directions ⟶

Head for Northwest Washington. From intersection of Connecticut and Nebraska avenues, head northeast on Nebraska for 0.4 miles. Turn easy (not sharp) right onto Military Road and drive east for 0.7 miles. Then turn right and south onto Glover Road to enter Rock Creek Park. Proceed for 0.4 miles, swinging left at fork and then taking first left to get to parking lot for Rock Creek Nature Center and Planetarium.

  Or use Metro and your feet: From either Friendship Heights Metro station (Red Line) or Fort Totten Metro station (Red, Green lines), take Metrobus E2 or E3 along Military Road. Get off at Oregon Avenue (opposite Glover Road). From southeast corner of intersection, walk uphill on paved path for 0.2 miles to reach trailhead. Contact Metro, (202) 637-7000 or www.wmata.com.

KEY AT-A-GLANCE INFORMATION

LENGTH: 7.3 miles

CONFIGURATION: Loop

DIFFICULTY: Easy–moderate

SCENERY: Rolling woodlands, creek valley, city streets, historic sites

EXPOSURE: Over 50% shady; less so in winter and on the streets

TRAFFIC: Generally very light–light

TRAIL SURFACE: About half dirt, half pavement; rocky and rooty in places

HIKING TIME: 3.5–4.5 hours (including historic-site time)

SEASON: Year-round

ACCESS: Rock Creek Park, Fort Stevens, cemetery open daily, dawn–dusk

MAPS: USGS Washington West (USGS); PATC Map N; sketch map in free NPS Rock Creek Park brochure

FACILITIES: Toilets, water, phone at nature center (open Wednesday–Sunday, 9 a.m.–5 p.m.); toilets, water near Miller Cabin

FOR MORE INFORMATION: Contact Rock Creek Park, (202) 895-6000 or www.nps.gov/rocr; read Gail Spilsbury's *Rock Creek Park* and Benjamin Franklin Cooling III and Walton H. Owen II's *Mr. Lincoln's Forts: A Guide to the Civil War Defenses of Washington*

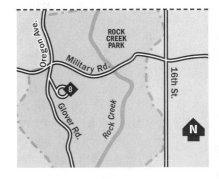

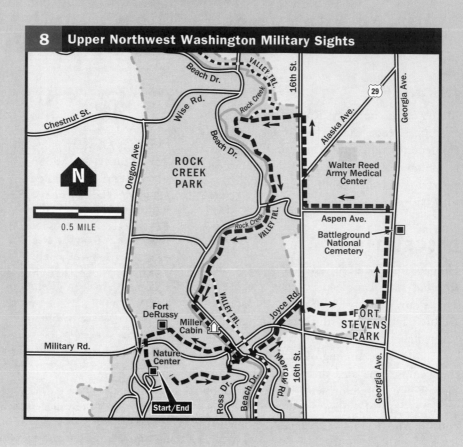

8   Upper Northwest Washington Military Sights

out of the park to wind through city streets, with stops at Fort Stevens, a Union cemetery, and Walter Reed Medical Center. Back in the park, it visits Fort DeRussy.

While in the park, don't go astray. The hike route mostly uses horse trails. Oddly, they're not signposted or blazed, but may be marked with no-bike symbols. Also, they're muddy when wet, so choose wisely if faced with on-trail mud versus off-trail poison ivy. And do be careful when crossing streets. To get started from the nature center's parking lot, walk south to the lot's entrance. There, turn left onto the road leading to the park's horse center. Then turn left again to cross the horse center's parking lot and reach a short paved road leading to a fenced riding ring. At the fence, turn left and head for an unpaved path that enters the woods. Follow it downhill for half a mile.

After carefully crossing Ross Drive, follow the trail that swings right alongside an unnamed ramp road. Then leave the trail and take the bridge across Rock Creek. After crossing Beach Drive, head uphill on Joyce Road, which swings left at a fork, glides under Military Road, and ascends to reach a T-junction. There, turn right, keep walking, and leave the park at 16th Street and Rittenhouse Street NW, in a mostly residential area.

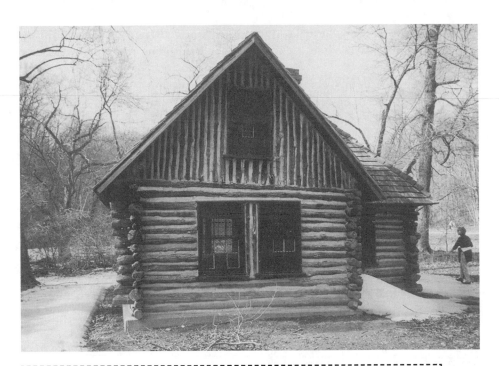

This log cabin has been linked to poetry since the 1880s, when it was on 16th Street and the bearskin-lined abode of poet Joaquin Miller.

Turn right and walk south for one block to Fort Stevens Drive. Turn left and east onto the drive and follow it gently uphill for three blocks to Piney Branch Road. There, carefully cross over and climb the grassy rampart to enter Fort Stevens Park. Managed by the National Park Service as part of Rock Creek Park, the fort site is now a grassy open area partially rimmed by a reconstructed and cannon-dotted parapet. A scale model depicts the original fort, and a streetside display board provides related information.

The fort was one of the Civil War hilltop defenses built around Washington. In July 1864, it was attacked by a small force under Jubal Early, sent north to draw off the Union troops around the Confederate capital, Richmond. After two days of fighting, Early's troops were driven off, and Washington was saved. But the episode may have prolonged the war by six months or more. On the parapet, locate a plaque commemorating Abraham Lincoln's visit to the besieged fort. It shows Captain (later Justice) Oliver Wendell Holmes grabbing Lincoln's arm after a surgeon standing nearby was fatally wounded. Holmes is supposed to have yelled, "Get down, you damned fool!" But a more reliable story has the fort commander telling the president to keep down.

Return to Piney Branch Road, turn right, walk north to the next corner, and turn right (east) onto Rittenhouse Street. At the end of the block, turn left onto Georgia Avenue and head north. After crossing Van Buren Street, watch for and turn right to enter Battleground National Cemetery. A one-acre burial ground for

Union soldiers who fought at Fort Stevens, it was dedicated by Lincoln on the conflict's second day. While walking around, try reading the much-weathered headstones.

Continue north on Georgia Avenue until you reach Aspen Street and Walter Reed Army Medical Center. The 110-acre campus is worth visiting. Named for a medical hero, it's a military facility dedicated to saving lives. It has attractive gardens, a remarkable medical museum (which has fragments of Lincoln's skull and the fatal bullet), and a Fort Stevens connection. On weekdays, enter at the Aspen security gate (carry a photo ID). A hundred yards in, pause at a "Lincoln under Fire" plaque on the right. It marks the site of the Sharpshooter's Tree (later toppled by a storm) from which snipers shot at Fort Stevens. Then head west across the campus to the 16th Street gate. On weekends or holidays, when the gate is closed, skip the grounds and take Aspen across to 16th Street.

There, turn right and head north along the shoulder, with Rock Creek Park on your left. At Holly Street, you'll be at the hike's halfway mark (3.7 miles). Just south of the intersection, look for a trail sign and a dirt trail. Follow them downhill into the woods.

At a trail junction, walk straight ahead on the Pine Trail. At the next one, turn left onto the Valley Trail. Stay on it for 1.5 miles as it follows Rock Creek downstream. Although not always close to the water, it's the hike's loveliest segment. After passing Rolling Meadow Bridge, the trail may be churned-up muddy, thanks to horse traffic. At the next fork, where a trail sign points left and warns, "Foot Travel No Horses" (making one wonder what grows at the ends of horses' legs), turn right and leave the Valley Trail. At the next fork, turn left and then cross a paved road (Beach Drive).

Then swing left onto a paved and parallel path. Walk about 200 yards and turn right to circle a dark and sinister-looking log cabin with a pitched roof, as I did one gray winter afternoon with Brigitte Savage. There's no explanatory sign, but she explained: "It's the witch's house!" (as in Hansel and Gretel). Later, I learned that it's the Miller Cabin. Now almost forgotten, poet Joaquin Miller—born Cincinnatus Hiner Miller—was very popular in the post–Civil War era and was lionized in both the United States and Europe as the Poet of the Sierras. But when he lived in the cabin in the 1880s, it was located on 16th Street. Decades later, the cabin was moved to the park as a gift to the nation.

From there, walk back upstream on the paved trail and take the bridge across the creek. Then, turn left to ease down an embankment. Turn left again onto an old road running into the creek at Millhouse Ford. But stay dry by turning right beforehand onto a horse trail heading downstream. At a junction, turn right onto another horse trail. After trekking uphill and roughly west through the woods, turn right onto a side trail marked by a "No Horses Permitted" sign. Then walk a few yards to reach ruined Fort DeRussy. As a trailside plaque says, the fort "commanded the deep valley of Rock Creek." Perched about 350 feet above sea level (the site is now the park's highest point), it did just that. During the Confederate attack, its guns were fired almost 200 times. Go just beyond the plaque and walk atop the now-overgrown earthen ramparts.

Then return to the main trail and turn right to continue. At a signposted junction, go straight, on the Western Ridge Trail. Ignore a paved path coming in from the left. Turn left at the next junction, next to a display board about Fort DeRussy. Then head downhill, cross Military Road, and proceed uphill to the trailhead.

NEARBY/RELATED ACTIVITIES

Attend Rock Creek Park's Civil War–related and other ranger-led programs. Attend summer evening poetry readings at the Miller Cabin; for details, visit **www.wordworksdc.com**. Also see and sample the activities listed in Hike 10, page 57.

09 ROCK CREEK PARK: Wild Northern Section

KEY AT-A-GLANCE INFORMATION

LENGTH: 9.3 miles (with shorter options)

CONFIGURATION: Modified loop

DIFFICULTY: Moderate

SCENERY: Gently rolling woodlands, stream valleys

EXPOSURE: Mostly shady; less so in winter

TRAFFIC: Usually very light to light; heavier on warm-weather evenings, weekends, holidays

TRAIL SURFACE: Mostly dirt or stony dirt; some pavement; rocky, rooty in places

HIKING TIME: 4.5–5.5 hours

SEASON: Year-round

ACCESS: Open daily, dawn–dusk

MAPS: USGS Washington West; PATC Map N; ADC Metro Washington; sketch map in free NPS Rock Creek Park brochure

FACILITIES: Toilets, water, phone at nature center (open Wednesday–Sunday, 9 a.m.–5 p.m.); toilets near Riley Spring Bridge (warm season only)

FOR MORE INFORMATION: Contact Rock Creek Park, (202) 895-6000 or www.nps.gov/rocr; read Gail Spilsbury's *Rock Creek Park*

IN BRIEF

The hilly and little-used woodlands of Rock Creek Park's northern section rank as one of Washington's best venues for off-street hiking in a wilderness-tinged setting.

DESCRIPTION

The same year that Congress accorded national park status to the three big chunks of California known as Yosemite, Sequoia, and Kings Canyon, it also preserved a piece of its own backyard. It decreed that Rock Creek's valley would become "a pleasuring ground for the benefit and enjoyment of the people of the United States." That was in 1890. Today, covering about 2,100 acres, the park consists largely of woodlands and stream valleys that protect the environment and provide habitat for assorted flora and fauna. Most visitors head for the picnic areas or other recreation facilities. But

----

Directions ⟶

Head for Northwest Washington. From intersection of Connecticut and Nebraska avenues, head northeast on Nebraska for 0.4 miles. Turn easy (not sharp) right onto Military Road and drive east for 0.7 miles. Then turn right and south onto Glover Road to enter Rock Creek Park. Proceed for 0.4 miles, swinging left at fork and then taking first left to get to parking lot for Rock Creek Nature Center and Planetarium.
  Or use Metro and your feet: From either Friendship Heights Metro station (Red Line) or Fort Totten Metro station (Red, Green lines), take Metrobus E2 or E3 along Military Road. Get off at Oregon Avenue (opposite Glover Road). From southeast corner of intersection, walk uphill on paved path for 0.2 miles to parking lot. Contact Metro, (202) 637-7000 or www.wmata.com.

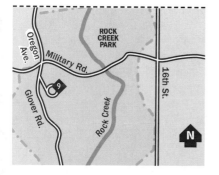

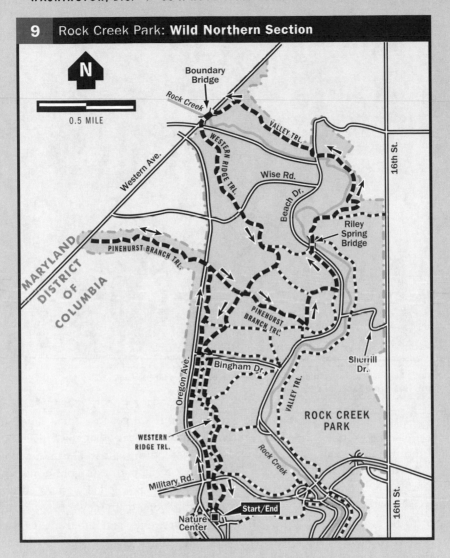

9 Rock Creek Park: Wild Northern Section

N

0.5 MILE

Boundary
Bridge

Rock Creek

VALLEY TRL.

WESTERN RIDGE TRL.

Western Ave.

Wise Rd.

Beach Dr.

Riley
Spring
Bridge

PINEHURST BRANCH TRL.

MARYLAND

DISTRICT
OF
COLUMBIA

PINEHURST
BRANCH TRL.

Oregon Ave.

Bingham Dr.

Sherrill
Dr.

VALLEY TRL.

ROCK CREEK
PARK

WESTERN
RIDGE TRL.

Rock Creek

Military Rd.

16th St.

16th St.

Start/End

Nature
Center

informed hikers head for the hills and trails—and some also consult Gail Spilsbury's heavily illustrated and history-rich *Rock Creek Park.*

This 9.3-mile hike consists of a modified loop that undulates enough to accumulate about 1,600 feet of elevation change. The major trails are blazed, named, and signposted. And there are several well-marked cross-park trails that you can use to create shorter hikes for yourself (see the map). Rain makes the unpaved trails muddy; horses make them even muddier. Beware occasional flooding and winter iciness, and do stay out of the poison ivy.

To get started from the nature center's parking lot, pick up the nearby nature trail at the north end, at an "Edge of the Woods" sign. Bear right onto a paved

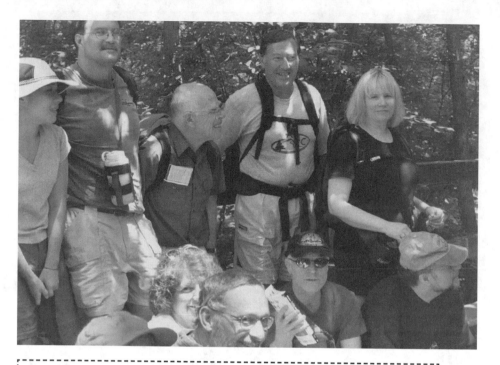

Hikers like to regroup at Boundary Bridge. Here (in back, from left) are veteran leaders Frank Turk, Ernie Bauer, and Paul Ray.

path next to a labeled chestnut oak. Proceed until you get to a small blue sign opposite a labeled spicebush. There, turn left onto a dirt path that takes the nature trail through the woods. At a paved woodland path, turn right and head downhill.

At Military Road, carefully cross and stay on the path as it goes uphill and back into the woods. For about 2 miles, follow the well-wooded western edge of the park northward. Watch for bikers; the path is one of the few off-road trails open to them in the park. The path gently curves, dips, and climbs as it passes through regal stands of mature tulip trees. After passing a fenced community garden on the right, cross a paved access road and jog to the left to pick up the path again and ignore whatever unpaved trails tempt you. Go through the same moves again when crossing a busier road (Bingham Drive). Then watch for a small yellow post next to trail junction. There, turn left for a side trip on the lovely Pinehurst Branch Trail.

The dirt trail follows Pinehurst Branch upstream for about 0.75 miles in a woodland corridor. Within 20 yards, cross Oregon Avenue, carefully, and look for the trail a few yards up on the right side of a driveway. Follow the yellow blazes as the trail winds through thickets and crisscrosses the stream. When the blazes end, you'll emerge in a residential area along Western Avenue, on the District-Maryland line. Look around, and then return to the yellow-post junction, but then keep going straight on what is the Pinehurst Trail for about 0.75 miles. Go straight through where the trail intersects the Western Ridge Trail. Then twice cross the stream—Pinehurst Branch—to reach a point where several trails merge just upstream from the stream's mouth on Rock Creek. That's roughly the hike's halfway point.

Cross the stream and turn left and then left again onto an unblazed dirt trail that goes uphill. At the top, turn right and descend on another unblazed trail, staying to the right at two successive forks. At an intersection just before a paved road (it's Beach Drive), turn left onto an unblazed trail heading north. To the right, just across the drive, you'll see and maybe hear the park's northernmost picnic area. The trail stays in the woods and close to the drive. At a junction (past the toilets), turn right, carefully cross the road, and take Riley Spring Bridge across Rock Creek.

At a trail junction about 50 yards on, turn left onto the blue-blazed Valley Trail, the major north–south trail on the park's eastern side. This northernmost segment is mostly a broad woodland path that curves westward across the park for almost 1.5 miles. In places, the nearby creek gives the impression of being a wilderness stream. Heading uphill, watch for an intersection overlooking a bend in the creek. Detour to the left (but not sharp left) and walk down about 40 yards to a rocky, off-the-beaten-trail spot where the slope is steep and the view is splendid. Then return to the main trail and continue.

The trail flattens out as it leaves the bluffs and eases across the creek's wooded floodplain. After crossing a wooden bridge over a tributary (Fenwick Branch), either turn left to take the trail along the creek bank and under a road (West Beach Drive), or go straight and cross the road with due care (and dry feet, if the underpass is flooded). Then continue on the reunited trail, staying with the blue blazes but off the side trails.

If it's spring, bear in mind that the stretch of trail leading to the Boundary Bridge passes through one of the District's richest displays of wildflowers. So either soak up the color as you hike by, or slow down to savor whatever takes your fancy. At the bridge, pause to take in the view, and then move on.

A short paved path will take you to a small parking lot adjoining Beach Drive. Carefully cross the drive and, having just spent a few minutes in Maryland, head uphill on a narrow dirt trail marked with greenish blazes. It's the Western Ridge Trail, the major north–south trail along the western side of the park, your route back to the trailhead, and near which you may see deer (but probably not the nocturnal coyotes known to be in this part of the park). On the 2.5-mile southbound journey, you'll pass through mature woodlands. Along the way, watch on the left for a remarkable tulip tree with five full-sized trunks. At Wise Road, cross wisely. Then press on, past a couple of cross-park trails, the first of which leads to Riley Spring Bridge. After that, you'll reach Pinehurst Branch and its trail—again. This time, cross both.

Walk through another intersection to reach Bingham Drive—again. Then take the paved path route back to the access road near the community garden. But this time, on emerging from the trees, turn left to walk along the blazed road. Just before reaching a "Do Not Enter" sign, turn right and follow a dirt trail alongside a fenced paddock. At the far corner, turn left onto the reassuringly signposted Western Ridge Trail. Proceed into the woods and mostly downhill. Turn right at a junction (to the left is another cross-park trail) and continue, mostly upward. At the next junction, turn right (again, to the left is a cross-park trail), and then right again onto a paved trail leading a short distance to the paved trail on which you started out. Turn left and head for the trailhead.

To shorten the hike by 1.5 miles, don't do the side trip on the Pinehurst Branch Trail. Another shorter-hike option is to make use of the cross-park trails shown on the map.

NEARBY/RELATED ACTIVITIES

See and sample the activities listed in Hike 10, page 57. Consider joining the still-new advocacy group called the Friends of Rock Creek Park's Environment (FORCE), **www.friendsofrockcreek.org.**

ROCK CREEK PARK: Rocky Central Section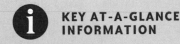

IN BRIEF

As this easy hike in Northwest Washington reveals, the chief natural attraction of Rock Creek Park's central section is a rocky stream valley set amid hilly woodlands.

DESCRIPTION

Rock Creek Park forms a big wedge that follows its namesake creek from Washington's northern apex down to the creek's mouth on the Potomac River. The park's central section features a rocky and superbly scenic creek valley that seems out of place in the middle of a city. This easy woodland loop consists of 4.5 miles of horizontal tromping and about 1,000 feet of elevation change (you can shorten the loop by using one of the several cross-park trails shown on the map). It's intended to provide you with a restorative dose of outdoor activity, plus a sampling of the park's natural

----

Directions ⟶

Head for Northwest Washington. From intersection of Connecticut and Nebraska avenues, head northeast on Nebraska for 0.4 miles. Turn easy (not sharp) right onto Military Road and drive east for 0.7 miles. Then turn right and south onto Glover Road to enter Rock Creek Park. Proceed for 0.4 miles, swinging left at fork and then taking first left to get to parking lot for Rock Creek Nature Center and Planetarium.

Or use Metro and your feet: From either Friendship Heights Metro station (Red Line) or Fort Totten Metro station (Red, Green lines), take Metrobus E2 or E3 along Military Road. Get off at Oregon Avenue (opposite Glover Road). From southeast corner of intersection, walk uphill on paved path for 0.2 miles to reach trailhead. Contact Metro, (202) 637-7000 or www.wmata.com.

KEY AT-A-GLANCE INFORMATION

LENGTH: 4.5 miles (with even shorter options)

CONFIGURATION: Loop

DIFFICULTY: Easy

SCENERY: Gently rolling woodlands, rocky creek

EXPOSURE: Mostly shady; less so in winter

TRAFFIC: Usually light; heavier on warm-weather evenings, weekends, holidays

TRAIL SURFACE: Mostly dirt or stony dirt; some pavement, grass; rocky, rooty in places

HIKING TIME: 2.5–3 hours

SEASON: Year-round

ACCESS: Open daily, dawn–dusk

MAPS: USGS Washington West; PATC Map N; ADC Metro Washington; sketch map in free NPS Rock Creek Park brochure

FACILITIES: Toilets, water, phone at nature center (open Wednesday–Sunday, 9 a.m.–5 p.m.)

FOR MORE INFORMATION: Contact Rock Creek Park, (202) 895-6000 or www.nps.gov/rocr; read Gail Spilsbury's *Rock Creek Park*

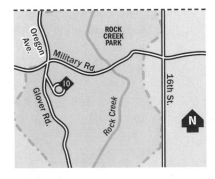

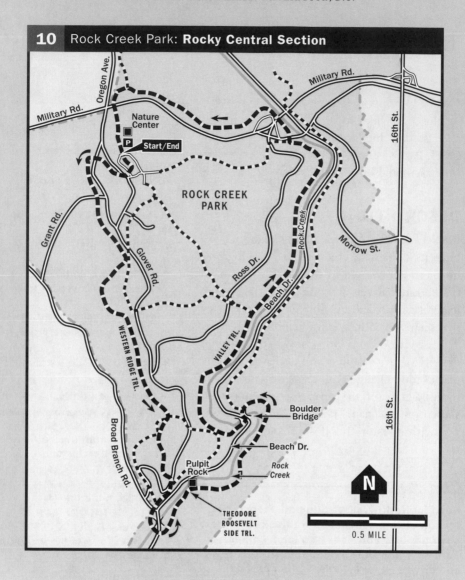

10 Rock Creek Park: **Rocky Central Section**

charms. Follow my directions closely, because some trails are unmarked, unblazed, and unnamed. Bear in mind that wet weather leads to puddling and muddiness, especially on trails used by horses, such as the one along the west bank of Rock Creek. And be sure to stay on the trail and out of the poison ivy.

To get started on the counterclockwise loop, leave the nature center's parking lot by the exit road (at the south end). Turn right onto the short side road connecting it to a nearby spur of Glover Road. Walk about ten yards and then cross the spur road carefully. Turn right on the grass and follow the edge of the woods away from the road and downhill past a picnic area. At an information board close

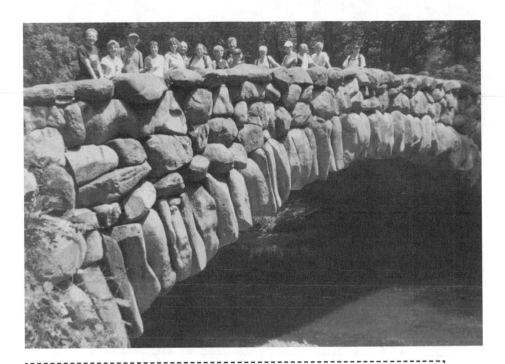

Hikers sometimes adorn Boulder Bridge, which has spanned Rock Creek since 1902.

to a road (Glover Road proper), look for greenish blazes on a tree and stumpy post. Turn left to carefully cross the road. Then swing half-left across the grass and toward the woods. There's no signpost, so look for a double greenish blaze on a beech tree about 40 yards from the road and head for the adjacent dirt trail.

The green-blazed Western Ridge Trail will take you south and mostly downhill to Rock Creek, along the flanks of a well-wooded ridge that falls away to the right. If the area seems wild, it's partly because there's a buffer of up to 400 yards of thickly wooded parkland between the trail and the nearest residential areas. Watch for mature oaks, tulip trees, and hickories, some of which may antedate the park's founding in 1890. And don't be surprised to see deer. Soon, on reaching a paved road (Grant Road), cross prudently to a trail junction. There, swing right onto a broad, stony trail on which horses are allowed. Then, at a "No Horses" sign, swing right onto another narrow dirt trail. Nearing a road (Glover, again), you'll find that the trail broadens into a stony path flanked by picnic areas and then recombines with a horses-allowed trail segment. Emerging from the woods, it passes the Equitation Field, a large fenced area that includes a horse-jumping ring. Follow the edge of the woods to the end of the fence, and then turn right, at a maple, and reenter the woods.

The trail slopes stonily downhill. Stay left at a fork. Then, at a parking lot, turn left and head for the nearby road (Glover, again). Cross it with care, turn right, and proceed along the edge for less than 50 yards to get to a steep, unmarked trail on the left. Follow it downhill. The trail bottoms out near where Broad Branch Road runs into Beach Drive. Head to the left and cross Beach Drive onto a bridge spanning Rock Creek. On the far side, turn left onto the sign posted Theodore Roosevelt Side Trail (TR himself liked to take friends on fast jaunts in the park), a charming and hilly woodland trail with good views of the creek. But watch your step; the trail is narrow, rocky, rooty, and sometimes slippery. At a signposted Pulpit Rock, detour a few yards to the left to visit a cliff-top cluster of rock spires. Clamber down among them and see if you feel like you're in a rock pulpit high above the creek—and have a sudden urge to declaim.

Then continue northward on the blue-blazed Valley Trail, which roughly parallels Beach Drive, a major park thoroughfare. The trail gets very close to the creek, which itself is quite rocky, with both boulders and underwater ledges causing audible riffles that blend well in summer with the cicada serenade. It's like being in a remote mountain valley. And that attractive ambience is enhanced on weekends, when Beach Drive is mercifully closed to motorized traffic. Follow the trail as it turns away from the creek and then forks. Turn left there to leave the Valley Trail and reach a nearby road (Beach Drive). Turn left to take the road—carefully—across Boulder Bridge. As you go, see if you think the bridge is rustically lovely or aesthetically repellent. And before or after, consult Gail Spilsbury's *Rock Creek Park* for an interesting account of the structure.

On the far side, walk about 40 yards and turn right onto an inconspicuous dirt trail heading uphill into the woods. It'll level off atop a ridge, show you the creek, and then intersect a broad, stony path—the hike's halfway point. There, turn right onto a creekside trail. At the next junction, turn right again. At the one after that, go straight through to stay close to Rock Creek at its rockiest. Continuing northward, you'll eventually swing left alongside a paved road that's part of the ramp system linking Military Road to Beach Drive. Watch for three short white posts along the ramp road. There, turn right and carefully cross the road. On the similarly decorated far side, proceed on the dirt trail ahead of you to start the hike's final mile. After passing under Military Road, turn left at the next intersection. Then head west and uphill across the park on a paved woodland path that parallels Military. On reaching the Western Ridge Trail, turn left, walk downhill to Military, cross safely, and proceed uphill to the trailhead.

To do a hike that's even shorter than this one, just use one of the lateral trails shown on the map to cut across the basic loop.

NEARBY/RELATED ACTIVITIES

Visit the vast and intriguing stone pile I call the Lost City. It consists of most of the Capitol's 1828 east portico, which was replaced in 1958 (to see more of the portico, head for the U.S. National Arboretum—see Hike 5, page 31). Drive or walk to the park's fenced maintenance yard—off the spur road just south of the nature center—and ask to see the site (the yard closes at 3 p.m.). Roam the stacked assemblage and speculate about what future archaeologists may make of it (old stones that cannot be deciphered?). Also keep in mind what blind Sen. Thomas P. Gore (Gore Vidal's grandfather) said long ago to a visitor smitten with the city's architectural treasures: "They will make wonderful ruins."

In late spring, treat yourself to the Shakespeare Theatre's Free for All at the park's nearby Carter Barron Amphitheater, 202/547-1122 or **www.shakespeare theatre.com;** the venue is outdoors, so you can attend in your trail togs.

After leaving the park, stop by at Politics and Prose, (202) 364-1919 or **www.politics-prose.com,** a well-stocked and cafe-equipped independent bookstore on Connecticut Avenue just south of Nebraska Avenue.

11 ROCK CREEK PARK:
Arboreous Southern Section

KEY AT-A-GLANCE INFORMATION

LENGTH: 9.4 miles (with shorter options)

CONFIGURATION: Loop

DIFFICULTY: Moderate

SCENERY: Parklands, street scenes

EXPOSURE: Mostly shady in parks; less so on streets and in winter

TRAFFIC: Light–moderate on Rock Creek Trail but can be heavy on warm-weather evenings, weekends; light elsewhere

TRAIL SURFACE: Roughly half pavement; rest mostly dirt

HIKING TIME: 3.5–4.5 hours

SEASON: Year-round

ACCESS: Parks open daily, dawn–dusk; zoo grounds (gated) open daily, 6 a.m.–8 p.m. from spring to early fall, 6 a.m.–6 p.m. at other times (but closed December 25)

MAPS: USGS Washington West; PATC Map N; ADC Metro Washington; sketch map in free park brochure

FACILITIES: Toilets, water, phones near Pierce Mill, at eateries on major streets

FOR MORE INFORMATION: Contact Rock Creek Park, (202) 895-6000 or www.nps.gov/rocr; contact National Zoological Park, (202) 673-4800 or www.si.edu/natzoo

IN BRIEF

Rock Creek Park's tree-rich southern section and ribbony western outliers enable hikers to loop through Northwest Washington on mostly shady trails.

DESCRIPTION

This 9.4-mile excursion loops through the well-wooded parklands and residential areas of Northwest Washington in celebration of the leafy heritage of what has long been called the City of Trees. Despite a net tree-cover loss of roughly 60 percent since 1980, the name still applies. The city's parks remain mostly wooded. Its residential streets, yards, and gardens sport canopies of leaves. Vacant lots, rights-of-way, and nooks quickly follow suit if left alone. The mostly deciduous trees along the hike route include oaks, hickories, maples, dogwoods, tulip trees, beeches, and sycamores. Of course, you'll also encounter other, more exotic varieties, with wildflowers and birds adding further color and interest to the trail-side parklands.

Directions ⟶

Head for Northwest Washington. Park near trailhead—Woodley Park–Zoo/Adams Morgan Metro station entrance on Connecticut Avenue (just north of Connecticut and Calvert Street NW). Heed posted parking regulations. Arrive early on warm-weather weekends and holidays. On weekdays, consider starting hike at no-time-limit parking lots at Pierce Mill or zoo.

Or use Metro to do hike: Woodley Park–Zoo/Adams Morgan Metro station is on Red Line (as are close-to-hike-route Cleveland Park and Tenleytown-AU stations); Metrobuses operate on nearby streets. Contact Metro, (202) 637-7000 or www.wmata.com.

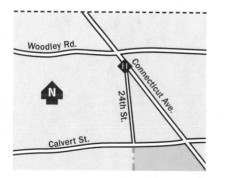

Woodley Rd.

Connecticut Ave.

24th St.

N

Calvert St.

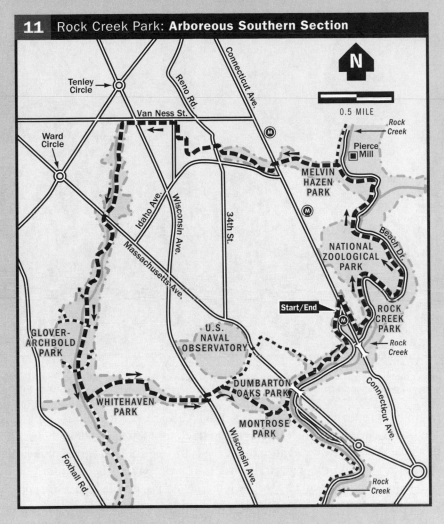

11 Rock Creek Park: **Arboreous Southern Section**

Administratively, the parklands are part of the National Park Service's Rock Creek Park. However, like the hike, they also include four separate units— Melvin Hazen, Glover-Archbold, Whitehaven, and Dumbarton Oaks parks. The hike route is only partially signposted and blazed, so pay attention to my directions. Although most of it is fairly level or gently undulating, it also has a few steep but short uphill stretches (slippery in icy weather)—and about 1,600 feet of elevation change. Stay to the right when you're on the busy, multiuse Rock Creek Trail, and be careful when crossing streets.

To get started from the Woodley Park–Zoo/Adams Morgan Metro station, walk over to 24th Street as it angles downhill from Connecticut Avenue to Calvert Street. Cross Calvert and head down into Rock Creek Park on the grassy left-hand verge. After crossing a side road, turn left onto the paved Rock Creek

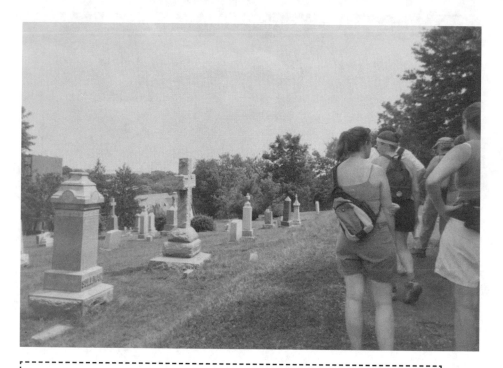

Detour through Holy Rood Cemetery, which is just off Wisconsin Avenue (the gate is to keep out cars, not appreciative walkers).

Trail to head generally north, alongside Rock Creek Parkway and the southward-bound creek. Just before reaching a road tunnel, turn left and follow the trail for half a mile through the gated grounds of the National Zoological Park. Emerging, swing left to stay on the main trail. At a trail fork, stay to the right and follow the trail downhill and under a low green bridge. At a signposted junction, take the Valley Trail, which crosses Rock Creek on a bridge and continues upstream next to the parkway. After a third of a mile, another bridge will take you back over the creek and into an open field.

Off to the left is the signposted Melvin Hazen Trail. Before taking it, detour to the other end of the field to see the restored Pierce Mill, dating from 1820 and now the creek's only surviving gristmill. Also walk over to the dam to see the fish ladder that's part of an ambitious project that, starting in the spring of 2006, made it possible for spawning blueback herring, white perch, and rockfish to ascend the creek for the first time in a century.

On the Melvin Hazen Trail, in a narrow wooded park of the same name, you'll follow a rocky stream valley uphill and generally westward for half a mile. You'll also be on the hike's first stretch of dirt trail, so be careful when the weather is cold or wet. At Connecticut Avenue, turn right to cross it at Sedgwick Street. On the far side, turn left and proceed back down the avenue. At a "Dead End Street" sign, turn right into an alley. At the end of the alley, descend some steps to rejoin the Melvin Hazen Trail. Proceeding across a mini-marsh by mini-boardwalk, turn right at the next junction onto a yellow-blazed trail. Then, stay right at a fork to follow a streamside trail to Tilden Road just before its junction with Reno Road.

Cross Reno and walk up Springland Lane. At the end, head up the steps and turn right onto a broad unpaved path that leads to Idaho Street. Proceed along Idaho and turn left at the next intersection onto Tilden Street. At the intersection after that, turn right onto 37th Street and proceed for two blocks. Then turn left onto Van Ness Street. Next, head for Wisconsin Avenue, a major thoroughfare with bathroom-equipped eateries. Cross Wisconsin Avenue, continue along Van Ness for about 100 yards, and then walk left onto a short paved road. At a stop sign, swing right onto a grassy area and cross to the northern end of both Glover-Archbold Park and its namesake trail.

From there, almost at the hike's halfway, 4.7-mile mark, head south on the blue-blazed woodland trail for 1.5 miles, crossing Massachusetts, Cathedral, and New Mexico avenues along the way and avoiding the side trails. Then, at a signpost pointing to the Whitehaven Trail, leave the Glover-Archbold Trail and turn left and east into wooded Whitehaven Park. Follow the buff-blazed trail uphill and then along the edge of an athletic field, staying close to the boundary fence. At the end of the fence, turn right and then bear left. Then descend with the trail and cross a picnic area to reach 37th Street. Cross the street carefully. On the far corner, go left and then right to ascend a steep but short flight of ungainly steps. At the top, stay to the right and continue along the Whitehaven Trail to the corner of 35th Street and Whitehaven Parkway. Follow the parkway to nearby Wisconsin Avenue, and turn left for a mini-detour.

First, head up Wisconsin Avenue for less than a block and turn left into the regrettably untended Holy Rood Cemetery, which has some 7,000 graves, including those of slaves. Circle through the cemetery to sample both history (the oldest grave is dated 1834) and the sweeping views (locals gather on the Fourth of July to watch the fireworks display on the Mall, and developers covet the property). Then leave and contemplate the nearby bathroom-equipped eateries (including Sam's, which has super-rich homemade ice cream). Then cross Wisconsin Avenue to head east and downhill on Whitehaven Street. At the end, swing right and downhill on the signposted Dumbarton Oaks Trail. You'll be in the park of the same name, which adjoins the renowned estate called Dumbarton Oaks (worth a separate visit). Designed originally as part of the estate by the remarkable Beatrix Farrand, the park has both touches of wilderness and slopes aglow with forsythia yellow and dogwood white in the spring (linger on the nearby bench).

Stay on the park's main trail. Where that gets somewhat faint, in an open area, swing right, cross a small stream, and continue along the trail on the far side. Leaving the park, pass a stone gatepost and start the hike's final mile at a trail junction. There, take the buff-blazed trail (marked with a no-bikes sign) that heads downhill toward Rock Creek Park proper. Follow the trail as it turns to the left and goes upstream alongside the creek. Cross a small bridge and stay to the right. Then turn left onto the Rock Creek Trail. Just past some exercise stations, swing left and uphill to reach and cross Calvert Street. Then walk up 24th Street to the trailhead. As this hike is a loop, consider selecting your own trailhead, such as Pierce Mill (see under Directions).

NEARBY/RELATED ACTIVITIES

Tour the fully restored Pierce Mill, (202) 426-6908, and the nearby Rock Creek Gallery (long known popularly as the Art Barn). After the hike, sample the Connecticut Avenue restaurants near the trailhead; try Tono Sushi, (202) 332-7300, or the Lebanese Taverna, (202) 265-8681. Or walk or ride one Metro stop north to Cleveland Park to try pan-Asian Ivy's Place, (202) 363-7802.

GLOVER-ARCHBOLD AND OTHER NORTHWEST WASHINGTON TRAILS

IN BRIEF

Using a network of parkland trails, hikers can semicircle semi-secretly through upscale neighborhoods of Northwest Washington, closing the loop along the riverfront.

DESCRIPTION

Ribbons of National Park Service parkland carry this diversified, pleasant, and mostly off-street hike through well-to-do Northwest Washington neighborhoods. It's an 8-mile counterclockwise loop that starts and ends on level trails along the Potomac River. The trails in between provide about 1,400 feet of elevation change on a moderately hilly woodland and inland excursion.

From the trailhead at Fletcher's Boathouse upper parking lot, head downriver on the unpaved C&O Canal towpath, between the restored canal and the Potomac. After almost a mile, pause to read a plaque about

- -

Directions

From Georgetown end of Key Bridge in Northwest Washington, drive west on M Street NW/Canal Road for 0.5 miles. At third traffic light, turn left to stay on Canal Road. Go 1.6 miles to Fletcher's Boathouse, on left. If upper parking lot is full, use lower and larger one. To get to Fletcher's from Chain Bridge, go east on Canal Road for 0.4 miles and make extreme right turn into Fletcher's upper parking lot. *Note:* Canal Road is a weekday rush-hour route that's one-way inbound in morning and one-way outbound in afternoon.

Or use Metro and your muscles to get to trailhead. From Foggy Bottom Metro station (Blue, Orange lines), take Metrobus D5 along MacArthur Boulevard, get off at V Street, and walk down to Canal Road and Fletcher's. Contact Metro, (202) 637-7000 or www.wmata.com.

KEY AT-A-GLANCE INFORMATION

LENGTH: 8 miles

CONFIGURATION: Loop

DIFFICULTY: Easy–moderate

SCENERY: Woodlands, river views, street scenes

EXPOSURE: Mostly shady; less so in winter

TRAFFIC: Generally light; heavier along river on warm-weather evenings, weekends, holidays

TRAIL SURFACE: Mostly dirt; some pavement

HIKING TIME: 3–4 hours

SEASON: Year-round

ACCESS: Trails open daily, dawn–dusk

MAPS: USGS Washington West; PATC Map N; map in free NPS Rock Creek Park brochure

FACILITIES: Toilets, water, phone, warm-weather snack bar at Fletcher's; toilets, water inside rec center; emergency phone at canal tunnel

FOR MORE INFORMATION: Contact Rock Creek Park, (202) 282-1063 or www.nps.gov/rocr, and C&O Canal NHP's headquarters office in Sharpsburg, (301) 739-4200 or www.nps.gov/choh.

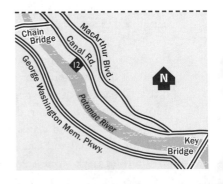

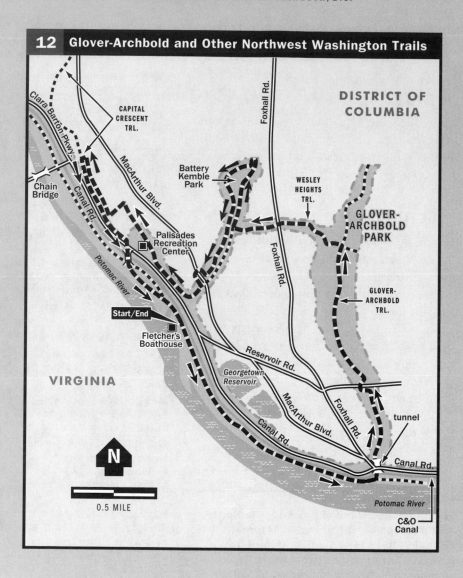

12 Glover-Archbold and Other Northwest Washington Trails

the ingenious inclined-plane system used in 1876–1889 to transfer boats between the canal and river. Then take the nearby steps down to the paved Capital Crescent Trail (CCT). Turn left onto the CCT and continue downriver for about three-quarters of a mile. Then swing right onto a curving concrete bridge that provides views of the river and the canal's spillways. At the end of the bridge, take a short dirt trail back to the towpath. Then turn right onto a 40-yard dirt trail leading to a lovely off-the-beaten-trail viewing spot on the riverbank.

Go back to and cross both the CCT and towpath. Take the lighted tunnel beneath the canal and Canal Road, and emerge to follow a signposted detour up to the road (past stone steps in disrepair). Then turn right to walk under an old trestle (once part of the trolley line to the Glen Echo amusement park) onto the Glover-Archbold Trail. Follow the blue-blazed, mostly dirt trail gently uphill and northward through the woods and alongside Foundry Branch. As you go, be thankful that the trail route was rescued in 1962 from becoming a multilane parkway. After about half a mile, you'll emerge onto open parkland and swing left to reach Reservoir Road at 44th Street. Cross Reservoir carefully (the traffic doesn't stop) and follow the trail downhill and through woodlands dominated by mature tulip trees. At a stream and T-junction, cross on the stepping-stones and turn left. Proceed along the trail, even when the surface becomes a large-diameter sewer pipe.

At a four-way intersection, turn left onto the yellow-blazed Wesley Heights Trail and head west through the woods. Crisscross a small stream three times, and then turn right at the next T-junction. Follow the trail gently uphill to 44th Street (no street sign there), cross, and turn right onto the sidewalk. After 50 yards, turn left to descend some wooden steps back to the trail at a yellow-blazed post. The trail pitches uphill to reach Foxhall Road at Edmunds Street—the hike's halfway point. Cross Foxhall carefully, descend some wooden steps, and keep going, generally downhill. Cross 49th Street (no street sign there) and then a wooden footbridge to enter Battery Kemble Park.

At the end of the bridge, turn right and head uphill and into the open. Continue to the summit, once occupied by a Civil War gun battery. Descend 30 yards from the summit and turn right onto a narrow dirt trail. Follow it downhill and across the park's access road. Go left at a fork and then swing right to continue through the woods. You'll emerge at MacArthur Boulevard (no street sign visible), opposite an old schoolhouse. Turn right onto the sidewalk and walk to the corner of Nebraska Avenue to cross MacArthur carefully (the traffic doesn't stop). Follow the far sidewalk to just past the schoolhouse, and turn right onto a narrow dirt trail going downhill along Battery Kemble Run. Near the bottom, stay on the trail as it curves right and away from the stream. Go left at a fork. Stay on the trail as it follows the former trolley-line right-of-way for 1.5 miles, taking you past many backyards and the Palisades Recreation Center.

Then cross Arizona Avenue on a plant-festooned footbridge, and proceed. On reaching Galena Place, turn left and go three blocks to where Galena ends at Potomac Avenue (no street sign visible). Cross Potomac and turn right onto the shoulder. Follow it for three blocks, looking to the left for views across the Potomac. Just past Manning Street, take a wooden stairway on the left down to the CCT. Turn left, walk along the CCT for half a mile to cross the bridge spanning the canal and Canal Road. At the end of the bridge, descend some steps, turn right, and do a final towpath half mile back to Fletcher's.

NEARBY/RELATED ACTIVITIES

Explore the river or canal in a Fletcher's rental boat (available during warm-weather months). Picnic at Fletcher's spacious riverside park.

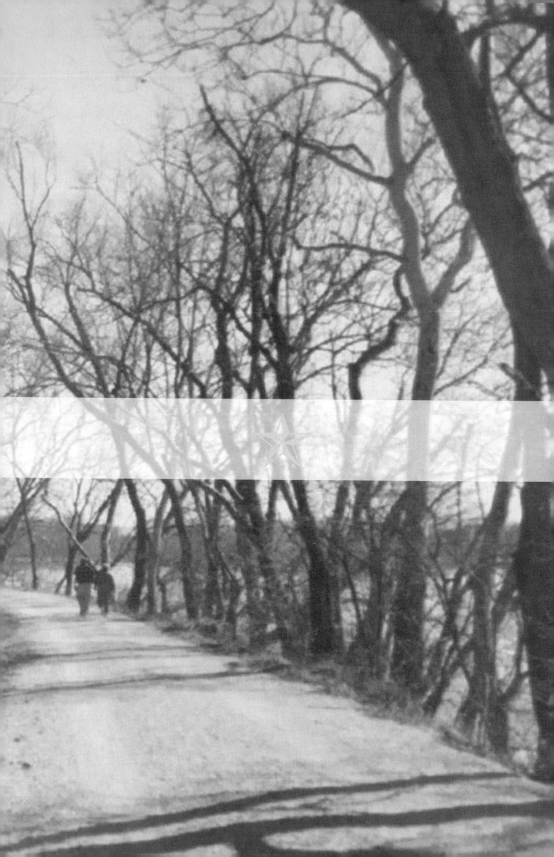

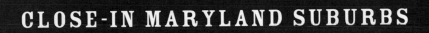

CLOSE-IN MARYLAND SUBURBS

13 CAPITAL CRESCENT TRAIL

KEY AT-A-GLANCE INFORMATION

LENGTH: 10.1 miles (with shorter, Metro-aided option)

CONFIGURATION: Modified out-and-back

DIFFICULTY: Moderate

SCENERY: Woodlands, parklands, street scenes, river glimpses

EXPOSURE: Shady; less in winter

TRAFFIC: Mostly light–moderate; moderate–heavy on warm-weather evenings, weekends, holidays

TRAIL SURFACE: Pavement, gravel

HIKING TIME: 4–5 hours

SEASON: Year-round

ACCESS: Open daily, dawn–dusk

MAPS: USGS Washington West; map in CCCT brochure (available from CCCT or from trailside boxes); map on display boards at rest areas

FACILITIES: Toilets, water, phone, warm-season snack bar at trailhead; water at rest areas near reservoir and Bradley Boulevard

FOR MORE INFORMATION: Contact Coalition for the Capital Crescent Trail (CCCT), (202) 234-4874 or www.cctrail.org

SPECIAL COMMENTS: On warm-weather weekends and holidays, stay to right while on trail to avoid speeding cyclists and in-line skaters

IN BRIEF

A former railroad right-of-way, the multiuse Capital Crescent Trail (CCT) curves through close-in suburban Maryland and Northwest Washington. Its paved lower segment provides hikers with a good workout and scenic outing in a parkland setting.

DESCRIPTION

The CCT is a narrow, parkland-encased pathway that arcs smoothly through affluent neighborhoods for 11 miles between Maryland's Silver Spring and Washington's Georgetown waterfront. The country's most-used rail trail, it has been heralded by the International Project for Public Places as one of the world's "21 great places that show how transportation can enliven a community." I can't vouch for that claim because I didn't know the area before it was enlivened. But the CCT definitely is an attractive and easy-to-follow recreational pathway that beckons to hikers year-round.

Directions ———————————————▶

In Washington, from Georgetown end of Key Bridge, drive west on M Street NW/Canal Road for 0.5 miles. At third traffic light, turn left to stay on Canal Road. Go 1.6 miles to Fletcher's Boathouse, on left. If upper parking lot is full, use lower and larger one. To get to Fletcher's from Chain Bridge, go east on Canal Road for 0.4 miles and make extreme right turn into Fletcher's. Note: Canal Road is a weekday rush-hour route that's one-way inbound in morning and one-way outbound in afternoon.

  Alternatively, from Foggy Bottom Metro station (Blue, Orange lines) take Metrobus D5 along MacArthur Boulevard, get off at V Street, and walk down to Canal Road and Fletcher's. Contact Metro, (202) 637-7000 or www.wmata.com.

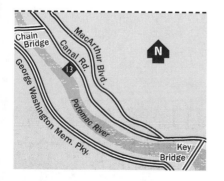

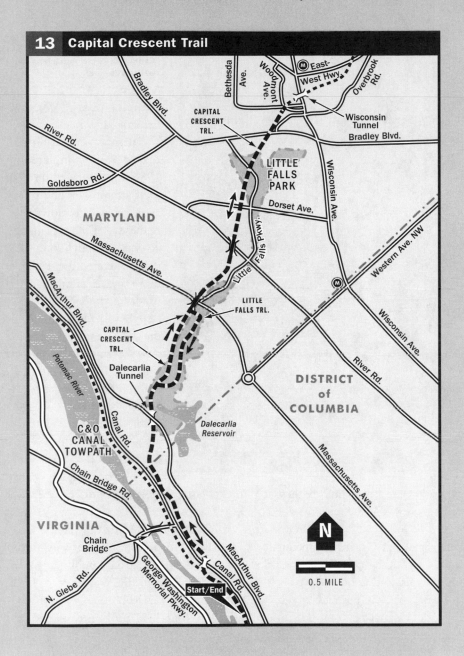

13 Capital Crescent Trail

I like using the trail's lower and paved segment for a 10.1-mile out-and-back hike that starts at Fletcher's Boathouse (about 2 miles above Georgetown), includes a streamside side trip, and winds gently uphill to restaurant-rich Bethesda. This trail segment is popular year-round, mostly as a neighborhood recreational trail. At least half of the users seem to be cyclists, with hikers, in-line skaters, joggers, strollers, and dog walkers making up the balance. On weekdays, some of the

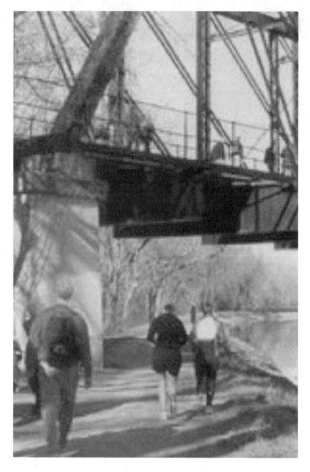

A former railroad bridge carries the Capital Crescent Trail across the C&O Canal and its towpath (steps connect both trails here).

traffic consists of commuting suits on wheels.

It may seem a bit odd that a trail completed in 1996 can go right through such a built-over and pricey area, as well as downtown Bethesda. The explanation is that, although the CCT itself is new, the route is more than a century old and predates modern suburban expansion. For much of the 20th century, it was the right-of-way of a railroad spur line that delivered coal and building supplies to the industry-cluttered Georgetown waterfront. That fact also explains the route's gentle grades, with only 350 feet of elevation change between Georgetown and Bethesda. When its last coal customer switched to truck delivery in 1985, the rail line was closed.

The following year, volunteers organized the Coalition for the Capital Crescent Trail (CCCT) to campaign for converting the private right-of-way into a public multiuse trail. With the help of assorted organizations, public agencies, individuals, and good luck, the effort succeeded. Today, the Washington, D.C., portion of the CCT is managed by the National Park Service as part of the adjoining C&O Canal National Historical Park. The Maryland portion is owned and maintained by Montgomery County.

Now a thriving membership organization, the CCCT continues to press for completion of the 4-mile section between Bethesda and Silver Spring. That section, called the Georgetown Branch Trail, is passable but currently is only a crushed-stone "interim trail" with on-street detours. Although the section is a key link to trails in and beyond Maryland's Rock Creek Regional Park, completion remains complicated by various political and funding issues.

To get started from the upper parking lot at Fletcher's, head upriver on the paved CCT (rather than the adjoining dirt-surfaced C&O Canal towpath). Keep the Potomac River on your left, although you won't see much of it thanks to the thickly wooded floodplain. Watch for a distinctive brown sign bearing the number 8. It's one of the half-mile posts that count down the CCT from Silver Spring. About a half mile from Fletcher's, the trail gently ascends, and then crosses the canal and Canal Road on a refurbished ex-railroad bridge. It then angles up the bluffs and, when the trees are bare, provides panoramic glimpses of the Potomac valley.

Climbing very gradually, the trail crosses into Maryland and then swings northward and away from the river. Just after passing half-mile post 6.5 and a rest area decorated with boards, it crosses a water-treatment facility and then ducks into the Dalecarlia Tunnel, built in 1910 to carry the railroad line under both Conduit Road (now MacArthur Boulevard) and the pipes carrying river water to Dalecarlia Reservoir. Read the informative plaque on the tunnel wall.

Beyond the tunnel, watch on your right for a glimpse of the reservoir, still one of Washington's chief water-storage units. Just after half-mile post 6, leave the CCT and turn right onto a 40-yard gravel path that ends at a T-junction. There, turn left to follow a paved path for more than a mile through Little Falls Branch Park. Emerging wildflowers, re-leafing trees, and flitting migratory birds can make this park a springtime delight. When you reach heavily traveled Massachusetts Avenue, turn left to get onto the sidewalk, go 70 yards, and then climb a short slope on the left to return to the CCT (at the hike's 3.3-mile mark). Then turn right, and keep going. Over the next 1.8 miles, you'll cross River Road (overpass, with a Whole Foods off to the left at the far end), Dorset Avenue (pedestrian crossing), Little Falls Parkway (pedestrian crossing), and Bradley Boulevard (overpass). Then you'll pass an informative rest area and half-mile post 3.5 and reach Bethesda Avenue, the hike's turnaround, at the 5.1-mile mark.

That's a fine location for giving in to gustatory temptation, in that the area is rich in ethnic restaurants (try the Delhi Dhaba Indian buffet on Woodmont Avenue, [301] 718-0008). Feel free to have seconds, too, because your return trip to Fletcher's will be a 5-mile glide downhill on the CCT (skip the Little Falls side trip).

Alternatively, have thirds and walk instead to the nearby Bethesda Metro station (Red Line), and find your way back to Fletcher's by train and bus. If you do that, also use the Metro to get to Fletcher's at the outset (see Directions). Parking at the Bethesda turnaround and doing the hike in reverse—long a convenient option—will no longer be possible in universally metered downtown Bethesda as of the spring of 2007. That's when the lone free-on-weekends parking lot is scheduled to become a construction site for at least two years.

NEARBY/RELATED ACTIVITIES

In the early spring, detour to see the glorious cherry blossoms of Bethesda's Kenwood area, just west of the CCT. At peak blossom time, the area is very crowded, but mostly with cars, so you can walk around freely under the pink-and-white canopy. To get started, leave the trail at Dorset Avenue and circle westward.

At any time of year, consider joining the CCCT (see page 72).

14 BLACK HILL REGIONAL PARK

KEY AT-A-GLANCE INFORMATION

LENGTH: 11.3 miles (with shorter option)

CONFIGURATION: Modified loop with out-and-back addition

DIFFICULTY: Moderate–hard

SCENERY: Woodlands, meadows, stream valleys, lake views with and without houses

EXPOSURE: Mostly shady; less so in winter

TRAFFIC: Usually light; heavier on warm-weather weekends, holidays, especially on hiker/biker trail and near visitor center

TRAIL SURFACE: Mostly pavement; some dirt, grass

HIKING TIME: 5.5–6.5 hours

SEASON: Year-round

ACCESS: Open daily, 6 a.m.–sunset, March–October (7 a.m.–sunset in other months)

MAPS: USGS Germantown; sketch map in free park brochure

FOR MORE INFORMATION: Visit or call visitor center (open daily 11 a.m.–6 p.m.), (301) 972-3476

FACILITIES: Toilets, water in visitor center, at boat dock, parking lot 5, picnic shelters (warm season); phones at entrance kiosk, visitor center

IN BRIEF

Black Hill Regional Park features a large lake, rolling woodlands, meadows, and a seasonal variety of views. Situated in northern Montgomery County, it's an attractive locale where hikers can vigorously roam suburban parkland.

DESCRIPTION

Located about 21 miles northwest of Washington, Black Hill Regional Park covers 1,854 acres of rolling woodlands, meadows, and water. In fact, water is the park's dominant physical feature, with Little Seneca Lake accounting for almost a third of the acreage. The lake, the metro area's largest, clearly ranks as the multiuse park's chief attraction for most visitors.

The 505-acre lake's presence makes the park doubly attractive for hikers. The irregularly shaped body of water (it resembles the head of a trident) provides one part of a fine hiking venue. The other part consists of hilly woodlands and meadows away from the lake. And the popular appeal of the lake and nearby recreational facilities tends to minimize traffic on the park's trails. For hikers, therefore, the

---

Directions

From junction of Capital Beltway (Interstate 495) and I-270 spur in Maryland, head northwest on I-270 (toward Frederick) for about 18.5 miles. Get off at Exit 18 and turn left onto Clarksburg Road (MD 121). Proceed generally southward for about 1.6 miles. Then turn left onto West Old Baltimore Road. Go east for 1 mile, and turn right into park. Take Lake Ridge Drive for 2 miles to visitor-center parking lot. Arrive early to beat the warm-weather crowds.

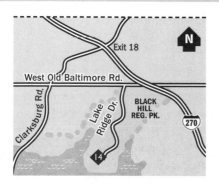

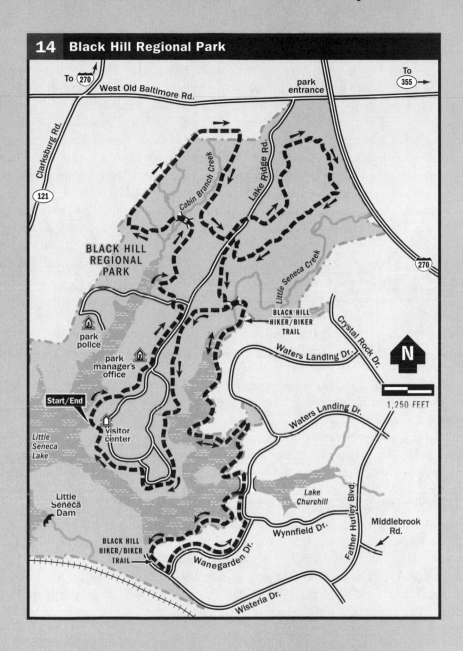

14   Black Hill Regional Park

park usually seems uncrowded, with most of the few other trail users being on bikes or horses.

Four decades ago, the area consisted of privately owned fields, woods, and streams. Then the metro area's water authority and Montgomery County agreed to create a dual-use emergency water-supply reservoir and park. Little Seneca

Creek was dammed, stream valleys filled up, and farmers left. When opened in 1987, the park was still enveloped in farmland. But since then, residential development spreading westward from Germantown has reached the park boundary. However, some two decades of protective park status have helped Black Hill nurture a rich population of plants and animals. Woodlands predominate, with oaks, hickories, beeches, maples, tulip trees, and conifers being seasonally complemented by bloom-laden bushes and wildflowers. Deer are plentiful, as are smaller animals. Seasonally, myriad birds contribute color, song, insect control, and seed dispersal. In winter, fish-hungry bald eagles and ospreys enhance the lake view.

The 11.3-mile hike route I've devised has about 2,200 feet of elevation change and makes use of the park's main trail network, both near and away from the lake. There's also a 6.9-mile version, which omits an out-and-back addition (as indicated below). The trails are unblazed but generally well signposted (except at the hike's start). Use the signs in conjunction with my trail directions, and stay on the trails to protect the habitat and avoid the poison ivy.

To get started, face the visitor center and look for a white trellis on the left. Take the paved trail nearby. Heading downhill, quickly turn right and then right again to get onto the paved Black Hill Trail, and keep in mind that it's a hiker/biker trail. It will take you between the visitor center on a knoll to your right and the lake to your left. For the next half mile, stay on the unshaded and undulating trail as it pulls away from the lake. In spring, it's a bushy avenue of color and fragrance, thanks in part to such domineering alien species as honeysuckle and multiflora rose.

At the park office, take a 30-yard detour to the left to see the site of a one-time gold mine. George Chadwick bought the land in 1947 as a summer retreat, dubbing it Gold Mine Farm. In the 1950s, as the Cold War escalated, he converted the mine into a bomb shelter. From the present-day look of it, he must have had in mind a very small bomb.

Retrace your steps to the main trail and continue to the nearby road (Lake Ridge Drive). Turn left and proceed along the open grassy shoulder for almost half a mile. Then turn left onto the shoulder of Black Hill Road and walk downhill. After 200 yards, cross the road carefully and head across the grass onto a woodland trail at a "Hiking Trails" sign. Note the droll nearby sign promising that, "You can take a walk around this trail and turn it into a voyage of purist discovery."

The dirt-and-grass surfaced trail winds gently downhill and then levels off close to the lakeshore. Continue until you get to a trail junction. There, turn left onto the Cabin Branch Trail, and go left again at the next junction. The half-mile-long, sometimes muddy trail undulates as it curves through the woods and crosses several small streams. A mini–suspension bridge spans the largest one, Cabin Branch Creek.

When you reach an unsignposted junction, stay left and on the descending main trail. At an orange pole, turn right onto a utility right-of-way. Stay on the broad, pole-dotted, and dirt-and-grass woodland path for more than half a mile as it crosses several small streams. The path forms part of the park's boundary line, and even wanders out of the park, as you'll see when you turn right at the next signpost onto another part of the Cabin Branch Trail (2.3 miles into the hike).

The mostly level trail parallels Cabin Branch Creek, off to the right. When you reach a trail fork, stay left and head for the signposted park entrance road. There, at Lake Ridge Drive again, turn left and walk along the shoulder for about 200 yards. When you're abreast of a yellow and dark-green gate, check for traffic, and then cross the road back into the woods and onto the Field Crest Spur. You'll be on the mostly shadeless trail for nearly half a mile. It follows the edge of the woods, and then swings to the right to cross overgrown fields dotted with bluebird boxes. Stay or go left at the first two trail junctions you reach. At the third one, turn right onto the Hard Rock Trail and follow it into the woods.

The trail is aptly named (here is no water, but only rock, and it's all hard), and it traces an undulating semicircle before returning to the fields. It's also scenic, but the traffic noise from nearby I-270 can be intrusive. Stay left at the next two intersections to remain on the trail. At the third intersection, go straight and slightly uphill (ignore the signpost). Stay on the trail as it dips into and out of a stream valley and reaches a trail junction very close to Lake Ridge Drive. There, turn left, in the direction of the Black Hill Trail (as the signpost says). Cross a utility right-of-way and tilt gently downhill. Go left at the next junction, and then follow a short trail section steeply down to Little Seneca Creek. Finally, you'll reach the Black Hill Trail.

Take the bridge across the creek (the hike's 5.1-mile mark), and think about detouring down-creek to a nearby rock outcrop for lunch. Then head away from the bridge, and go sharply right at a fork onto a short side trail. Where that trail starts uphill, look on the right for a skinny path leading a few yards to the nearby mossy ruins of an old gristmill and sawmill. The mill was abandoned a century ago, after almost a century's service. Walk around carefully to avoid slipping on the moss—and into the poison ivy. Return to the side trail, and then turn right to rejoin the main trail. But to do the hike's 6.9-mile option, turn left instead and recross the bridge, and follow the directions below for the last part of the full hike.

To do the out-and-back, stay on the main trail for about 200 yards and then turn right onto the paved and mostly sunswept Black Hill Trail to start a 4.2-mile out-and-back. It follows the creek and then hugs the shore of a large lake arm for a little more than 2 miles. Admire the lake views, but also notice, on your left, the houses lining the trail. Anytime you reach an intersection, turn right. Also turn right after crossing the causeway, which separates the lake arm from privately owned Lake Churchill.

I like to return to the causeway by looping through a stylish residential area. To do that, turn left along Wisteria Drive, left onto Wanegarden Drive, left onto

Wynnfield Drive, and then reach the causeway (see the map). Alternatively, skip the detour and just go straight back on the hiker/biker trail.

After you recross the Little Seneca Creek bridge, stay to the left and head uphill on a rocky path. At the hilltop intersection, turn left to begin the last leg of the hike—a 1.8-mile stretch of the Black Hill Trail. The first part, unpaved, is an old road through the woods. Stay to the left at each intersection. The road gives way to a narrow and undulating dirt trail with intermittent lake views.

Just after the trail swings to the right and pitches steeply downhill, detour on a short side trail to a lovely spot at the water's edge. Back on the main trail, you'll arrive at a paved section. Turn left there and keep asphalt underfoot for the hike's remaining 0.75 miles. On reaching the dock area, head uphill to the visitor center and trailhead.

NEARBY/RELATED ACTIVITIES

At any time of year, explore the visitor center and linger with binoculars on the center's always-open observation deck for panoramic views of the lake. In winter, watch for bald eagles and ospreys. In warm weather, explore the lake by rental boat (available Wednesday through Sunday); call (301) 972-6157. Also explore the park's separate western portion (not covered here).

C&O CANAL TOWPATH:
Carderock to Great Falls

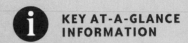

15

IN BRIEF

The C&O Canal towpath provides hikers with scenery, exercise, and glimpses of history—and is completely on the level. This close-in segment in Montgomery County, features great falls, wide water, and spectacular cliff trails.

DESCRIPTION

What is now the C&O Canal National Historical Park ranks as one of the metro area's prime recreational resources. It preserves the land, flora, fauna, and many historic sites along 185 miles of the Potomac River's left bank between Washington, D.C., and Cumberland, Maryland. It is rich in opportunities for humans to locomote vigorously on the restored canal towpath, now a popular multiuse trail, as well as to savor nature and find solitude. Because the park traverses a landscape that has been shaped in different ways by both natural and human forces, I have devised four separate towpath-based hikes. This particular hike, located just outside the beltway, also features several side trails and part of the restored canal.

Directions ———————————➤

Starting from American Legion (or Cabin John) Bridge on Capital Beltway (Interstate 495), proceed north on beltway in Maryland for about 100 yards and take Exit 41. Bear left at fork at small "Carderock" sign onto Clara Barton Parkway heading west. Go 0.9 miles to first parkway exit. Ascend short ramp, turn left at stop sign, and cross over parkway. Follow road as it swings right into Carderock Recreational Area and then swings left and goes through underpass. Turn right at T-junction. Then take first left into parking lot, 0.4 miles from parkway.

ⓘ KEY AT-A-GLANCE INFORMATION

LENGTH: 11.7 miles (with shorter options)

CONFIGURATION: Modified, semiloopy out-and-back

DIFFICULTY: Moderate

SCENERY: Water, woodlands

EXPOSURE: Mostly open

TRAFFIC: Usually light; heavier on warm-weather evenings, weekends, holidays

TRAIL SURFACE: Hard-packed dirt on towpath; asphalt on Berma Road; dirt, rocks, roots on side trails

HIKING TIME: 7.5–9 hours

SEASON: Year-round

ACCESS: Open daily, dawn–dusk

MAPS: USGS Falls Church, PATC Map D

FACILITIES: Toilets, water, phone at trailhead, off-trail at Great Falls (plus warm-season snack bar); toilets off-trail near milepost 11; phone, toilets near start of Berma Road and Old Angler's Inn

FOR MORE INFORMATION: Call Great Falls visitor center, (301) 299-3613; visit www.nps.gov/choh; call park's headquarters office in Sharpsburg, (301) 739-4200

SPECIAL COMMENTS: Billy Goat Trail can be dangerous when wet or icy

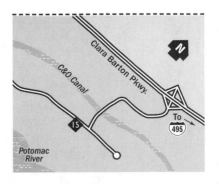

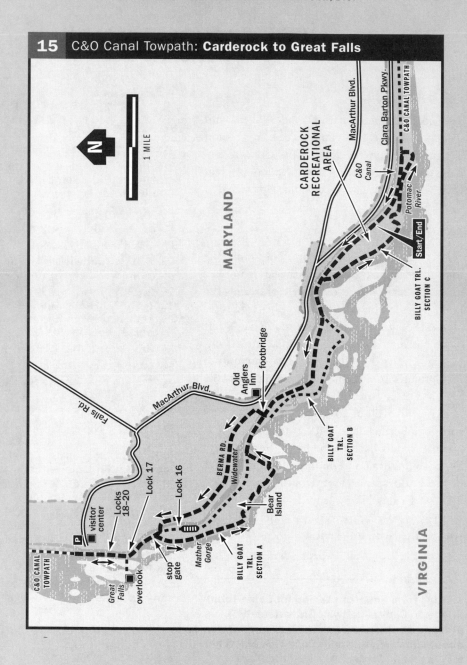

15   C&O Canal Towpath: Carderock to Great Falls

The Chesapeake and Ohio Canal had its origins in a grand ambition voiced by Thomas Jefferson, George Washington, and other early American leaders to make the Potomac navigable and link it to the Ohio River valley. The Potowmack Company, chartered in 1785 with Washington as its first president, announced it would clear a channel and build skirting canals around the rapids. It took almost 20 years just to complete the canals, the channel was never cleared, boat travel was severely limited by fluctuating water levels, and the company eventually collapsed.

The Chesapeake and Ohio Canal Company, launched in 1828, inherited its predecessor's charter and property. Its plan was to stay out of the river and build an on-land canal dotted with locks and paralleled by a towpath for the mules and horses that would provide the motive power for the boats. The canal was not finished until 1850—eight years after the Baltimore & Ohio Railroad had reached Cumberland—so the canal was already largely obsolete commercially. The Civil War and recurrent floods further damaged the canal and its toll-based business. After a devastating 1889 flood, the waterway was bought by the B&O. It remained in sporadic and local use until 1924, when another flood led the B&O to abandon it. In 1938 the railroad gave it to the federal government to settle a $2 million debt.

The National Park Service managed to restore the canal's lower 22 miles before World War II intervened, but did little else for a long time thereafter. In 1954 a public campaign launched by Supreme Court justice and outdoorsman William O. Douglas saved the canal route from being paved over as a parkway. Congress made the property a national monument in 1961 and a national historical park in 1971.

The full hike I have devised is a challenging, 11.7-mile, modified out-and-back hike with about 500 feet of elevation change and much rockiness in places. However, you have the option of making it much easier—8 miles, almost no up-and-down, and rock-free—by skipping the five off-towpath segments (see the last paragraph in this section). The full hike starts with about 2 miles of towpath alongside the restored, water-filled canal, followed by an inland mile on low bluffs overlooking a lake, and a final mile close to the Potomac. The return leg of 7.7 miles includes a close look at thundering Great Falls and two sections of the rugged and justly famous Billy Goat Trail.

From the parking-lot trailhead at Carderock, opposite the toilets, cross a grassy strip and a nearby road to get onto a woodland trail (marked by a notice to cyclists) that leads about 150 yards to the towpath. There's no signpost there, so mark or memorize the spot for your return journey. Then turn left and head northwest on the broad and level towpath, keeping the canal on your right.

Half a mile up-canal (thick woods hide the Potomac here), you'll pass milepost 11 (the towpath is studded with mileposts, starting in Washington). Then, about 0.3 miles past milepost 12, turn right to cross the canal by footbridge and begin the hike's first off-towpath segment. It was long an official detour around a closed towpath section, and I have come to prefer it to the now-reopened section. To get started, ascend some steps (off to the right is historic Old Angler's Inn), turn left, and proceed along an old and tree-shrouded paved road—Berma Road. En route, watch for a short side trail leading left to a lovely overlook high above

Widewater, a natural, mile-long lake that was incorporated into the canal route. Eventually, turn left and descend some steps to recross the canal on a wooden walkway. That's the upper part of a reconstructed stop gate, designed to divert floodwater out of the canal and into the river—and still used during floods.

Descend from the walkway to rejoin the towpath (about 0.75 miles past milepost 13), and proceed up-canal. For the next half mile, look to your left for dramatic views of the river's rapids-filled side channels. Arriving at Lock 20, which is the hike's 4-mile mark, step across a short wooden bridge spanning the canal to reach Great Falls Tavern. The building, parts of which date from the late 1820s, long served as a lock house, hotel, or both. It's now a visitor center, and includes museum exhibits.

Recross the canal, turn left, and head back down the towpath for 0.3 miles, to the signposted Great Falls Overlook trail and your second off-townpath detour. Using a 0.25-mile-long walkway, the detour crosses narrow gorges often choked with flood debris or filled with deafening torrents. At the spray-flecked mid-river overlook, discover just how great the falls are—not so much from their height as from the sense of brute force conveyed by water crossing the fall line.

Continue down the towpath. At Lock 17, embark on your third detour by turning right onto a side trail that pitches steeply downhill. Two wooden steps from the bottom, take a narrow dirt trail to the right and clamber about 50 yards up to a rocky knoll that provides a splendid view down a narrow gorge. Small clam shells wedged in rock crevices are a stark reminder of both the river's high flood levels and the presence of the invasive Asian clam that has displaced the native freshwater mussel.

Return to the narrow trail, turn right, and follow the undulating trail a couple of hundred yards to a lovely, off-the-beaten-trail spot featuring a rock-rimmed pool, a sand-and-shell beach, and—if it's off-season or a weekday—utter tranquility. Leaving the beach, stay to the right and take a narrow trail leading uphill. Turn right when you reach a retaining wall, and follow it to a low crossing place, and then turn right onto the towpath.

Just before reaching the stop gate, turn right at a sign for the blue-blazed Billy Goat Trail. The sign doesn't say so, but it's the trail's section A and your fourth and most challenging detour. For most of its roughly 2 miles, section A follows the perimeter of Bear Island. It includes a rocky cliff-top route along the Potomac's narrow, mile-long Mather Gorge. The blue blazes lead through a wild and beautiful landscape dominated by steep rocks and scraggy vegetation. Wend your way around huge boulders, over smaller ones, and past huge potholes and rockbound ponds (some with water lilies). After several chances to see the river below, perhaps you'll also gaze into the abyss to see if it gazes back. Eventually, after the trail curves left again, you'll reach the towpath, near the southern end of Widewater.

Continuing down-canal on the towpath, ignore the various Billy Goat Trail signs (I prefer to skip section B) until you pass milepost 11. Then watch for a sign that puts you on the trail's section C, your final detour, at the "West End." It will take you on a scenic 1.7-mile woodland trek along the edge of a side channel and then the main channel. It has its ups and downs, but it's a lot easier than section A. Follow the blue blazes. Eventually, the towpath appears again at the "East End," near the ruins of a swing bridge built in 1941 for the use of the Civilian Conservation Corps workers who restored the canal. From there, head up-canal for half a mile, passing milepost 10. Then, soon after crossing an overpass, turn left onto the inconspicuous woodland path you marked or remembered, and return to the trailhead.

Here are four ways to shorten the full hike: Omit section A to save almost 1 mile and 2 hours; omit section C to save almost 2 miles and 1.25 hours; omit the overlook to save 0.5 miles and 0.75 hours; and omit the rock pool detour to save 0.1 mile and 0.5 hours. If you omit section C, take the Berma Road detour to get back to the towpath and trailhead.

NEARBY/RELATED ACTIVITIES

Do the C&O Canal Association's springtime Justice Douglas Annual Hike (the association started as a small group formed by Douglas on a save-the-canal hike he led in 1954). Contact the association, (301) 983-0825 or **www.cando canal.org.**

16 C&O CANAL TOWPATH:
Rileys Lock to Swains Lock

KEY AT-A-GLANCE INFORMATION

LENGTH: 13.2 miles

CONFIGURATION: Out-and-back

DIFFICULTY: Moderate

SCENERY: Woodlands, river and canal views

EXPOSURE: Mostly open

TRAFFIC: Light to moderate; heavier near trailhead, Swains Lock on warm-weather weekends, holidays

TRAIL SURFACE: Chiefly hard-packed dirt or pebbly dirt; some grassy, sandy patches; muddy when wet

HIKING TIME: 5–6.5 hours

SEASON: Year-round

ACCESS: Open daily, dawn–dusk

MAPS: USGS Seneca, Vienna

FACILITIES: Toilets, water, phone at trailhead; toilets at Violettes Lock, Pennyfield Lock; toilets, water, phone, warm-season snack bar at Swains Lock

FOR MORE INFORMATION: Call Great Falls visitor center, (301) 299-3613; visit park's Web site, www.nps.gov/choh; call park's headquarters office in Sharpsburg, (301) 739-4200; read canal history in Hike 15, page 81

IN BRIEF

This scenic C&O Canal towpath outing in Montgomery County, features woodlands and wildflowers, a water-filled canal, an aqueduct, locks, and lock houses.

DESCRIPTION

This 13.2-mile out-and-back hike will acquaint you with what I think is the loveliest stretch of the C&O Canal National Historical Park south of Monocacy. This stretch of parkland envelops the milepost-dotted canal towpath between Rileys Lock, 0.2 miles below milepost 23, and Swains Lock, 0.4 miles below milepost 17. The hike starts at Rileys. I like the novelty of doing the downriver part first. Also, Rileys has ample parking, whereas Swains's small lot can fill up quickly. Strangely, the towpath in between is almost always uncrowded.

Before or after the hike, explore the trailhead area, commonly called Seneca. Adjoining Rileys Lock (Lock 24) is Seneca Aqueduct, a 126-foot-long structure that carried the canal across the mouth of Seneca Creek. Completed in 1833 as a single unit, the lock and aqueduct were built of red Seneca sandstone from nearby quarries, as were the other locks on

Directions

From Capital Beltway (Interstate 495) in Bethesda, Maryland, just north of the Potomac River, take Exit 39A and follow 0.7-mile exit ramp to get onto River Road (MD 190) heading west. Proceed for about 11.6 miles toward and through Potomac to reach stop sign where MD 190 ends. Then turn left to continue west on River Road for 0.7 miles, and turn left onto Rileys Lock Road. Go 0.7 miles to end of road at Rileys Lock parking lot.

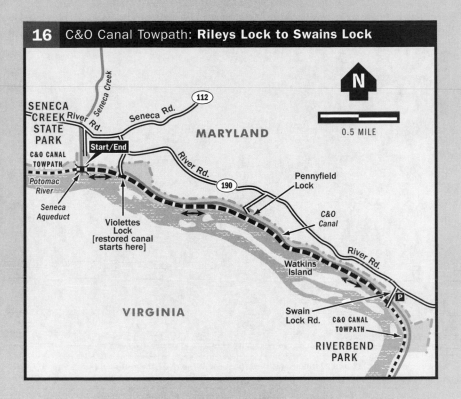

letter labels from map:

16 C&O Canal Towpath: **Rileys Lock to Swains Lock**

N

0.5 MILE

SENECA CREEK STATE PARK

C&O CANAL TOWPATH

Seneca Creek

Seneca Rd.

River Rd.

112

MARYLAND

Start/End

River Rd.

190

Potomac River

Seneca Aqueduct

Violettes Lock [restored canal starts here]

Pennyfield Lock

C&O Canal

River Rd.

Watkins Island

VIRGINIA

Swain Lock Rd.

C&O CANAL TOWPATH

P

RIVERBEND PARK

this hike. Next to the lock is the restored lock house once occupied by lockkeeper Riley and his family. Originally, the aqueduct had three arches, but now has only two, thanks to being battered by debris-laden floodwaters in 1971. For good views across the Potomac, walk over to the nearby flared wing wall of the aqueduct. Also note the stone pillar etched with a short line and a date. The line marks the height reached by floodwaters on June 2, 1889, the canal's second-to-last ruinous flood.

To get started, step onto the towpath, turn left, and head downriver. The woodland path is next to a dry and overgrown canal—but only for about 0.75 miles. After that, the scenery changes to an open area close to the river that's dominated by two restored locks. Violettes Lock (Lock 23), on the left, was a regular move-the-boats-through lock. Look closely at the top of the downstream wing wall on the towpath side to see the grooves worn by straining towropes. The other lock, now closed, supplied the canal with water and enabled boats to enter and leave the canal. Violettes Lock (disappointingly, perhaps, Violettes was a male lockkeeper's surname) was as far as the canal restorers got in the 1940s (see Hike 8). For the rest of your way down-canal, you'll be following a water-filled canal under an open sky.

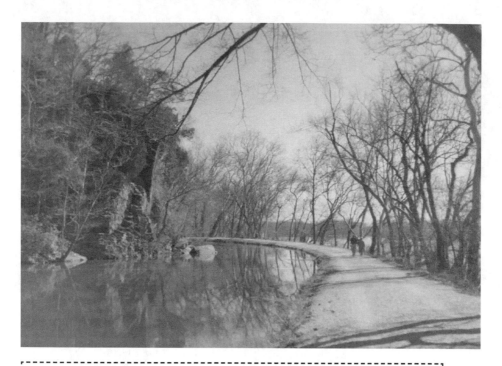

Between mileposts 22 and 21, hikers get superb views of the river, the restored canal, and the wooded cliffs at Blockhouse Point.

About half a mile beyond milepost 22 lies an area that is lovely, if not gorgeous. The canal winds along the foot of a line of cliffs, and the towpath faithfully follows its curves. In places, the canal and river are scarcely 30 feet apart. At milepost 21, turn right onto a dirt side trail to start the first of four short and scenic off-the-beaten-trail detours. The first detour is a 300-yard round trip to the riverbank, where huge red maples lean over the water.

Then, back on the towpath, you'll find that, over the next 1.5 miles, the cliff walls subside into hilly woodlands as the canal pulls away from the river. After that, you'll reach Pennyfield Lock (Lock 22), with its towrope-grooved wing wall and reputation among birders as a springtime hot spot. The side trail adjoining the nearby old lock house is the start of the second detour. Follow the dirt trail to the water, turn left, and walk along the wooded shore across a narrow channel from Watkins Island. At a small clearing containing a large maple festooned with poison ivy, turn left. Then take a ten-yard trail to return to the towpath. Continuing, you'll once more be in a picturesque setting of cliffs rising above the canal and towpath, plus a low stone wall along the river's edge. You'll have a mile of this scenery, passing milepost 19 on the way.

Then, about 0.5 miles beyond milepost 18 and just after passing under a concrete bridge, take a short passageway to your right—the third detour. Walk out onto an overlook atop a concrete water-intake-and-treatment structure for a view of the undiverted river tumbling through a narrow channel hemmed in by

Watkins Island. And read the plaques about the Potomac River valley and its floods. Continuing on the towpath for 0.75 miles, you'll pass milepost 17 and reach Swains Lock (Lock 21), with its signature towrope grooves. A wooden bridge spans the lock. On the far side is the original lock house, still home to the Swain descendants of the last lockkeeper. Linger a bit (the nearby riverbank is a picnic area), and then start on the 6.2 miles back to Rileys. On the way back, watch for milepost 20, and turn left there for the fourth detour. A short dirt-and-grass side trail leads about 200 yards to a riverbank wildlife sanctuary. In the summer and fall, the trail is a sea of yellow as it passes through a large patch of wingstem, and is often colorfully alive with birds.

NEARBY/RELATED ACTIVITIES

Tour Riley's lock house, which is filled with period furnishings. Tours are offered on weekend afternoons, March to November, by Girl Scouts in period costume. Rent a canoe at Swains and explore the canal by water.

17 McKEE-BESHERS WILDLIFE MANAGEMENT AREA

KEY AT-A-GLANCE INFORMATION

LENGTH: 7.9 miles (with shorter option)

CONFIGURATION: Modified loop

DIFFICULTY: Easy

SCENERY: Crop and fallow fields, hedgerows, woodlands, tree reservoirs, other wetlands, river views

EXPOSURE: Mostly open

TRAFFIC: Usually very light

TRAIL SURFACE: Mostly dirt or grass, some gravel and old pavement

HIKING TIME: 3–4 hours

SEASON: Late fall–early spring (to avoid vicious mosquitoes and flies)

ACCESS: Towpath open daily, dawn–dusk; elsewhere, no restrictions (but see text)

MAPS: USGS Seneca, Poolesville

FACILITIES: Toilets, water near trailhead (at temple), toilet at towpath campground

FOR MORE INFORMATION: Visit www.dnr.state.md.us/public lands/central/mb.asp#sa; call DNR's Gwynnbrook Center, (410) 356-9272 (weekday mornings only)

SPECIAL COMMENTS: Beware of hunters, January–September, mid-April–mid-May (see text); don't park on temple grounds, especially on weekends

IN BRIEF

Wedged between the Potomac River and River Road in western Montgomery County, lies a little-known wildlife management area where careful hikers can roam a splendid expanse of bird-rich crop fields, wetlands, woodlands, and hedgerows.

DESCRIPTION

It's easy to overlook the state-owned McKee-Beshers Wildlife Management Area (WMA), located on the Potomac River floodplain roughly 15 miles northwest of Washington. I did so many times before deciding to explore it. And what I found was a secluded, 2,200-acre expanse of former farmland managed as habitat for game species and other wildlife. So I devised this 7.9-mile loop that samples the WMA's fields, woodlands, and hedgerows, and adjoining areas, but only skirts the wetlands.

Follow my directions carefully in that the C&O Canal towpath and other peripheral route segments are easy to find and follow, but the WMA segments are unblazed and unsignposted. And remember that the WMA is seasonally popular with both vicious insects and hunters. Avoid the bugs by staying away during,

----

Directions

From Capital Beltway (Interstate 495) in Bethesda, Maryland, take Exit 39 to get onto River Road (MD 190) heading west. Proceed for 11.8 miles to T-junction, where MD 190 ends but River Road turns to left. Continue on River Road for 3 miles. Just after passing Hunting Quarter Road on left, park in gravel turnout on south shoulder about 100 yards before Buddhist temple's flag-bedecked driveway on left (at 18400 River Road).

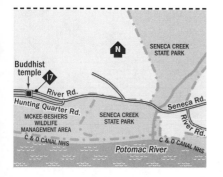

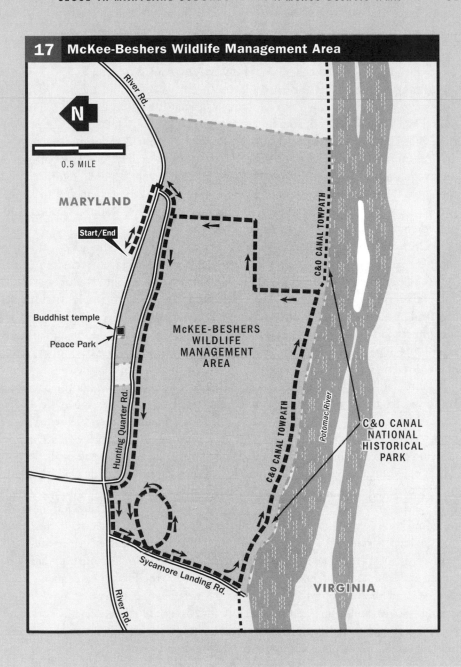

17 McKee-Beshers Wildlife Management Area

N

0.5 MILE

MARYLAND

Start/End

Buddhist temple

Peace Park

Hunting Quarter Rd.

River Rd.

McKEE-BESHERS
WILDLIFE
MANAGEMENT
AREA

C&O CANAL TOWPATH

C&O CANAL TOWPATH

Potomac River

C&O CANAL
NATIONAL
HISTORICAL
PARK

Sycamore Landing Rd.

River Rd.

VIRGINIA

say, May to October, or use protective clothing and insect repellent. Avoid the
hunters by staying away when they're active (visit **www.dnr.state.md.us/wildlife**
for details) or by hiking in-season only on Sundays, when Maryland's no-hunting
law is in effect. Also beware of periodic field trials, when, bizarrely, hunters are
allowed to shoot birds for their dogs to retrieve, even on Sundays. And take along

field glasses and reference books, especially *A Birder's Guide to Montgomery County, Maryland* (Maryland Ornithological Society, Montgomery County Chapter), which has a detailed chapter on the WMA by Paul Woodward.

To get started from the roadside trailhead, walk back along the road for 200 yards, and turn right onto Hunting Quarter Road. Proceed on what is a woodland, rough-surfaced, sometimes muddy, and usually (alas) garbage-strewn road that curves right to parallel River Road for about 2 miles and marks the WMA's northern boundary. You'll soon pass on your left a yellow-bar–gated unpaved road leading south into the WMA. That's where you'll return to the road near the hike's end. Continuing, you'll pass two more such gates. Also notice two of the WMA's so-called green-tree reservoirs, which are flooded seasonally to provide habitat for wood ducks and other birds.

On reaching River Road, turn left and head west along the grassy shoulder for 0.4 miles, and then turn left again to get onto gravel-surfaced Sycamore Landing Road heading southwest. After going 0.3 miles, turn left at a yellow-bar gate, and walk along a curving grassy road for about 200 yards to reach a field trials area and pavilion. If you see armed men with dogs there, just retrace your steps to the gravel road and do the hike's 6.9-mile version. Otherwise, do the agricultural mini-loop. Start by heading east across the field to the left of the pavilion. On the far side, swing left at a thick hedgerow to follow the edge of that field—and then two more fields—in a counterclockwise direction until you're back at the pavilion. En route, try to identify the growing or harvested crops. Some WMA fields are used to grow corn, sorghum, and other crops for humans (under a lease arrangement), and sunflowers, millet, and other crops for wildlife, as well as native grasses to furnish habitat for wild turkeys and other ground-nesting birds.

Then return to Sycamore Landing Road, turn left, and resume walking south for 0.5 miles to reach the C&O Canal National Historical Park and the Potomac River across from Maddux Island, at the hike's 4.4-mile mark. Turn left and east to tromp for 1.7 miles along the former canal's restored and tree-shrouded towpath, which parallels the WMA's southern boundary. You'll get river views to your right (best in winter) and abundant trailside wildflowers on both sides in spring and summer. You'll pass towpath milepost 27, the Horsepen Branch campground, and then milepost 26. About 200 yards beyond milepost 26, turn left onto a narrow and unmarked dirt trail that crosses the ruined canal, leaves the park, and disappears into the WMA's woods. You'll soon reach an open area and be on a broad, fields-flanked dirt road heading north.

Keep going north for 0.6 miles and then turn right at the first conspicuous four-way intersection to head east on a sometimes-overgrown farm road that passes through more crop fields (also note the handsome wall of pines on the right). After another 0.6 miles, you'll reach a three-way junction next to a lone tree. Turn left there to head north for 0.4 miles on another often-overgrown farm road, which becomes a dirt-surfaced woodland road. At a familiar yellow-bar gate, turn right onto Hunting Quarter Road and hike the last 0.2 miles back to the trailhead.

NEARBY/RELATED ACTIVITIES

Combine this hike with a 2-mile hike in the temple's nearby Peace Park. It's a lovely, wooded, and gently hilly area dotted with small meditation gardens and two of the traditional sacred Buddhist structures known as stupas. Pick up a trail map at the temple and also visit the temple's Web site, **www.kpc-md-tara.org.** And if you do the WMA hike on a Sunday, try the temple's inexpensive buffet lunch. Also explore the temple itself. Sunday afternoon is also when the nearby Seneca Schoolhouse Museum (at 16800 River Road) is open to the public. Stop by to see the restored 19th-century one-room schoolhouse and its authentic McGuffey Readers.

18 LAKE ARTEMESIA NATURAL AREA AND NORTHEAST BRANCH TRAIL

KEY AT-A-GLANCE INFORMATION

LENGTH: 10 miles

CONFIGURATION: Modified out-and-back

DIFFICULTY: Easy–moderate

SCENERY: Parklands, water views, glimpses of suburbia

EXPOSURE: Mostly open; more so in winter

TRAFFIC: Usually very light to light; heavier on warm-weather weekends, holidays

TRAIL SURFACE: Mostly pavement; some dirt

HIKING TIME: 4.5–5.5 hours

SEASON: Year-round

ACCESS: Open daily during daylight hours

MAPS: USGS Washington East, Beltsville

FACILITIES: Phone at trailhead; toilets, water, phone at lakeside building; warm-season–only toilet in Riverdale Park; toilets in other trailside parks

FOR MORE INFORMATION: Contact Prince George's County Department of Parks and Recreation, (301) 699-2407 or www.pgparks.com

IN BRIEF

This flat hike is a refreshing excursion through suburban Maryland just northeast of Washington. It features landscaped parklands, a man-made lake, and a streamside trail.

DESCRIPTION

A hole is to dig, as Ruth Krauss explained in a book so titled. Once dug, it's also a fine thing to use for a lake, especially one that's to be the centerpiece of a park. That's the story of Lake Artemesia, located in Prince George's County near College Park. The Washington Metropolitan Area Transit Authority needed sand and gravel to build a nearby section of Metrorail's Green Line. So it dug a huge hole in some county land. It then paid to have the hole and environs transformed into an area of landscaped county parkland enveloping a 38-acre lake.

Opened in 1992, Lake Artemesia Natural Area (named for Artemesia N. Drefs, a local resident) has a healthy animal population, including

----

Directions ———————→

From Capital Beltway (Interstate 495 and I-95) in Maryland, take Exit 23 and head south for 0.5 miles on Kenilworth Avenue (MD 201). Turn right onto Greenbelt Road (MD 193), head west for about 0.7 miles, and turn right onto Branchville Road. Follow it for 0.7 miles as it traverses industrial park, U-turns under Greenbelt Road, and crosses Berwyn Road to become Bellew Road. Once on Bellew, turn left into parking lot.

Or use Metro to do hike: Take Green Line train to Greenbelt station, Metrobus C2 along Greenbelt Road to Branchville Road, and then shank's mare for about 0.7 miles to trailhead. Contact Metro, (202) 637-7000 or www.wmata.com.

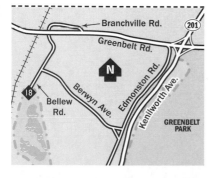

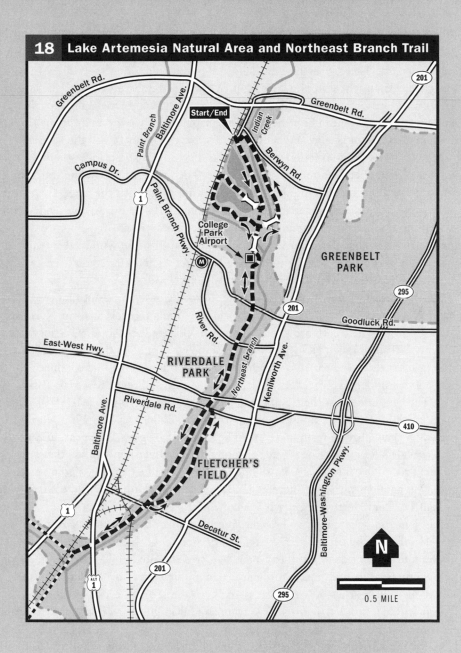

18 Lake Artemesia Natural Area and Northeast Branch Trail

deer, beavers, amphibians, and (during warm weather) too many bugs. The area is also popular with humans, especially on warm-weather weekends and holidays. Its paved trails are part of an evolving multiuse trail network known as the Anacostia Tributary Trail System. This modified out-and-back hike of 10 miles uses the system's Northeast Branch Trail. Trail signs are somewhat sparse, so follow my directions.

From the parking-lot trailhead, head south on the paved trail that parallels Bellew Avenue to quickly reach the natural area's gated entrance. Walk to a nearby bulletin board. There, bear left and take the paved trail along the willow-fringed shoreline, keeping the water on your right. Warm weather brings color to the lake in the form of blossoming irises and water lilies. When the wind kicks up in the fall, the willows sway and you can hear the lake water lapping with low sounds by the shore. In winter, a glaze of lake ice and a dusting of snow can eerily bleach the lakescape.

At a five-way intersection, turn right and cross a rustic bridge spanning the narrow channel between the lake's two lobes. Turn right to follow the trail along the curving shoreline. Continuing, swing left and away from the lake. Then turn right just before reaching the natural area's lakeside building. At the next intersection, turn left. Stay to the left and follow the lakeshore until just before reaching the rustic bridge. Then turn right and disappear into the woods. Bear right at the next junction, about 1.75 miles into the hike. Thereafter, you'll be on the mostly flat Northeast Branch Trail for just over 3.5 miles.

The first bridge you'll cross, in a lovely wooded glen, spans Paint Branch. When water reappears, it'll be where Paint Branch joins Indian Creek to form Northeast Branch. The trail then curls around the runway of College Park Airport. Passing under a highway (Paint Branch Parkway), you'll reach a junction near the Denis Wolf Rest Stop (just a sheltered bench). Go straight, across a wooden bridge, and continue. Then take another underpass (River Road), leave the woods, and reach Riverdale Park.

The next underpass shelters the trail from East-West Highway (MD 410). After that, you'll start to see houses and apartment buildings, along with Northeast Branch, a channelized stream in a sunken bed flanked by grass. Then carefully cross underpass-less Riverdale Road. After passing through Riverside Park, do the same at the next road (Decatur Street). Pass under a railroad bridge, and keep going to pass under yet another highway (Alternate US 1) and reach the junction of the Northeast Branch Trail and Northwest Branch Trail, the hike's turnaround point. Nearby is the stream junction, where the two branches merge to form the Anacostia River.

Heading back northward, recross Decatur Street, but then turn right to take the sidewalk to the far side of Northeast Branch. Turn left onto a mile-long dirt trail that follows the stream and passes through a community park called Fletcher's Field. When the trail reaches a paved access road, continue on the grassy shoulder. At Riverdale Road, turn left, recross the stream, and turn right to get back on the Northeast Branch Trail. Remember to turn right near the Denis Wolf Rest Stop. At the lake area, forget the rustic-bridge intersection. Instead, stay to the right, and watch for a bridge spanning another stream. Cross it and then turn left onto the Indian Creek Trail. Follow that northward for about half a mile. At paved Berwyn Road, turn left onto the sidewalk and keep going for about 200 yards, to the parking-lot trailhead.

NEARBY/RELATED ACTIVITIES

Tour the College Park Aviation Museum, (301) 864-6029, at the airport. Drive there, or add a 1.4-mile detour to your hike, starting near Paint Branch Parkway (see map).

GREENBELT PARK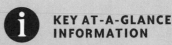

IN BRIEF

Secreted in Prince George's County, well-wooded Greenbelt Park is a great place to get fresh air and exercise, take in seasonal color, walk with friends, and contemplate life.

DESCRIPTION

Located a dozen miles northeast of the White House, Greenbelt Park ranks as the second largest nature preserve (after Rock Creek Park) within the Capital Beltway. Covering 1,100 acres, it nestles amid a grid of major highways and suburban streets. Most of it remains undeveloped, with picnic areas and a campground being its major attractions. But it's also an attractive—if little-used—hiking locale. This hike is an easy 6-mile loop through the woods, with little elevation change. Each season offers

----

Directions ➞

From Capital Beltway (Interstate 495 and I-95) in Maryland, take Exit 23 and head south for 0.5 miles on Kenilworth Avenue (MD 201). Turn left onto Greenbelt Road (MD 193), head east for about 0.3 miles and turn right into park. Alternatively, from Baltimore-Washington Parkway, head west on Greenbelt Road for about 1 mile and turn left into park. Within park, follow winding entrance road for 200 yards and turn right onto Park Central Road (park's chief artery). Follow it for 1.6 miles around Sweetgum picnic area and south through park. Just before the end of that road, turn right onto paved side road (leading to campground) and park at ranger station about 100 yards ahead on right.

Or use Metro to do hike starting near park entrance. Take Green Line train to Greenbelt station, Metrobus C2 along Greenbelt Road, and 100-yard walk into park. Contact Metro, (202) 637-7000 or www.wmata.com.

ℹ KEY AT-A-GLANCE INFORMATION

LENGTH: 6 miles (with shorter option)

CONFIGURATION: Loop

DIFFICULTY: Easy

SCENERY: Woodlands, stream valleys

EXPOSURE: Lots of shade; less in winter

TRAFFIC: Usually very light to light; heavier near picnic areas, especially on weekends, holidays

TRAIL SURFACE: Basically hard-packed dirt; rocky, rooty, or grassy in some places (watch out for poison ivy); boardwalked and bridged in wet places

HIKING TIME: 2.5–3 hours

SEASON: Year-round

ACCESS: No restrictions

MAPS: USGS Beltsville; ADC Prince George's Co.; sketch map in free park brochure

FACILITIES: Toilets, water, phones near trailhead; toilets at Sweetgum picnic area near park entrance

FOR MORE INFORMATION: Contact park's on-site headquarters office, (301) 344-3948, or visit www.nps.gov/gree

SPECIAL COMMENTS: Call park to check on current condition of boardwalks and bridges on western parts of Perimeter Trail

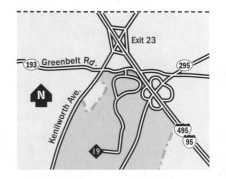

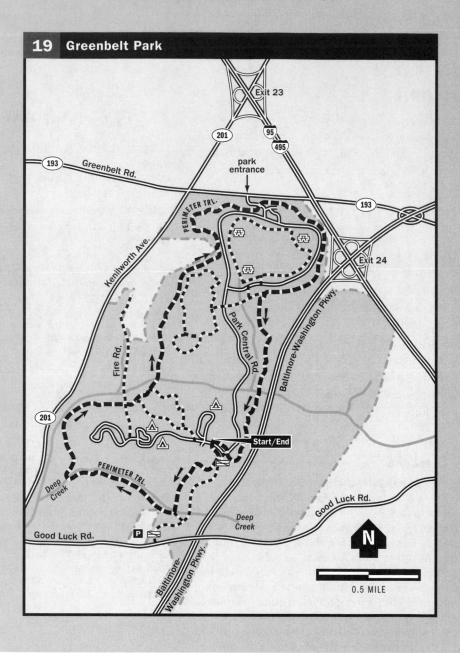

19   Greenbelt Park

an array of phenomena to observe. Only in a few places does the outside world intrude and that's mostly in the form of traffic noise near the park boundaries.

The park is not a wilderness that has thwarted developers. Rather, it derives from an ambitious federal attempt at large-scale social engineering in the 1930s. Inspired by the international "garden city" movement, the Roosevelt administration bought up marginal and abandoned tobacco fields in Prince George's County. It planned to create an experimental community shielded from Washington by a green belt of open land. But the plan was modified. The city of Greenbelt was duly built. Most of the open space, though, was incorporated into a sprawling U.S. Department of Agriculture research center. That left Greenbelt Park—formally taken over by the National Park Service in 1950—as the chief buffer zone. The park remains a work in progress. Over six-plus decades, the hemmed-in but well-protected tract has gradually evolved into a thriving woodland area that is rich in plant life. It also serves as a haven for such four-footers as deer, foxes, and groundhogs, and scores of bird species.

The hike begins at the ranger station (open every day except Christmas). Start the first leg by walking back along the side road to Park Central Road. Turn right onto that road and go around the vehicle barrier that protects the bike trail beyond. Take the dirt trail to the right and then quickly turn left onto the yellow-blazed Perimeter Trail. You'll be on that trail for the rest of the hike, following the yellow blazes around the park in a clockwise direction. (The park's major trails are color coded and well marked.)

Head south to a boardwalk spanning a marshy area along a shallow stream called Deep Creek. At the next intersection, turn right and stay on the trail as it curves westward close to the stream. At the next intersection, leave Deep Creek and embark on the hike's second leg by following the Perimeter Trail to the right and north, close to the park's western flanks. Anytime you reach an intersection, take the yellow-blazed option. After crossing a fire road and passing two side trails on the right (the second of which is the Blueberry Trail), you'll cross another stream, Still Creek (which lives up to its name about as much as Deep Creek does). That's the hike's 2-mile mark.

The next leg of the hike is a 2-mile segment that curves past a residential area and turns east roughly parallel to the park's northernmost boundary. There it intersects the entrance road. Cross carefully, then swing past the Holly and Laurel picnic areas. After that, on the fourth leg, follow the yellow blazes south, cross Still Creek again, and hike roughly parallel to the Baltimore-Washington Parkway. Eventually the trail curves to the right and away from the parkway. At Park Central Road, turn right onto the side road leading back to the ranger station.

You can use the Blueberry Trail to shorten the hike by about a mile: start at the ranger station, but follow the paved road west and then turn right onto the 0.8-mile Blueberry Trail, which joins the Perimeter Trail just south of Still Creek. There, turn right onto the Perimeter Trail and do the rest of the hike as described above.

NEARBY/RELATED ACTIVITIES

Attend some of the park's annual events held in the fall and also in the spring on Earth Day. Explore the park's birth twin—the nearby city of Greenbelt—and see what's left of the 1930s experimental community, including the Greenbelt Museum, (301) 474-1936, housed in one of the community's original buildings on Crescent Road.

20 | PATUXENT RESEARCH REFUGE

KEY AT-A-GLANCE INFORMATION

LENGTH: 11 miles (with shorter options)

CONFIGURATION: Modified loop

DIFFICULTY: Moderate

SCENERY: Woods, wetlands, meadows

EXPOSURE: Mostly open; less so in months when sun is low in sky

TRAFFIC: Generally very light; heavier on weekends, holidays

TRAIL SURFACE: Dirt, gravel, pavement

HIKING TIME: 3.5–5 hours

SEASON: Year-round, but best in spring and fall, especially for birders

ACCESS: Open daily, 8 a.m.–4 p.m. November–March (until 5:30 p.m. on March weekends), 8 a.m.–7:30 p.m. April–August, 8 a.m.–6:30 p.m. September, 8 a.m.–6 p.m. October (closed Thanksgiving, Christmas, and New Year's); register and get access pass at North Tract contact station

MAPS: USGS Laurel; sketch map of North Tract (get at contact station)

FACILITIES: Toilets, water at contact station

FOR MORE INFORMATION: Visit patuxent.fws.gov; call (301) 497-5580, (301) 776-3090 (contact station)

SPECIAL COMMENTS: Note Maryland's no-hunting-on-Sunday law; know what "UXO" means (see text)

IN BRIEF

Hidden away in suburban Maryland between Washington and Baltimore lies a huge wildlife refuge where hikers can find a diverse and spacious landscape, open skies, many wild birds and animals, a few vestiges of the past, and much tranquility.

DESCRIPTION

As Megalopolis relentlessly gobbles up open space between Washington and Baltimore, it's reassuring to know that 12,750 acres of land near Laurel, remain—and will remain—gloriously undeveloped. Located mostly in Anne Arundel County (the rest is in Prince George's County), the acreage makes up Patuxent Research Refuge, which is run by the U.S. Fish and Wildlife Service as the nation's only national wildlife refuge devoted to wildlife and wildlife-habitat research. The refuge, which consists of deciduous and coniferous woodlands interspersed with wetlands and meadows, is a haven for myriad birds and land animals. It's also a safe and delightful place for hikers who like solitude and tranquility while communing with nature.

Directions

From Capital Beltway (Interstate 495) in Greenbelt, Maryland, take Exit 22 and head northeast on Baltimore-Washington Parkway. Proceed for 5 miles, and then turn right, or east, onto MD 198 (Fort Meade Road). Proceed eastward for 1.9 miles (starting with 0.5-mile exit ramp), and then—at prominent sign for Patuxent Research Refuge—turn right onto mostly unpaved road (Bald Eagle Drive). Keep going for 1 mile to reach contact station and parking lot.

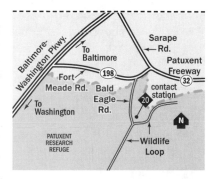

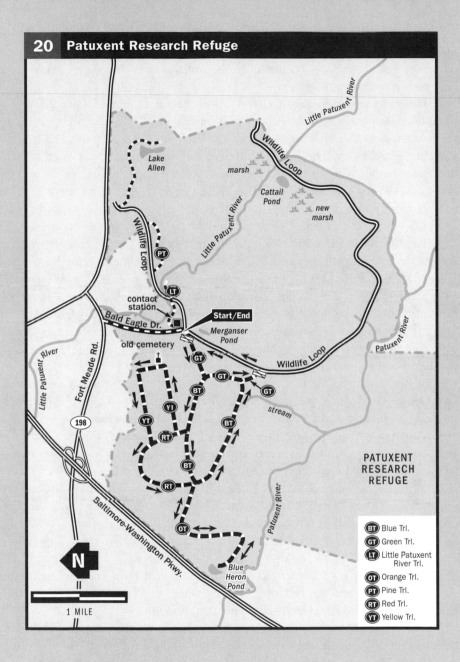

20 Patuxent Research Refuge

Little Patuxent River

Lake Allen

marsh

Cattail Pond

new marsh

Wildlife Loop

Little Patuxent River

PT

Wildlife Loop

LT

contact station

Bald Eagle Dr.

Start/End

Merganser Pond

old cemetery

Patuxent River

Wildlife Loop

GT

GT

GT

stream

BT

Little Patuxent River

Fort Meade Rd.

YT

Y!

BT

198

RT

BT

PATUXENT RESEARCH REFUGE

RT

OT

Patuxent River

Saltimore-Washington Pkwy.

Blue Heron Pond

N

1 MILE

BT Blue Trl.
GT Green Trl.
LT Little Patuxent River Trl.
OT Orange Trl.
PT Pine Trl.
RT Red Trl.
YT Yellow Trl.

The refuge was established in 1936 on mostly marginal farmlands and cutover woodlots bought up by the federal government (for as little as $30 an acre). Subsequently more than quadrupled in size, the refuge now consists of three contiguous tracts. The open-to-the-public South Tract, which has an impressive visitor center and a few short and easy trails, attracts most of the refuge's human visitors. The closed-to-the-public Central Tract accounts for most of the research facilities. The open-to-the-public North Tract gets very few human visitors, has about 20 miles of trails, and, as I have discovered, serves as a very satisfying close-in hike venue.

The hike I've devised consists of an 11-mile (easily shortened if needed) modified loop, with less than 400 feet of elevation change, that gently circles through the northwestern sector of the North Tract. The trails are mostly broad dirt-and-gravel or gravel roads. They're color named, color coded, and signposted (watch for circles marked with arrows atop redwood-colored posts, but ignore the mysterious signs bearing such letters as "U" or "X"). Officially, they're open not only to people on foot (including hunters, seasonally), but also to people on bikes, horses, and even skis (so far, though, I've encountered only my own hiking companions).

The North Tract is worth visiting at any time of year, but the greatest wildlife activity occurs in the spring and fall. More than 200 animal species have been recorded at the refuge, so I suggest you take along field glasses and a bird book (or an expert birder)—plus the refuge's own bird checklist (available at the contact station). A wildflower book (or an expert friend) also can be seasonally helpful.

My standard advice about staying on the trail and not bushwhacking holds very true for the North Tract, but not for the customary reasons (poison ivy, plant destruction, trail erosion). In this case, the reason is UXO. The North Tract was incorporated into the refuge only in the early 1990s. Previously, as part of Fort George G. Meade, it had been used as a military training facility. UXO stands for "unexploded ordnance," and I also surmise that tank maneuvers and exploded ordnance may help account for the scarcity of mature trees.

To get started on the hike, step out the contact station's front door, swing left, and follow Bald Eagle Drive to a nearby stop sign. There, turn right and continue along the paved road for 140 yards to the point where it curves left and an unpaved road goes straight ahead. Go around the vehicle barrier and get going on the unpaved road. You'll be on the Green Trail, which ascends very gently through scrubby and mostly deciduous woodlands. On arriving at a T-junction after 0.7 miles, go straight, access the Blue Trail (the Green Trail continues to the left), and follow it for 0.5 miles to a fork. There, turn right and slightly uphill onto the Red Trail and stay red for 350 yards to the next T-junction, where you'll make another trail-color switch—this time to yellow.

Follow the Yellow Trail for 1.9 miles as it swings (as though following three sides of a rectangle counterclockwise) and gently undulates through mostly young woodlands. En route, soon after making that trail's first 90-degree left turn, pause to walk through a small, old, tree-shaded, and fenced cemetery on the right. Recorded as the Biggs (Anderson)–Waters Cemetery, it is one of seven family graveyards dotted around what is now the North Tract, and it serves as one of the few visible and visitable reminders of the refuge's pre-1930s history. You'll find burial dates there ranging from 1771 to 1968 (just be sure not to disturb the area in any manner).

Continuing beyond the cemetery, you'll make another sharp left turn and eventually arrive at another T-junction. There you should turn right to leave the Yellow Trail and access another stretch of the Red Trail. Continue for 0.6 miles to the next T-junction, and turn left there to stay on the Red Trail (that turn will be obvious because the third trail is closed). After a final 0.7 red miles and almost at the hike's 5-mile mark, reach a four-way and three-color intersection. Turn right there to begin a 3-mile out-and-back excursion on the Orange Trail, which curves and very gently undulates westward through open woods to terminate at Blue Heron Pond.

Set within an expanse of meadowland that's yours for the visual scanning and admiring, but not for the walking (remember "UXO"), the pond is often a great place to see ducks and other waterfowl (although I've yet to see a heron there). And if you have the time and interest, make use of the bird blind perched next to the pond. Then, when you're ready, take the Orange Trail back to the four-way intersection. There, turn right onto the gently rolling southern leg of the Blue Trail (the northern leg goes straight ahead), and keep going for 1.6 miles.

On reaching a fork, go straight ahead so that you'll be on the southern part of the Green Trail. Then follow the green for 350 yards until you reach a paved road (the Wildlife Loop). There, turn left and north to follow the road for 1.3 miles through open countryside back to the contact station, taking care to watch for occasional passing motor vehicles. On the way, pause at Merganser Pond on the right side of the road. In my experience, mergansers and other ducks seem to favor this pond, and a variety of common land birds often flit along the shoreline and catch not only the observant human eye but also the occasional hawk eye. On returning to the contact station, detour to check out the bird-feeding area and butterfly garden just across the road.

To shorten this 11-mile hike to 9.6 miles, stay on the Red Trail and skip doing any of the Yellow Trail, and to further shorten it to 6.6 miles, omit the Orange Trail altogether.

NEARBY/RELATED ACTIVITIES

After the hike, explore the other accessible parts of the North Tract. Use the Little Patuxent River Trail, a dirt trail that starts on the north side of the contact station parking lot, to hike for 1.5 miles out and back on a floodplain riverbank that's well decorated with birds and wildflowers in the spring. Hike around the ponds at New Marsh, which is 5 to 6 miles by car down the Wildlife Loop from the contact station. Hike around 13-acre Lake Allen, which is 2 miles the other way on the loop road—and pause to sample the short and sandy Pine Trail and visit St. Peters P. E. Church Cemetery.

I recommend that, after leaving the North Tract, you tour the huge and exhibit-rich National Wildlife Visitor Center (open daily, 10 a.m. to 5:30 p.m., except on Thanksgiving Day, December 25, and New Year's Day). It's about

11 miles away, in the refuge's South Tract. To get there, return to the parkway; go south for 5.1 miles, and then turn left to take the Powder Mill Road exit heading east; follow that road for 1.9 miles, turn right onto the entrance road (the Scarlet Tanager Loop), and proceed for 1.5 miles to the center's parking lot.

After you're through at the center, step outside to sample the adjoining and signposted woodland and meadowland trails (you can pick up a sketch map at the center). But note before starting that part of the lovely trail around 53-acre Cash Lake is closed during the winter and spring to protect wintering and nesting waterfowl.

Consider returning to participate in some of the refuge's public programs, which include bird walks and occasional evening hikes, including an "Owl Prowl."

COSCA REGIONAL PARK 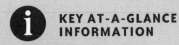 21

IN BRIEF

For hikers, multiuse Cosca Regional Park serves as a delightful, trail-laced nature preserve tucked away in suburban Maryland just southeast of Washington.

DESCRIPTION

Cosca Regional Park, one of only two hiking venue's in this book named for women (see Hike 18 for the other), is a small gem of a little-known nature preserve that lies near Clinton, in suburban southern Prince George's County. When opened in 1967, it was called Clinton Regional Park and was surrounded by farmlands. It was later renamed Louise F. Cosca Regional Park in memory of a member of the Maryland–National Capital Park and Planning Commission who had played a key role in its creation. Today, although some farms remain, houses abound along the park's perimeter, and the park is best known for its playing fields, man-made lake, nature center, and other amenities. Nevertheless, the park's 700 acres are maintained mostly as a nature preserve of woodlands where savvy hikers can enjoy nature, exercise, and solitude year-round.

Directions ——————————————➤

From Capital Beltway (Interstate 495 and I-95) in Maryland, take Exit 7 and drive south on Branch Avenue (MD 5), heading toward Waldorf. After about 3.5 miles, turn right onto 0.4-mile exit ramp leading to Woodyard Road (MD 223). Turn right onto Woodyard south. Stay to right and go 0.8 miles, and turn left onto Brandywine Road. Go 0.9 miles and turn right onto Thrift Road. Go 2 miles and turn right at "Clearwater Nature Center" sign. Follow park entrance road for 0.2 miles to parking lot nearest nature center.

KEY AT-A-GLANCE INFORMATION

LENGTH: 5.5 miles

CONFIGURATION: Modified loop

DIFFICULTY: Easy

SCENERY: Rolling woodlands, lake views, stream valleys

EXPOSURE: Mostly shady; less so in winter

TRAFFIC: Usually light–very light; heavier close to nature center, lake, picnic areas, and on warm-weather weekends, holidays

TRAIL SURFACE: Mostly dirt; some pavement, grass

HIKING TIME: 2.5–3 hours

SEASON: Year-round

ACCESS: Open daily, 7:30 a.m.–dusk

MAPS: USGS Piscataway

FACILITIES: Toilets, water inside nature center; warm-season-only toilets, snack bar at boathouse; warm-season-only toilets at pavilion and off-trail at camping area; water at picnic area

FOR MORE INFORMATION: Contact park, (301) 868-1397, or nature center, (301) 297-4575

SPECIAL COMMENTS: Remember that park's entrance gates close at dusk

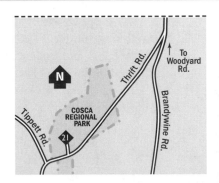

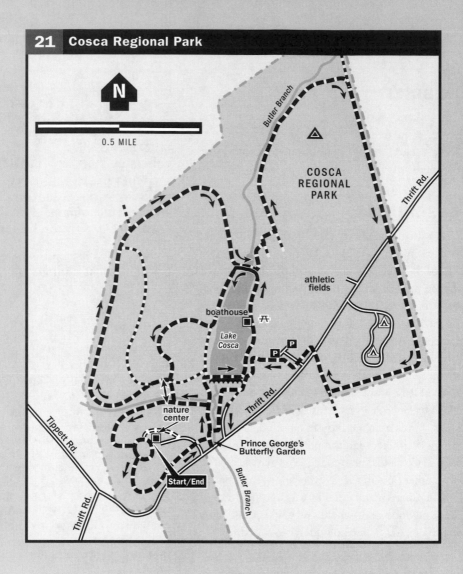

21   Cosca Regional Park

This hike consists of an easy 5.5-mile loop that uses most of the park's trails and has only 700 feet of elevation change. The woods are deciduous, with a scattering of pines and hollies. Wildflowers dapple the woods with color over three seasons. Migratory songbirds do the same in spring. Butterflies follow suit in a special garden in summer. Oaks, hickories, beeches, maples, tulip trees, and gums add to the park's palette in the fall. Deer and squirrels are the most frequently seen four-footed creatures, but others are also present, as beaver-chewed trees attest.

The trails are well maintained, but not well marked or signposted. So be alert, stay on the trail and out of the poison ivy, and follow my directions carefully

Cosca's woodlands form a trail-laced nature preserve where hikers are surprised by fearless residents.

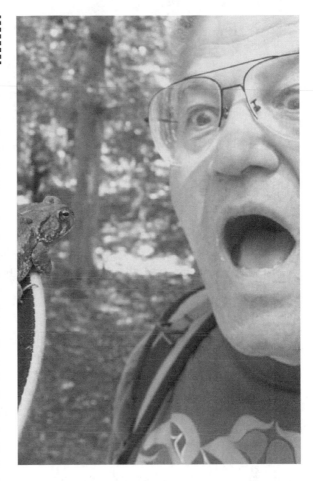

because the route has many turns. For most of the way, you'll see only a few direct signs of encroaching suburbia—mostly a few perimeter houses, plus some ominous signs of streambank erosion. You're likely to encounter other visitors (mostly neighborhood folks) only in the vicinity of the nature center, lake, and picnic areas.

To get started from the parking-lot trailhead, head uphill on a service road that goes past the nature center. At a circular paved path, go either way around until you see a lopped-off beech tree. There, turn onto a red-blazed dirt trail. Follow this trail downhill through the woods, staying to the right at the first T-junction, to reach and cross a paved road (the entrance road). On the far side, pass a large inanimate turtle and a "butterfly garden" sign and proceed along the dirt trail. At a streambank junction, turn right and proceed to Prince George's Butterfly Garden. With its labeled wildflowers and domesticated plants, the oak-rimmed garden is charmingly colorful in spring—and doubly so in summer, when butterflies abound. Then return to the streambank junction.

From there, walk alongside the stream and stay on the trail as it crosses an intersection next to a footbridge and turns sharply left to follow a tributary. At the next intersection, turn right, cross the culverted tributary, and proceed to what I call the "Five Trails intersection." There, take the green-blazed farthest left-hand trail, which goes uphill past several graffiti-ridden beeches. At the first fork, turn left and head downhill. The trail levels off near the tributary stream, on the left. It then climbs and curls to the right, passing a large clump of bamboo on the left. As the main trail levels off again, ignore a side trail on the right and then another on the left. Proceed past an orange trail marker and continue on a mostly level trail close to the edge of the woods.

Then the trail angles downhill and curves to the right. When you reach a faint fork, take the main trail to the right, which leads to a T-junction at the north end of man-made Lake Cosca. There, turn left and follow the trail across two bridges, pausing to take in the view. If you're there on a warm-season weekend or holiday, you'll probably see boaters and other visitors, as well as mostly domesticated geese and ducks.

Continuing, turn left at the next T-junction to start the hike route's most scenic portion, a half-mile-plus section mostly along Butler Branch, the lake's chief feeder. Follow the stream out from under the trees and across a power-line right-of-way, and then turn right and then left, cross a tiny stream, and turn right at the next T-junction to re-enter the woods. Twenty yards farther on, at a T-junction marked by a defaced beech, turn left onto a trail that goes uphill and then levels off to become a winding trail that stays mostly close to Butler Branch. Stay left at a T-junction marked by a short and signless signpost.

As you proceed, you'll find that the trail swings right, leaving the stream, proceeds uphill, and then crosses a mini-plateau to reach another T-junction. There, turn right onto a broad and undulating dirt trail—a utility right-of-way dotted with orange markers. Follow the markers for more than a mile along the park's eastern boundary. En route, cross another trail and also Thrift Road (the hike's 2.75-mile and halfway point). At a fence, abandon the markers, turn sharply right along the park's southern boundary and a line of backyards, and head downhill. After passing a camping area on the right and crossing another trail, you'll reach another part of the power-line right-of-way. Out in the open, cross to the far side to reach a T-junction. There, turn right onto a broad dirt-and-grass road and head uphill, staying to the left at a fork.

On reaching a paved road (Thrift Road again), turn left and walk along the shoulder for about 90 yards, then cross carefully and head down a paved entrance road. At the bottom, turn left and walk along the road to the second parking lot. Then turn right and walk toward the red-and-white sign at the lot's far end. There, enter the woods again on a paved path. Immediately take the next left-hand fork, which goes uphill and then curves right and swings gently downhill through the picnic areas. At the end of the pavement, turn left. Then turn right to take some steps down to a T-junction close to the dam. At the bottom, turn left to get onto a paved lakeside path, and follow it straight downhill. As it levels off, pass a group pavilion on the left and then turn sharply right onto a grassy trail leading to the looming dam.

Then turn left and uphill to angle up the dam's grassy slope to reach its west end. En route, you'll see below you a stream emerging from the dam—it's Butler Branch, reborn as the lake's outlet. At the top, turn right onto a gravel path and walk to the dam's far (east) side. There, at the T-junction you passed through earlier, turn left onto the lakeside paved path and continue northward along the east bank of the lake—and past the steps you came down. Continuing, you'll pass the boathouse and then circle around the lake's north end and then head south on the dirt trail along its west bank.

After passing one side trail, watch for another one just after a green bench directly across the lake from the boathouse. Take that second trail and head uphill and into the woods. At the top of the hill, swing right at the fork and descend steeply to the Five Trails intersection. Then cross the culverted tributary again, and turn right to follow the red-blazed trail uphill to the circular paved path near the nature center, and from there return to the trailhead.

NEARBY/RELATED ACTIVITIES

Explore the nature center, officially the Clearwater Nature Center, which houses exhibits, helpful staffers (ask them about the center's year-round programs and events), and various living creatures, including Tumbleweed, a black-tailed prairie dog. Outside, visit the herb garden and the caged hawks, owls, and eagle guarding it (they're maimed birds that couldn't survive in the wild).

Contact the park to learn more about the county's plans—announced in mid-2006—to add 10 miles of trails to Cosca's currently modest trail network.

22 HENSON CREEK TRAIL

KEY AT-A-GLANCE INFORMATION

LENGTH: 11 miles (with shorter options)

CONFIGURATION: Basically out-and-back

DIFFICULTY: Moderate

SCENERY: Mostly woodlands, burbling creek, suburban parkland

EXPOSURE: Mostly shady; less so in winter

TRAFFIC: Very light–light; usually much heavier in Tucker Road Park

TRAIL SURFACE: Pavement, with dirt on short side trail

HIKING TIME: 4.5–5.5 hours

SEASON: Year-round

ACCESS: No restrictions

MAPS: USGS Alexandria, Anacostia; ADC Prince George's County

FACILITIES: None at trailhead; toilets, water, phones at Tucker Road Park, Tucker Road Community Center

FOR MORE INFORMATION: Contact Prince George's County Department of Parks and Recreation, (301) 699-2407 or www.pgparks.com

SPECIAL COMMENTS: Complete the hike before dark

IN BRIEF

Lying just southeast of Washington, the little-used Henson Creek Trail gives hikers a delightful chance to walk through a tree-lined stream valley containing a string of small parks and flanked by a few kempt residential neighborhoods and many still-open areas.

DESCRIPTION

The mostly parkland-encased Henson Creek Trail ranks as one of the treasures of southern and suburban Prince George's County. It's a paved and easy-to-follow path that parallels a small Potomac River tributary for almost 6 miles in a developing area just south of the beltway. The county plans to eventually extend the trail at both ends as part of the Matthew Henson Greenway, named for a famous Arctic explorer and Maryland native.

This hike consists of an out-and-back 11-mile excursion that uses almost all of the existing trail. The out part includes a couple of minor detours, including a hill climb of less than 100 vertical feet that provides the hike's

----

Directions

From Capital Beltway (Interstate 495 and I-95) in Oxon Hill, Maryland, take Exit 4B and drive along 0.2-mile exit ramp to get onto MD 414 (St. Barnabas Road) heading roughly east. Proceed for 1.5 miles and turn right onto Hagan Road. Proceed for 0.5 miles and swing right at yield sign to get onto Temple Hill Road. Continue for 0.2 miles and then turn sharp left at traffic light to stay on Temple Hill Road. Stay on it for 0.8 miles to reach Henson Creek Neighborhood Park on right (just beyond "Henson Creek Trail" roadside sign). Park in parking lot near playground.

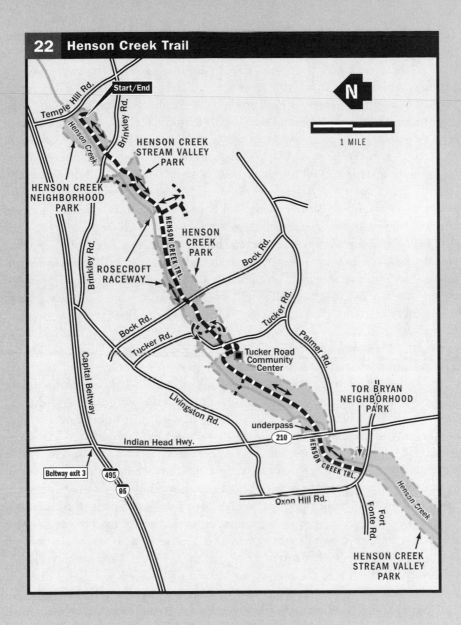

only vista and only exception to its universal flatness. Although you'll be on a designated multiuse trail, it's unlikely you'll encounter more than a few people, mostly strolling or biking locals. But you will pass some mushroom-shaped trailside signposts of a design that's ubiquitous in the Netherlands (if you're puzzled, visit **ohbike.org/facilities/anwb**). Use the signposts to gauge distances when shortening the hike to suit yourself. Use caution when crossing three major roads. And use your senses to enjoy the trail's flora and fauna and tranquility (away from those roads).

To get started, take the nearby paved path leading away from the trailhead parking lot and follow it for 100 yards across a level grassy field to a T-junction marked by signpost number 106. Turn left there onto the grass-bordered paved path that parallels canalized and tree-lined Henson Creek on the right. After a little more than half a mile, you'll pass signpost number 105 and then reach Brinkley Road. Cross carefully, and keep going through an open area flanked on the left by a low marshy area with a tangle of shrubs and trees. Beyond the open area, the path continues through the open woods and along the creek, where you'll see recurrent signs of both bank erosion and bank restoration. On reaching a trail junction (almost 1 mile into the hike), go straight to stay on the main trail.

Half a mile later, after crossing a little bridge and passing a yellow gas-pipeline pole on the left, watch for a cluster of cattails and a faint dirt trail, also on the left. There, leave the main trail and hike uphill on a 0.3-mile round-trip detour. Ascending on what is actually a gas-pipeline right-of-way, you'll reach a broad grassy ridge lined with town houses. There, leave the trail, and walk out along the ridge for about 80 yards. Pause to take in the view, which includes a church tower in Oxon Hill and also part of nearby Rosecroft Raceway, a harness racing facility. Then return to the main trail, turn left, and continue following the creek, passing close to the racetrack.

Soon after crossing a small bridge, you'll reach Bock Road (at the hike's 2.75-mile mark). Cross it carefully, follow the road downhill for 10 yards, and turn left onto a service road. Go about 40 yards and turn right at trail marker number 104 to get onto the trail proper. Over the next few hundred yards, the paved path wiggles through the woods and becomes part of a service road before entering landscaped Tucker Road Park. Just before reaching a small lake, swing right to get onto a paved fitness trail that curves around the lake. On reaching some tennis courts, turn right onto a side path that goes just to the right of a football field. Continue past a playground, cross the service road to continue on the fitness trail, and swing right at the next intersection to stay on that trail, which mostly parallels a large parking lot and then joins it. Turn left to walk 200 yards through the rest of the parking lot and out to Tucker Road. Cross the road carefully (3.25 miles into the hike) to get onto a narrow sidewalklike path.

Turn left on that path and walk along Tucker Road for 200 yards, and turn right onto Ferguson Lane, next to a "Tucker Road Community Center" sign. Go about 150 yards and turn right, at signpost number 102, onto a paved path near some tennis courts, and swing past the community center. Reaching a small traffic circle on the left, stay to the right, walk through a small parking area, and continue on the paved path. At the next T-junction, turn sharp left and continue. After passing a side trail and then some picnic tables on the right, you'll cross Henson Creek by dry footbridge (at the hike's 4.9-mile mark), and have the creek on your left. About 200 yards later, you'll get across heavily traveled Indian Head Highway by using the hike's only underpass.

Back in the woods, stay on the path as it passes some backyards and reaches Tor Bryan Neighborhood Playground at signpost number 101. That's the hike's 5.7-mile mark and turnaround spot, where there are also picnic tables, a covered shelter, and playground temptations. On the return trip along the trail, skip the fitness trail in Tucker Road Park and also the pipeline detour so you'll have to do only 5.3 miles.

NEARBY/RELATED ACTIVITIES

After the hike, head for almost-nearby Oxon Hill Farm, a 512-acre riverfront working farm run by the National Park Service. For information and directions, call (301) 839-1176 or visit **www.nps.gov/nace/oxhi.**

23 GREENWAY TRAIL:
Black Rock Mill to Long Draught Branch

KEY AT-A-GLANCE INFORMATION

LENGTH: 8.8 miles

CONFIGURATION: Out-and-back

DIFFICULTY: Easy–moderate

SCENERY: Stream valley, woodlands, rural views

EXPOSURE: About 50% shady; less so in winter

TRAFFIC: Usually very light, even on warm-weather weekends, holidays

TRAIL SURFACE: Hard-packed dirt; rooty in places

HIKING TIME: 4–5 hours

SEASON: Year-round, but best from fall through spring

ACCESS: Open daily, 8 a.m.–sunset (but closed Thanksgiving Day, December 25)

MAPS: USGS Germantown, Gaithersburg, Seneca; sketch map in free park pamphlet

FACILITIES: None

FOR MORE INFORMATION: Visit trail volunteers' Web site, www.seneca trail.org; contact Seneca Creek State Park, (301) 924-2127

SPECIAL COMMENTS: Beware of flooding (see text); consider becoming a trail volunteer

IN BRIEF

The unspoiled and little-used Greenway Trail in Seneca Creek State Park is one of the metro area's best close-in trails.

DESCRIPTION

Running the length of Seneca Creek State Park and beyond in west-central Montgomery County, the 25-mile-long Greenway Trail is one of the finest close-in hiking trails I know. It follows the creek from the Damascus area, where it connects with the Lower Magruder Trail (see Hike 38, page 186), down to the Potomac River at Rileys Rock (Seneca), where it meets the C&O Canal towpath. Officially called the Seneca Creek Greenway Trail, it was constructed over a decade-plus and mostly by a band of resolute volunteers, who still plan to link the Damascus end with Patuxent River State Park.

This out-and-back hike of 8.8 miles, with a modest 800 feet of elevation change, uses a section of the trail located about 20 miles northwest of Washington. It's a very scenic section, which mostly lies close to Great Seneca Creek, one of Seneca Creek's chief

----

Directions

From junction of Capital Beltway (Interstate 495) and I-270 in Maryland, proceed northwest for about 6 miles (toward Frederick). Get off at Exit 6B and proceed generally west on MD 28 (which becomes Darnestown Road in part). About 6.4 miles along MD 28 and 1 mile past Germantown Road (MD 118), turn right onto Black Rock Road. Proceed on narrow and twisty road for 0.7 miles. Turn left into small parking lot at Black Rock Mill. If lot is full, cross bridge and park on shoulder on right.

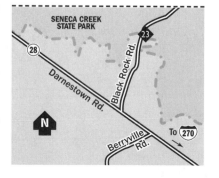

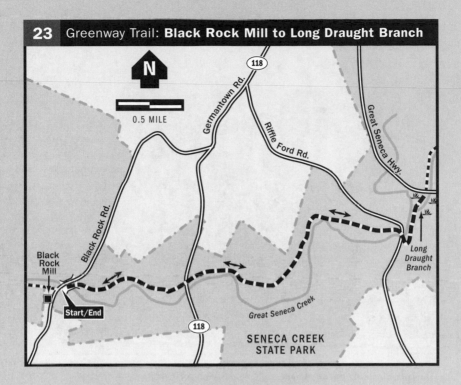

23 Greenway Trail: **Black Rock Mill to Long Draught Branch**

headwaters. You'll be in a serene and mostly pastoral landscape of wildflower-dappled floodplain areas, thickets, and wooded hills flanked by farmlands—although the town houses are creeping closer. You'll also be on one of the metro area's very few stream-valley trails that does not have a redolent companion sewer pipe. Deer, smaller four-footed creatures, birds, wildflowers, and trees are plentiful. But humans are not, maybe because the trail seems to remain little known. Check with the park on trail conditions beforehand, because the creek sometimes floods. Be aware that, although the trail is quite well blazed and sign-posted, some of the posted distances are inaccurate.

Before getting started, take a look at Black Rock Mill, now a roofless shell with thick fieldstone walls and glassless windows. Use the second-story walkway to peer into the interior. Read the chain-suspended display boards outlining the mill's century of operations starting in 1815, as well as the effects of flooding. Note the marked flood levels, some of them above your head. The hulking mill is a spooky sight at dusk. Rising tall and black against the western sky and topped by gallowslike rafters, it seems dark and satanic, in contrast with the green and pleasant land around it. Some scenes for the 1999 movie *The Blair Witch Project* were shot nearby.

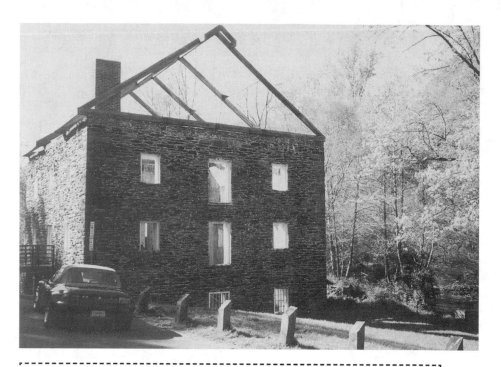

Starting in 1815, Black Rock Mill served for a century as a grist mill, sawmill, and local meeting place—until ruined by floods.

To get started from the mill, cross the creek bridge, bear right, and walk along the road for 50 yards. Pass a "Seneca Creek Greenway Trail" sign, and march between a pair of bluish-green blazes to head upstream and generally eastward on a floodplain where the oak and hickory woods are brightened by dogwood and red-bud blossoms—and warblers—in the spring. Half a mile into the hike, you'll leave the creek temporarily to negotiate some easy switchbacks. But then you'll be on the level for another half mile before turning right to descend alongside a stream gully. Following the bluish-green blazes, turn left to cross the gully by bridge and then head uphill through some pines. The trail then levels off and eases downhill through a large hemlock grove and out onto the open floodplain.

Then you'll reach busy Germantown Road, 1.6 miles into the hike. Cross carefully and proceed on a broad, flat, and more open floodplain area, heading mostly northeast along the edge of the woods. The trail stays quite close to the creek, except in the few places where it takes a shortcut across or around a low hill or ridge. It's flanked by woods on the right and by fields on the left. As you hike, listen for chattering kingfishers along the creek and the staccato calls of woodpeckers in the woods, and watch for beaver-felled trees. In muddy places, where deer tracks are common, look for the difference between males and females (female prints are more pointed).

At Riffle Ford Road, 4 miles into the hike, cross carefully. Then turn right to take the bridge over the creek, and turn left onto a broad and level dirt path.

It doubles as a stretch of both the Greenway Trail and Long Draught Trail, so you'll see both yellow and bluish-green blazes. Follow the path to an open wetland straddling Long Draught Branch near its mouth on Great Seneca Creek. There, at the hike's 4.4-mile mark, pause at a low observation deck to look around and listen. Watch in particular for waterbirds. In warm weather, also look for bluebirds, which make good use of the wetland's nesting boxes and insect population, and see if you see any evidence that bluebirds carry the sky on their backs. Then scurry back to Black Rock Mill before dark.

NEARBY/RELATED ACTIVITIES

Explore or sample other sections of the Greenway Trail. I recommend the Clopper Lake section, about 1.1 miles farther up the trail from this hike's turnaround spot (alternatively, contact the park for driving directions).

24 WATKINS REGIONAL PARK

KEY AT-A-GLANCE INFORMATION

LENGTH: 6 miles (with shorter options)

CONFIGURATION: Double loop

DIFFICULTY: Easy

SCENERY: Woodlands, wetlands, crop fields, old farm buildings

EXPOSURE: More than half shady; less so in winter

TRAFFIC: Light–moderate on Spice-bush Trail and in Largo-Lottsford Junction area, heavier on warm-weather weekends, holidays; generally light elsewhere

TRAIL SURFACE: Mostly dirt or grass; stretches of pavement on Spicebush Trail and in Largo-Lottsford Junction area; Wetland Trail muddy in places

HIKING TIME: 3–4 hours

SEASON: Year-round

ACCESS: Open daily, dawn–dusk

MAPS: USGS Upper Marlboro; sketch maps on display board near trailhead and in free park brochures

FACILITIES: Toilets, water, phone at nature center (open daily 8:30 a.m.–5 p.m. Monday–Saturday, 11 a.m.–4 p.m. Sunday and holidays), near picnic area, and in Largo-Lottsford Junction area

FOR MORE INFORMATION: See under Description

IN BRIEF

Watkins Regional Park, located in suburban Maryland just east of Washington, is best known for its bountiful recreational facilities. But most of the park consists of a gently rolling landscape of trail-laced and hiker-friendly woodlands, wetlands, and open farmlands.

DESCRIPTION

Although the remaining farmlands in the Largo section of central Prince George's County continue to give way to new houses and manicured yards, there are still some local areas where plants and wildlife predominate. One of them is Watkins Regional Park, opened in 1964 and named for Roger M. Watkins, a long-time park planner and advocate. It's little known as a hiking venue, but is worth exploring, especially in the cooler months.

The park's popular northern portion includes ball fields and other standard recreational facilities, plus a miniature railroad, a restored antique carousel, a small and specialized farm, and one of the metro area's

----

Directions

From Capital Beltway (Interstate 495) in Largo, Maryland, take Exit 15B to get onto Central Avenue (MD 214) heading east. Once on Central Avenue, proceed for 2.8 miles and then turn right onto Watkins Park Drive (MD 193). Proceed on drive for 0.8 miles, and then turn right into Watkins Regional Park. Continue through park for 1 mile as follows: Turn right at first T-junction; then turn left to get onto park's main road; pass through area signposted Largo-Lottsford Junction; turn left at T-junction and sign for nature center; proceed for about 0.1 mile to parking lot. Walk downhill on paved footpath for 90 yards to nature center.

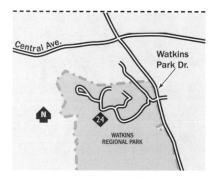

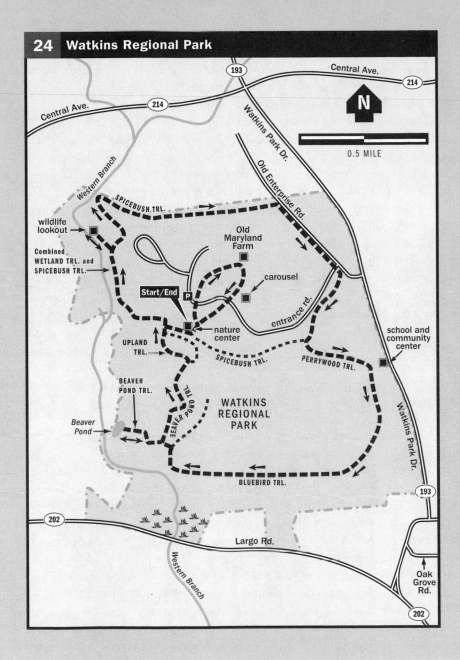

24 Watkins Regional Park

most attractive nature centers (see Related/Nearby Activities). The park's little-used-by-humans central and southern portions are mostly covered by deciduous woodlands dominated by oaks and hickories, with a scattering of such trees as tulip trees, dogwoods, beeches, and gums. There's also a sturdy understory of spicebush and other bushes, brambles, and seasonal wildflowers. But there are also extensive fields of soybeans and other crops, grown under lease by local farmers and serving as a tangible reminder of the area's rural heritage. Together, the woodlands and fields provide a diverse habitat for deer, birds, beavers, and other wildlife, and a scenic landscape for visiting hikers.

The park's trails are mostly named, signposted, and color coded. With Mike Darzi's help, I have devised a short and easy hike that consists of two clockwise loops—a 5-miler followed by a 1-miler—that together have trifling elevation change (less than 300 feet of up and down combined). To shorten the hike by a little or a lot, do only one of the two loops. A further option is to skip most of the Spicebush Trail and go directly east from the nature center to get onto the Perrywood Trail (see map) and follow the rest of my directions—for a 4-mile hike (including the second loop). Keep in mind that the trails in the southern part of the park tend to get overgrown in the warm season, so consider using bug repellent or wearing long pants, watch for poison ivy, and do a posthike tick check.

To get started on the hike, tear yourself away from the nature center and walk off the deck to the rear. Cross the small bridge spanning a turtle pond to get to a four-way intersection. There, ignore the confusing signs and turn right onto a woodland trail that goes slightly downhill and levels off. After crossing a small bridge, bear left at a fork onto a trail that's blazed blue and yellow. At the next T-junction, turn right and follow the blue and yellow blazes uphill for about 20 yards to a signposted T-junction. There, turn left to stay on the blue- and yellow-blazed trail (it's the combined Spicebush Trail and Wetland Trail).

On reaching a signposted Y-junction, detour by going straight for 50 yards to a wildlife lookout in a marshy area on the Western Branch floodplain. See and hear whatever birds are present. Then retrace your steps to the Y-junction and swing left to continue on the blue- and yellow-blazed trail. At the next T-junction, turn left to leave the Wetland Trail (yellow blazes) and continue on the Spicebush Trail (blue blazes) as it undulates through the woods. Where and when the trail reaches a parking lot for a picnic area, turn left and follow the edge of the lot until you reach, on your left, a rusty bridge leading to group pavilion number 3. Cross the bridge and, about 50 yards before reaching the pavilion, turn left onto the blue-blazed Spicebush Trail and once again undulate through the woods.

Continuing, cross a paved road to get onto a paved path that spans a power-line right-of-way and its down-the-center equestrian trail. At the path's end, turn right onto a narrow paved road—it's Old Enterprise Road—and proceed, watching for blue trail blazes and occasional passing vehicles. After you pass the park's entrance road (on the left) and a white-on-brown park sign (on the right), turn right at a signpost to slip back into the woods on a blue-blazed dirt trail (about 2 miles into the hike). Keep going, cross a paved side road leading to a campground, and turn right at a signposted T-junction to take a footbridge across a small stream.

At the next T-junction, turn left to leave the Spicebush Trail and get briefly onto the red-blazed Perrywood Trail and then onto the red-, white-, and blue-blazed

Bluebird Trail. The trail may be faint, so be prepared to bushwhack for less than 50 yards to get out of the woods and into an open and scrubby area of grasses and low bushes. Once there, head for a nearby red-, white-, and blue signpost, and walk past it, keeping a nearby fence to your left. Then swing to the right and cross an overgrown swale and swing left to get to the top of a low rise that curves to the left. There, peer ahead and walk toward the next trail signpost, keeping a large crop field to your right and noting more fields beyond that one. When you get to a point closest to the buildings on the left (a school and community center), swing slightly to the right and follow the edge of the field until you reach a grassy unpaved road.

Cross the road, swing right, note the reassuring three-colored trail sign nearby, and start walking along a farm road that will be your route westward for more than a mile as you cross crop fields and pass more trail signs and a series of bluebird nesting boxes. First, though, you'll go by several aging reminders of the area's prepark era—an ancient barn on the right and then a derelict house, a possibly occupied trailer, and an abandoned cottage on the left. And when you reach a vine-festooned old barn, follow the road as it jogs left and then right near bluebird nesting box number 6. Next, cross the power-line right-of-way again and stay on the farm road as it swings to the right along the field edge and toward some woods. On reaching a green trail sign on the left (3.9 miles into the hike), turn left and take a dirt trail—the green-blazed Overlook Trail—into the woods.

On reaching a fork, stay to the right and proceed along a trail that is initially level before it dips gently downhill (the left fork goes downhill from the start). When you get to a T-junction, turn left onto the Beaver Pond Trail (it should be blazed orange, but may still be colored green). Proceed to the pond, which lies on the Western Branch floodplain, and look for the beaver lodge and whatever birds are present. Then return to the T-junction, but turn left to stay on the Beaver Pond Trail. At the next and signpostless T-junction, turn left to get onto the green-blazed Upland Trail, which is modestly true to its name. After descending some steps, take the footbridge across a small stream to get to the same T-junction you passed through at the start of the hike. There, turn right and return to the nearby nature center.

Pause, and then do the hike's second loop. Go to the front of the nature center, swing right and walk past the butterfly and hummingbird garden to get onto the signposted and white-blazed White Trail. Follow the dirt trail through the woods (and across the park's main road) to Old Maryland Farm. Swing right to follow the farm's fence to the entrance, and then roam the enclosure for a close look at rare Hog Island sheep and other livestock. From there, take the paved path to Largo-Lottsford Junction (with its tempting carousel), cross the main road, and walk through the parking lot to bear right onto a paved path that leads gently downhill to the nature center.

To find out more about the park, visit the park's page on the Prince George's County Department of Parks and Recreation Web site, **www.pgparks.com/places/parks/watkins.html**; call the park at (301) 218-6700 (general-information line),

(301) 218-6702 (nature center), or (301) 218-6770 (Old Maryland Farm); and pick up the numerous free brochures available at the nature center.

RELATED/NEARBY ACTIVITIES

Linger at the nature center, which has live birds—both captive ones and permanently disabled birds of prey, other exhibits, an attractive outside deck (that serves as a fine lunch spot), lots of park information, and informative staffers. Ask about the center's nature-related programs, as well as about the park's summer-time concerts and other events. In summer, take a ride on the century-old Gustav Dentzel carousel, which is one of less than a dozen working carousels in the Washington-Baltimore area.

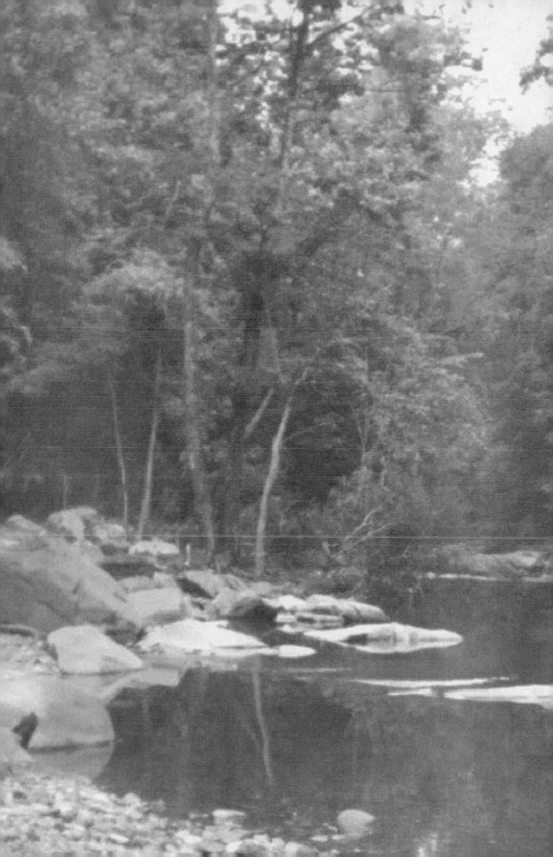

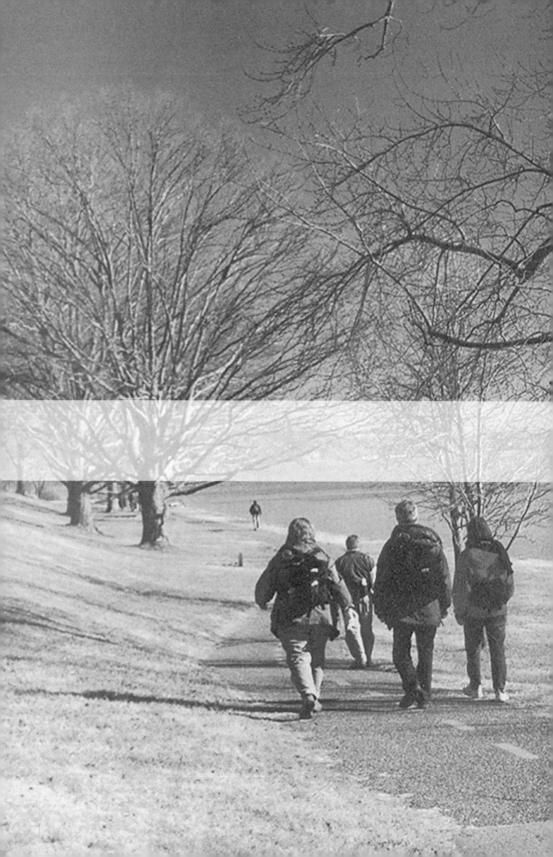

CLOSE-IN VIRGINIA SUBURBS

25 HOLMES RUN PARKLANDS

IN BRIEF

City-owned parklands along Holmes Run enable hikers to traverse built-up western Alexandria on a mostly off-street and tree-shaded route that's even somewhat scenic.

DESCRIPTION

On this easy-to-moderate, hill-less, 8.6-mile suburban hike you'll mostly follow the Holmes Run valley across Alexandria's non-touristy western section. Along the way, you'll encounter a string of small parks, a healthy marsh, both scenic and scruffy views, an oak older than the city, a baby waterfall, and a colorful off-trail spot—and but one significant street crossing. You'll start with a 4-mile circuit, followed by a 4.6-mile modified out-and-back. To shorten the hike, short-circuit the circuit or turn around sooner at the far end.

The hike route has no blazes and few useful signs, so follow these directions carefully. And before starting, check for flooding at a

- -

Directions ————————————————→

From Washington, cross Potomac River and head southwest on Shirley Memorial Highway (Interstate 395) for about 7 miles. Get off at Exit 3 in Alexandria, and drive east for about 1 mile on Duke Street. Then turn left onto North Pickett Street, go about 100 yards, and turn right onto driveway leading into parking lot of Charles E. Beatley Jr. Central Library (5005 Duke Street).

Alternatively, from King Street Metro station (Blue, Yellow lines), use either Metrobus system or local DASH bus system to get to library parking lot. Contact Metro, (202) 637-7000 or www.wmata.com, or DASH, (703) 370-3274 or www.dashbus.com.

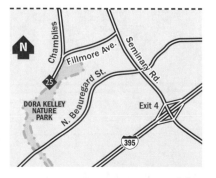

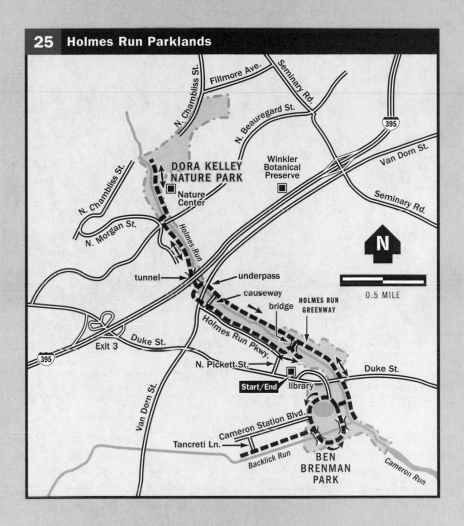

25 Holmes Run Parklands

critical spot: Return to North Pickett Street, turn right, and pick up and follow Holmes Run Parkway for 0.5 miles; just before Van Dorn Street, cross the parkway to scan the causeway below; if it's underwater, reschedule your hike.

To get started from the parking-lot trailhead, head for nearby Duke Street, turn left, and then take the first road on the left, which goes up and over Duke and into Ben Brenman Park. At the next intersection, across from a toilet-equipped building that's also a satellite police station, turn right onto Brenman Park Drive, using the walkway between the roadway and the fountain-equipped lake that's the 64-acre park's centerpiece. Then turn left on reaching Somerville Street, which marks the boundary between the open and landscaped park and the upscale condo-and-townhouse residential community called Cameron Station (for

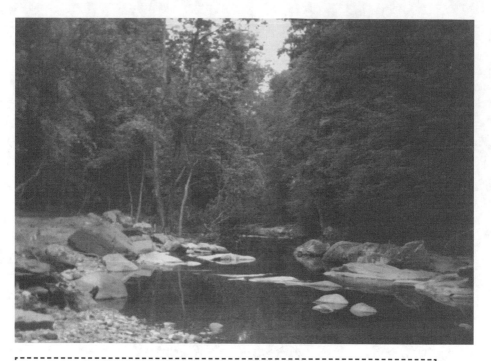

There are stretches upstream from North Beauregard Street, where Holmes Run could pass for a tranquil creek in the country.

its predecessor, an army base). Next, wind through the community by turning right onto Kilburn Street and then left onto Cameron Station Boulevard, the community's main thoroughfare.

Proceed for several blocks. Then turn left onto Tancreti Lane, walk one block, and then continue straight on a short walkway to reach a paved path that lies within a landscaped strip of land between channelized Backlick Run and a line of condos. Turn left and walk for 0.4 miles along what serves as a popular neighborhood mini-esplanade.

At the end of the path, at Somerville, turn right to cross the stream by footbridge to an untidy scrubland area bordered by railroad tracks. Turn left to traipse along the partly paved path paralleling the stream. Before swinging left to another footbridge, head for the nearby picnic pavilion on the right and then go a bit beyond it for views of the area and its waterways—and, in season, blackberry and wineberry bushes. Then return to cross the second footbridge and swing right to stay on the path as it curves around a ball field. Watch on the right for yet another footbridge, and take it across Holmes Run. Turn right, and proceed on a paved path, past a very modest waterfall, to that stream's junction with Backlick Run to form Cameron Run.

There, after pausing, turn around and head back along the path. Do not recross the footbridge on the left, but continue on the path. Follow it through an underpass beneath Duke Street and then bear left at the next trail junction to keep going on the Holmes Run Greenway. Pause to take note of a massive and healthy 300-year-old willow oak on the right. Then continue until you reach a concrete footbridge on the left, at the hike's 4-mile mark.

Cross the bridge and turn left into James Marx All Veterans Park. Follow the winding paved path to the end, continue on a short gravel path, and then descend the streambank to a lovely, off-the-beaten-trail spot. In summer, you'll find Virginia dayflowers and other plants in bloom there—and dragonflies, goldfinches, and chimney swifts in colorful aerial motion. Retrace your steps to the concrete footbridge, but don't cross. Instead, continue upstream on a mostly unpaved trail between the stream and Holmes Run Parkway. At the end of the trail, take the steps down to the causeway, turn left, eschew the causeway, and head upstream on a concrete waterside walkway that becomes an underpass beneath Van Dorn Street.

Continuing, you'll briefly be in a dank and dimly lit tunnel under Shirley Highway (I-395). Emerging, you'll be on a tree-lined paved path that leads through a garden-apartment area to North Beauregard Street at North Morgan Street. There, cross North Beauregard and walk uphill along North Morgan for about 200 yards. Then turn right onto a short path leading across Holmes Run and into heavily wooded Dora Kelley Nature Park. (*Note:* If the path is flooded, detour by going back to and up North Beauregard for a hundred yards and turning left onto the main path.) After crossing the stream, pause to take in the view upstream. Note both the smoothly worn rocks and the shoreline coating of sand and gravel that's evidence of Holmes Run's tendency to flood. Turn left at a nearby T-junction to get onto the park's main trail. Proceed upstream on the paved path. At the first side trail on the right, detour uphill to visit the renovated Jerome "Buddy" Ford Nature Center (usually open from 10 a.m to 5 p.m., Tuesday through Saturday). There, take a look at the park-related exhibits and ask for a free booklet keyed to the trail markers you'll find later in the hike.

Return to the main path and continue upstream. But pause to scan and listen to a small and picturesque marsh on the right that seems delightfully out of place in thickly populated suburbia. Its abundant plant forms include alders, willows, cattails, sedges, and grasses. It also has much wildlife, ranging from aquatic insects to frogs to turtles to waterbirds to muskrats.

At the path's end, at North Chambliss Street (the hike's 6.7-mile mark) in a residential area, turn around and go back. But diverge at the first intersection to turn left and go gently uphill, passing several numbered nature-trail markers. Just past marker number 17, turn right, descend some steps, and follow the dirt trail to see more of the marsh. Then turn left onto the main path and resume your return journey.

At the lower causeway, beyond the I-395 tunnel, cross the stream, ascend the short slope, and turn right to get onto the paved path that forms the spine of the manicured and mile-long stretch of parkland you will have encountered earlier (the Holmes Run Greenway). The hike's most heavily used trail segment, the greenway functions as a neighborhood park. When you reach the concrete bridge spanning Holmes Run, turn right to take it, and then keep going on North Pickett to get back to the trailhead.

NEARBY/RELATED ACTIVITIES

Visit the nearby and quite remarkable Winkler Botanical Preserve (see Hike 26, page 131). Consider adding it to this Holmes Run hike by detouring from the intersection of North Beauregard and North Morgan streets (see the map).

Tour the library, which is named for a former Alexandria mayor and was designed by Michael Graves, who also imaginatively sheathed the Washington Monument in blue fabric for its year of restoration. Bold and geometric outside and spacious inside, the library includes an unusual and lovely reading garden. See if you agree with me that the building ranks as one the metro area's best looking public libraries—and also that it's not nearly as central as its name claims.

WINKLER BOTANICAL PRESERVE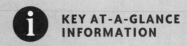

IN BRIEF

The Winkler Botanical Preserve is a private nature sanctuary hidden in western Alexandria. It's a lovely and unusual place to take a mini-hike both in the city and far from it.

DESCRIPTION

The Winkler Botanical Preserve is an extraordinary urban locale, especially for a first-time visitor. It's a tranquil place that seems to be part park and part wilderness, where the scenery changes every few yards (much as happens in Japanese formal gardens). Within its 44 acres lie gentle wooded hills, a full-sized mountain lodge, a small lake, a half-hidden pond, several little streams, a baby waterfall, a midget orchard, mini-meadows, a tiny covered bridge, a small-scale network of trails, and even a Hobbit House, along with the flourishing and full-scale flora that validate the preserve's name.

Directions ➤

From Washington, cross Potomac River and head southwest on Shirley Memorial Highway (Interstate 395) for about 5.4 miles. Get off at Exit 4 and turn right onto Seminary Road. Drive northwest for 0.2 miles and, at second traffic light, turn left onto North Beauregard Street. Proceed for 0.9 miles, counting off side streets on left, and then take fifth one, Roanoke Avenue. Follow it for 0.1 mile and drive through gated entrance into preserve's parking lot. If lot is full, park along avenue outside gates.

Or use local bus service and your feet to get to preserve—Metrobus and DASH operate along North Beauregard Street, and Roanoke Avenue has sidewalks. Contact Metro, (202) 637-7000 or www.wmata.com; or DASH, (703) 370-3274 or www.dashbus.com.

ℹ️ KEY AT-A-GLANCE INFORMATION

LENGTH: 1.9 miles

CONFIGURATION: Loop

DIFFICULTY: Very easy

SCENERY: Small-scale woodlands, meadows, lake, pond, streams

EXPOSURE: Shady; less so in winter

TRAFFIC: Very light to light; increases to moderate when school groups visit

TRAIL SURFACE: Mostly wood-chip mulch or mulch and dirt; some gravel, grass

HIKING TIME: 1–2 hours (including dawdling)

SEASON: Year-round, but best in warm-weather and leafy months; groups of up to 5 people can visit whenever preserve is open; larger groups are limited to weekdays and must call to make reservations

ACCESS: Open daily, 8:30 a.m.–5 p.m. (but closed on major holidays)

MAP: USGS Alexandria

FACILITIES: None

FOR MORE INFORMATION: Contact preserve, (703) 578-7888

SPECIAL COMMENTS: Remember that entrance gates close at 5 p.m.; stay on trails to avoid trampling vegetation; respect preserve's group requirements (see above); observe posted regulations

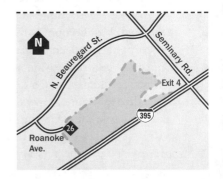

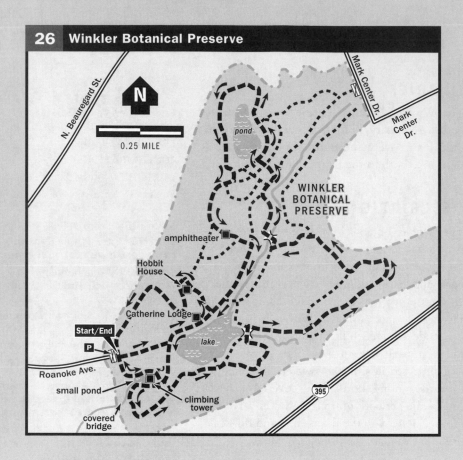

26 Winkler Botanical Preserve

It's astonishing to realize that, in the mid-1970s, the property was an overgrown and refuse-strewn tract of neglected land along Shirley Memorial Highway. Its transformation began later that decade, when the Mark Winkler family decided to create a private botanical preserve that would serve as both a sanctuary and a research and educational institution specializing in the trees and other plants native to the Potomac River valley.

It had to be built literally from below-ground up. The terrain itself was reshaped. Vast amounts of stone were trucked in to give the rock-poor tract some outcroppings and character. An integrated lake, pond, and stream system was created to control erosion and enhance the landscape. The Winklers decided that, as both a sanctuary and a research and educational institution, the preserve would specialize in plants native to the Potomac River valley. So, old trees were saved, alien plants removed, and a long-term effort was begun to plant hundreds of native species. Catherine Lodge (named for a Winkler) was built to serve as the preserve's headquarters and as a meeting place for nature-oriented classes and other programs aimed at both schoolchildren and families. Trails were added. The public was invited.

After close to three decades, the preserve is not yet finished, and may never be. But it's certainly an ecological triumph, and a reflection of what nature and conservation-minded humans can achieve in concert. And the numbers are encouraging. The preserve now has 70 species of trees and about 650 species of wildflowers and other plants. Its resident and transient wildlife population includes red foxes, small mammals and rodents, and red-shouldered hawks and lots of other birds. Because the wiggly hike route I have devised is only 1.9 miles long (making it this book's shortest excursion), I think you'll get the most out of it by practicing the great art of sauntering. It uses most of the preserve's trails, which, although well maintained, are neither signposted nor blazed. So here I focus on describing the hike route rather than on the details of what you will see. Nor are the plants labeled. So if you're botanically curious, take along some reference books. Do the same if you're also interested in birds, for they're not labeled either.

The preserve is at its best during the warm-weather months, when tree leaves hide the nearby looming buildings, and the frog and insect chorus masks some of the ambient traffic noise. At nearly all times, though, it's a wonderful place for introducing young children to both nature and hiking. But make sure that everyone stays on the trail—and that the family dog stays home.

To get started from the parking lot, step onto the preserve's gravel-surfaced main path, and follow it for about 200 yards to the lodge. Don't try to go in, but do try out the unusually comfortable wooden bench next to the path (I'm sure it's a sibling of two in the U.S. National Arboretum's Fern Valley). Also admire the traditional Adirondack chairs on the lodge's porch. Then continue along the path for 20 yards, and turn left to go through a wooden gateway and head uphill on a dirt trail. After passing a small rock pool, you'll reach a simple wooden structure that the preserve's staff calls the Hobbit House. I'm not very Tolkien on it, but pause to see for yourself.

Continuing uphill, turn left at a T-junction and then turn left again at a four-way intersection to follow the dirt trail downhill to a small stone bridge spanning a streamlet. Cross over and turn right at a fork to head uphill. You'll soon reach a dark brick wall that's 20-plus feet high. Follow the base of it along the preserve perimeter on a semi-overgrown dirt trail that winds through the wildest part of the preserve for almost 0.3 miles. Then stay on the trail as it eases downhill and away from the wall to reach the preserve's main path near the parking lot. Cross the path to get onto a grassy trail. Head downhill, cross a small gully, and then ascend on a mulch-covered trail to reach what looks like a Black Forest fire tower. The wooden tower is actually a climbing wall for young would-be mountaineers.

Then take a mulched trail down to a very small pond that's the source of a very small brook. Just before turning left to head uphill, pause to take a 20-foot detour on a covered bridge across the brook and back. It's the only covered

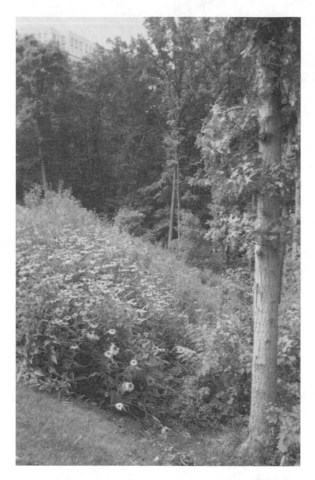

bridge I know of in Alexandria and this book.

Then clamber up the wooded slope, which makes up the steepest part of the entire hike, but, like all the other parts, also is short. At the top, turn left and proceed along a fairly level dirt trail. Where the trail forks, go right. At the next junction, turn left and walk about 15 yards to a mini-overlook above the two-acre lake. There, take in the mini-vista, including the far shore's Adirondack-style lodge. Also watch for birds. Prick up your ears, too, and listen for the sound of a waterfall. You will see the rock-girt pool from which the water leaves, but you won't see the fall or hear the pump.

Back on the main trail, turn left and follow a set of giant stone steps down to a stream. Cross on a rustic bridge, noting the tiered pools leading to the lake. On the far side, turn right and head gently uphill on a mulched wooded trail. Ignore a side trail on the left, swing left at the next fork, ignore two clearings on the left, and, at the top of the slope, turn sharply left. Continue on the next level, ignore another clearing on the left, and follow the trail downhill and through a four-way intersection (note the drywall stone bridge to the left). Near the bottom, turn right onto a dirt trail leading to a wooden bridge spanning a little stream. Keep going and then turn right onto the main gravel path.

Proceeding, walk across a small open area and pass an old apple orchard that was rescued from threatening bulldozers in the Leesburg area. Then continue gently uphill through the woods on the gravel path until you see a dirt side trail on the left marked by a small stone cube 12 feet up on the left. Ease gently uphill on that trail, and go straight through a four-way intersection to reach the end of the trail at a T-junction. There, just ahead, you'll see a lovely small pond dotted with lily pads and half-hidden by a border of trees, bushes, and cattails. In summer, it attracts butterflies and birds—and me. Turn left at that junction, and then go sharply left around a twin-trunked oak to continue counterclockwise on the dirt trail around the pond, albeit at a distance.

Swing right at the next T-junction. After that, turn right at each of the next two forks. Then go ten yards to turn sharply left at a T-junction, and head downhill. Go straight through the next two T-junctions, continuing downhill. Then bisect a woodland classroom—a small amphitheater with a stone stage and flattened-log benches. Continue down the trail to reach the main gravel path again. Turn right, and proceed to the lodge. Then swing left and cut across the grass to take a closer look at the lake.

Take in the view, including, at last, the waterfall. Then, turn right and walk along a grassy lakeshore trail. Swing left at a junction, and walk past a magnificent stand of staghorn sumac. Then head across the meadow to the tower. From there, return to the trailhead—and be sure to do so by 5 p.m.

As an option to doing the hike as I've described it, consider just wandering around freely, checking out the side trails and keeping reference books in hand and field glasses at the ready. But be sure to stay on the trails.

NEARBY/RELATED ACTIVITIES

Arrange to return to take a guided tour of the preserve. Also consider combining this short hike with my Holmes Run outing (Hike 25, page 126). You can easily tap into it by walking down North Beauregard Street to Morgan Street.

27 MOUNT VERNON TRAIL AND FORT HUNT PARK

KEY AT-A-GLANCE INFORMATION

LENGTH: 8.2 miles

CONFIGURATION: Modified out-and-back

DIFFICULTY: Easy–moderate

SCENERY: Parklands, woodlands, river views

EXPOSURE: Mostly open

TRAFFIC: Usually light; moderate–heavy on warm-weather evenings, weekends, holidays

TRAIL SURFACE: Pavement, dirt

HIKING TIME: 3.5–4.5 hours

SEASON: Year-round

ACCESS: Trail closes at dark; park open daily, 7 a.m.–sunset (when gates close)

MAPS: USGS Mount Vernon; ADC Northern Virginia; sketch map in free trail brochure

FACILITIES: Toilets, phones near trailhead, at Mount Vernon (cafeteria too); toilets, water, phones along trail

FOR MORE INFORMATION: Contact George Washington Memorial Parkway office, (703) 289-2500 or www.nps.gov/gwmp; Mount Vernon Estate and Gardens, (703) 780-2000 or www.mountvernon.org; River Farm (now headquarters of American Horticultural Society), (703) 768-5700 or www.ahs.org

IN BRIEF

Augmented by a turn through Fort Hunt Park, the Mount Vernon Trail in Fairfax County south of Alexandria provides hikers with a lovely parkland outing along the Potomac River.

DESCRIPTION

First, in the 19th century, George Washington's former Mount Vernon estate became a de facto national shrine. Then, in the 1930s, the federal government created the scenic George Washington Memorial Parkway to carry motor vehicles down to Mount Vernon from Key Bridge, across from his namesake city. Then, in 1973, it added the Mount Vernon Trail, a paved path in the parkway right-of-way for people who like to locomote by muscle power. Today, the 18-mile-long trail attracts hikers, bikers, runners, skaters, dog walkers, strollers, joggers, and runners. It's officially part of the Potomac Heritage National Scenic Trail (see Hike 29, page 143) and serves as the core segment of this hike.

This 8.2-mile, mostly out-and-back, level hike uses the trail's lowermost portion. That's where the southbound Potomac River turns west and the Virginia riverbank becomes a picturesque

----

Directions

From Capital Beltway (Interstate 495 and I-95) in Alexandria, Virginia, take Exit 177B to get on northbound US 1. At first traffic light, turn right onto Franklin Street, drive three blocks, and turn right onto South Washington Street, which becomes George Washington Memorial Parkway. At city's southern end, proceed on parkway for 5.6 miles, and take exit ramp to Fort Hunt Park. Enter park, turn right onto loop road at T-junction, and then take first left, into parking lot (about 7 miles from beltway).

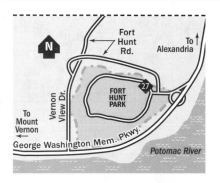

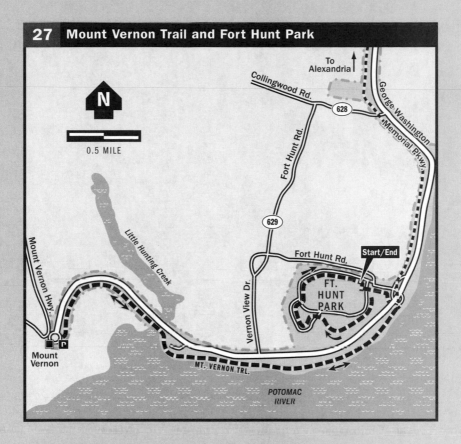

corridor of open parklands, woods, and across-the-water views. The hike also includes part of Fort Hunt Park. Located on former Washington-owned land, the fort existed from the 1890s to about 1920 to guard the river approach to the capital. It was converted into a park in the 1930s.

To get started from the trailhead parking lot, head back toward the park entrance. But at the T-junction, walk straight on the loop road, keeping to the right in the reserved-for-foot-traffic lane. Where the road curves right, swing left onto a dirt trail heading into the woods. Ignoring a side trail on the left, follow the main trail as it swings right and gently uphill. Where it levels off and becomes faint, keep bearing left along the edge of the woods until you're heading downhill on a well-defined trail. Continue across a small bridge. At the next junction, turn right onto an unpaved path that ascends gently to an abandoned paved road. Turn left and follow it to the end. There, turn left to walk clockwise around the loop road, staying to the right.

After passing the trailhead, turn left at the T-junction and head for the park entrance. En route, take an optional detour to look at an 1890s gun emplacement, on the right. Or visit another one, down a short trail just outside the entrance. In

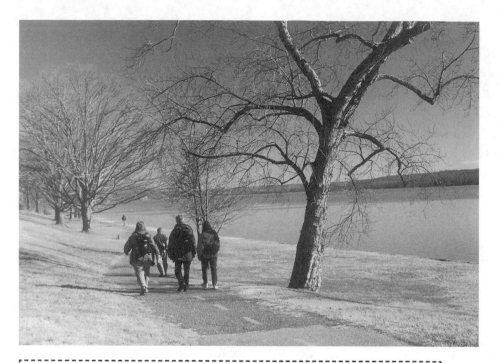

In winter, hikers on the Mount Vernon Trail often have the long stretch that hugs the river below Fort Hunt Park all to themselves.

both cases, there's no river view but much poison ivy. Outside the park, carefully head downhill and cross a traffic intersection to reach the Mount Vernon Trail at an information board. Turn right and follow the trail. Stay to the left where it joins a roadway to curve through an underpass (that's the parkway above). Then turn left to rejoin the trail at the hike's 2-mile mark. Just over half a mile later, pass milepost 2, one of the trailside markers that count down to Mount Vernon. Remember to keep to the right and safely away from other trail users.

Proceed on the riverbank trail and savor the views. Watch for geese and ducks on the water, ospreys on the hunt, and bald eagles on the wing. Pause to look for the resident eagles nicknamed George and Martha (the names stay the same but the birds occasionally get replaced by aggressors, as happened yet again in 2006). After Riverside, the trail leaves the shore and uses a long uphill slope to reach milepost 0 and the Mount Vernon parking lot. Traverse the lot, bear right, and head for the visitor center, 0.3 miles beyond milepost 0, at the hike's 4.8-mile mark. Then, when you're ready, walk back the 3.4 miles to the Fort Hunt trailhead.

NEARBY/RELATED ACTIVITIES

During the hike, visit Mount Vernon and River Farm (another estate of Washington's just up the parkway). In summer, attend a Sunday-evening concert at Fort Hunt. Finish hiking by 7 p.m., relax on the grass, and let the sounds of music creep in your ears.

HUNTLEY MEADOWS PARK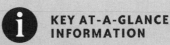

IN BRIEF

Huntley Meadows Park is a huge nature preserve located in southern Fairfax County. It's a great place to take a short hike and spend a lot of time observing wildlife, especially birds.

DESCRIPTION

Covering 1,424 acres just south of Alexandria, Huntley Meadows Park ranks as one of the metro area's largest close-in parks. Its centerpiece is a 500-acre freshwater marsh—the area's largest—enveloped by mostly deciduous woodlands. The result is a protected natural habitat with a remarkable array of plants and animals.

Huntley is an attractive year-round hiking venue, especially for people keen on natural history. But it has only a few maintained trails. Consequently, Huntley hikes tend to be short in distance, although not always so in time.

This very easy, 4.6-mile, and hill-less outing mostly uses the maintained trails. You'll find that they are in good condition (if sparingly signposted) and selectively dotted with useful information boards. I have also included in the hike a sampling of the park's "informal trails," which tend to be muddy but are worth exploring (as revealed to me by veteran hiker and Huntley aficionado Gary Kosciusko).

KEY AT-A-GLANCE INFORMATION

LENGTH: 4.6 miles

CONFIGURATION: Modified out-and-back

DIFFICULTY: Very easy

SCENERY: Wetlands, woodlands

EXPOSURE: Mostly shady; much less so in winter

TRAFFIC: Light save for birders and school groups on spring mornings

TRAIL SURFACE: Mostly fine gravel on main land trails; boardwalk across marsh; dirt on side trails—muddy when wet

HIKING TIME: 2–4 hours (including time spent looking, listening, inhaling)

SEASON: Year-round

ACCESS: Open daily, dawn–dusk

MAPS: USGS Alexandria, Mount Vernon

FACILITIES: Toilet at parking lot; toilets (inside), water, phone at visitor center

FOR MORE INFORMATION: Visit www.fairfaxcounty.gov/parks/Huntley; call or visit park's visitor center, (703) 768-2525 (free brochures available; open 9 a.m.–5 p.m. and noon–5 p.m. on holidays, closed on Tuesdays); contact Friends of Huntley Meadows Park, www.friendsof huntleymeadowspark.org

Directions

From Capital Beltway (Interstate 495 and I-95) in Alexandria, Virginia, take Exit 177A and follow long ramp to get onto Richmond Highway (US 1) heading roughly southwest. After 3 miles, turn right onto Lockheed Boulevard. Go 0.7 miles west to end of Lockheed at Harrison Lane. There, turn left into park's main entrance and go 0.2 miles to visitor-center parking lot.

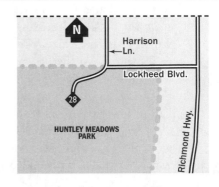

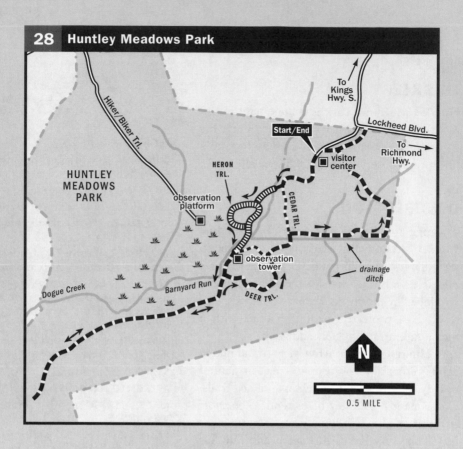

Be sure to stay on the trail to avoid both poison ivy and ticks, as well as to avoid getting lost (visitors sometimes do go astray). Carry insect repellent during the warm-weather months; Huntley is bug-rich and unsprayed. Also, take along binoculars and maybe a pocket reference book or two.

To get started from the parking lot, take the 100-yard paved trail to the visitor center. Step inside, or return later, to check out the exhibits and stock up on flora and fauna checklists and other materials. Also grab a seasonal trail guide from the outside dispensing box. Then get onto the broad and level Cedar Trail, which heads into the woods. With trail guide in hand, watch for the numbered trail markers. At the first trail junction, turn right onto the 0.6-mile-long Heron Trail. Just after that, and after marker 5, you'll reach the edge of the marsh. From there, staying right, take the wooden boardwalk across the wetlands to an observation tower equipped with information boards and great views.

See, hear, read, and even smell what the marsh has to offer. In spring, for example, look and listen for migrating songbirds and mating frogs. In summer, watch for water birds and dragonflies galore (sometimes they look like moving

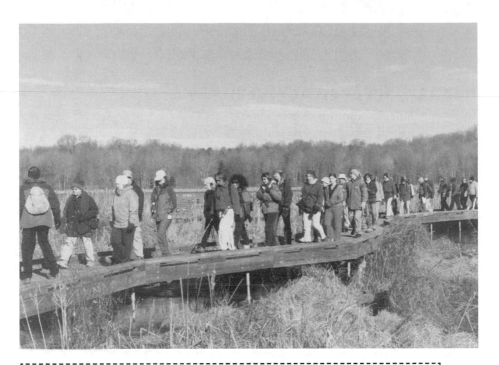

Huntley's birds usually outnumber humans, but they didn't on a winter 2006 hike led by
Gary Kosciusko (far left) and Marcia Wolf.

blossoms on the duckweed-carpeted water) and maybe catch the scent of a common
white-plumed plant called lizard's tail. In fall, watch for migrating raptors, warblers,
and waterbirds. In winter, ducks hang around if the marsh doesn't ice over.

At any time of year, look for beaver lodges and dams, but don't expect to
see the nocturnal builders. After the former farmland became federal property
in 1941, it was used by a succession of agencies. But beavers got a clawhold in some
unused areas, and their construction efforts went unchecked after the low-lying
land was sold to Fairfax County for $1 and converted into a county park in 1975.

Leaving the observation tower, step off the end of the boardwalk, walk about
15 yards, and turn right onto a dirt side trail. Then, at a junction with a broad
woodland trail, turn right and keep going on that trail—the park's longest informal
trail—while dodging the often-muddy patches for 1.1 miles. On reaching a dirt
road, turn around and return. After passing the dirt side trail, stay on the main trail
at the next junction, turn right at the one after that to get onto the gravel-surfaced
Deer Trail, and then turn right at trail marker 12 to get onto the Cedar Trail.

Next, just after trail marker 14, decide whether you're feeling adventuresome
and nimble—or not. If you are not, just stay on the Cedar Trail back to the visitor
center. But if you are, turn right onto a faint side trail that parallels an old drainage
ditch. Follow it through the woods for 0.6 miles. On the way, cross a couple of
side ditches by leaping, walking across logs, or sloshing. Next, turn left at the
park boundary, go 60 yards, and then swing left again to get onto an often-muddy

old farm road that will take you back another 0.6 miles to a paved path. There, turn left to walk a hundred yards to the trailhead parking lot.

NEARBY/RELATED ACTIVITIES

Explore Huntley's bountiful visitor center. Check out its nature exhibits and the photo-rich display about the park's history. Scan the visitor logbook for the latest bird finds and peek through the observation window at the outside bird feeder. Ply the friendly staff with questions. For instance, ask about the emu once found mentioned in the logbook. Take advantage of the park's naturalist-led tours and other year-round programs. Try the volunteer-led Monday morning bird walk. Explore the park's hiker/biker trail; get details at the visitor center.

POTOMAC HERITAGE NATIONAL SCENIC TRAIL: Scotts Run to Roosevelt Island

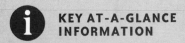

29

IN BRIEF

Fairfax and Arlington counties are the close-in home of a far-out trail endowed with river views, touches of wilderness, relics, and solitude.

DESCRIPTION

Here's your chance to both sample the second longest trail east of the Mississippi River (after the Appalachian Trail) and experience what proselytizer Bruce Glendening calls "one of the best urban-area hikes east of the Mississippi." The sample consists of the 10-mile-long Potomac Heritage Trail (PHT), secreted in the George Washington Memorial Parkway's broad right-of-way along the Potomac River between the Capital Beltway and Theodore Roosevelt Island. I present it here as a one-way, 11.4-mile hike with about 1,300 feet of elevation change (including a front-end piece in a nature preserve).

- -

Directions

Car shuttle is required, so first drive to car drop-off and then convoy to trailhead. From Washington's Mall area, use Constitution Avenue heading west to cross Theodore Roosevelt Memorial Bridge, staying to right. Then take first exit to right and then another right onto northbound George Washington Memorial Parkway. Take first exit (within 300 yards) into Theodore Roosevelt Island parking lot on right. Park there, at drop-off (see map on facing page). Then drive to trailhead as follows: Return to northbound parkway, proceed for about 9.5 miles to get on to outer southbound Capital Beltway (Interstate 495) lanes, and continue for 0.8 miles to reach Georgetown Pike (VA 193) at Exit 44; turn right and go 0.2 miles, and then turn right into nature preserve's satellite parking lot—the trailhead. (If lot is full, drive 0.4 miles west to main lot and walk back.)

KEY AT-A-GLANCE INFORMATION

LENGTH: 11.4 miles (with shorter options)

CONFIGURATION: One-way

DIFFICULTY: Moderate

SCENERY: River views, woodlands, waterfalls, sites of historical interest

EXPOSURE: Open; more so in winter

TRAFFIC: Very light–light

TRAIL SURFACE: Mostly dirt, with extensive rooty, grassy, rocky, muddy stretches; one rocky gorge, with handrails; pavement

HIKING TIME: 5.5–6.5 hours

SEASON: Year-round

ACCESS: Open daily, dawn–dusk

MAPS: USGS Washington West, Falls Church

FACILITIES: Toilets, water, phone off-trail at Turkey Run Park; toilets, water off-trail on Roosevelt Island

FOR MORE INFORMATION: Contact NPS's George Washington Memorial Parkway, (703) 289-2500 or www.nps.gov/gwmp, and Potomac Heritage National Scenic Trail office, www.nps.gov/pohe; Potomac Heritage Trail Association, www.potomactrail.org; Potomac Appalachian Trail Club, (703) 242-0693 or www.patc.net; Potomac Trace, www.potomactrace.org

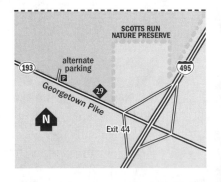

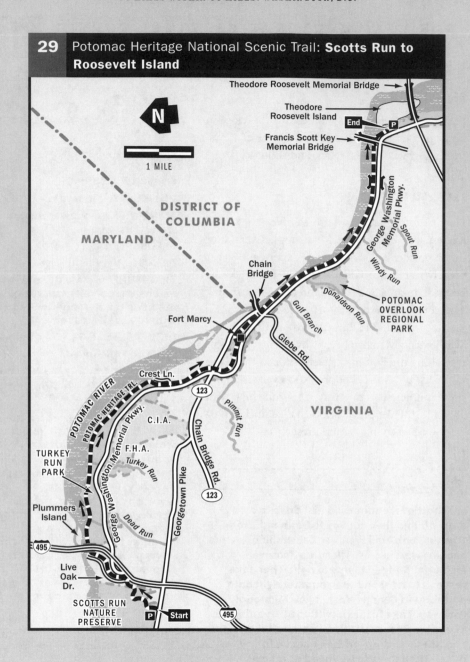

29 Potomac Heritage National Scenic Trail: **Scotts Run to Roosevelt Island**

The long trail, officially called the Potomac Heritage National Scenic Trail (PHNST), is actually a designated network of trails extending from Pennsylvania's Laurel Highlands to Chesapeake Bay. It includes more than 800 miles of trails, including many existing trails. Although authorized by Congress in 1983, it remained mostly a grand and little-known concept until significant progress began to be made recently, thanks to the efforts of the National Park Service (NPS), other government agencies, and some zealous private organizations and individuals. Even so, the PHNST and PHT names still get used interchangeably (albeit not here).

The PHT lies mostly on bluff-flanked floodplain sections separated by a wooded bluff-top section looming some 200 feet above the Potomac. In warm-weather months, the bottomlands are a colorful tangle of trees, bushes, blooms, and darting birds. At the water's edge in spring, watch for the silvery glint of migrating shad and for the black wings of hungry cormorants that follow them upriver.

The Potomac Appalachian Trail Club maintains the trail, which it built for the NPS in the mid-1980s after a storm wrecked an informal riverside path. Much of the trail tread is narrow, rocky, and rooty. Although also faint in places, the trail is well marked by once-blue and now-turquoise blazes and by signs at key junctions. Be careful on the rocks, and be ready for muddy patches. Also, do not attempt this hike in wet or icy weather or at flood times (check "River Stages" on the Washington Post's daily weather page, and stay away if the water level at Little Falls is higher than 4 feet).

To get started from the preserve's satellite parking lot, get on a broad dirt trail that heads gently uphill through the woods. At an intersection marked by an imperfect trailside map, turn right to proceed on a fairly level dirt trail that's been designated as a PHNST segment; turn right at the first T-junction and go straight through at the second one; then leave the preserve to turn left onto Live Oak Drive, and head downhill to the end. Then turn right to get onto the PHT proper (at the hike's 1.4-mile mark), and descend steeply to the riverbank, passing beneath the American Legion Memorial Bridge.

Just beyond the bridge, scan the far shore and take note of Plummers Island, even if you won't be able to see much. The 12-acre, NPS-owned island is renowned for its remarkable biodiversity and may be North America's most thoroughly studied island (to learn more, visit **www.pwrc.usgs.gov/resshow/perry/bios/History.htm**). Continuing downriver, you'll traverse a thick wedge of woodlands and cross Dead Run. If it's spring, linger near Turkey Run Park (about 4.4 miles into the hike), which Bruce Glendening ranks as "premium bluebell territory." Unseen off to your right will be the Central Intelligence Agency's large campus. In the 1960s, according to "BG," an unnamed stream in that vicinity was known informally as Pulp Run or CIA Run because it would sometimes be turned white by its load of shredded paper.

After that, you'll move away from the river for a couple of miles as the parkway property narrows to curve around some private riverfront estates and impassable bluffs. You'll have several short, steep woodland trail segments to negotiate. Then you'll be on a fairly level segment very close to the parkway. Eventually you'll reach Fort Marcy (at the hike's 6.6-mile mark). The well-preserved Civil War fort is now equipped with replica artillery pieces, information boards, and picnic tables, so that hikers can both rest and educate themselves. Then head downhill to Pimmit Run. There, use a fair-weather crossing of large rocks, and

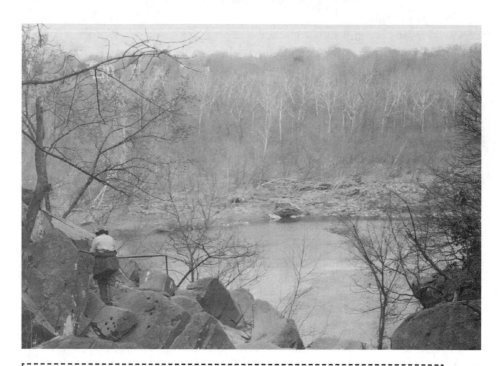

Descending through the rocky mini-gorge at Gulf Branch, use the handrails, watch your step, and pause to admire the river view.

enjoy the charming view as the trail follows Pimmit Run down to the Potomac at Chain Bridge.

Just before reaching the river, you and the stream will pass beneath Glebe Road (at the hike's 7.1-mile mark). On the other side, turn right to ascend some stone steps leading to a dirt trail that winds upward beneath the parkway to eventually flatten out as a ridgetop trail. Continuing downriver for 0.5 miles, watch for river views (superb in winter), and then tilt leftward and downhill. You'll pass through a rocky mini-gorge that is equipped with handrails and steps and will take you—and a small stream, Gulf Branch—down to the base of the bluffs.

At the bottom, turn right, step across Gulf Branch, and proceed along the blazed trail that winds across the bottomlands. Over the next 4 miles, you'll variously be walking along the riverbank, hopping over the rocks at the water's edge, and hugging the rock walls. And you'll cross Donaldson Run and Windy Run, the upper reaches of which can range from paltry trickles to mist-shrouded waterfalls. You'll also pass some rusting mementos of the days when the bluffs were quarried. Also note the tiny islands known as the Three Sisters, where a cross-Potomac bridge was planned but not built.

Next, as you near Francis Scott Key Memorial Bridge, ease inland, again get close to the parkway, take a footbridge across Spout Run, and pass beneath the high bridge. Then cross a grassy area to reach the Roosevelt Island parking lot—and decide whether Bruce is right about this hike.

Also see if you agree with the Potomac Heritage Trail Association's eloquent notion (written by Ric Francke) that the PHNST's "ultimate gift . . . is one of connections between tidewater and mountain ridges; between the colonial past and the technological present; and among individuals who acknowledge and appreciate our varied environments, our heritage and the opportunity for self-propelled travel along natural and historic pathways and who are willing to work toward its completion."

For a shorter one-way PHT hike, start from other places along the parkway, such as Turkey Run Park for a 7.8-miler, Fort Marcy for a 4.8-miler, or Chain Bridge for a 4.3-miler. And to sample the PHT as part of a circuit hike, start at Roosevelt Island and do the 9.3-mile "Key-Chain Hike," which involves Chain Bridge, Key Bridge, and the C&O Canal towpath—and was my PHT offering in this book's first edition.

NEARBY/RELATED ACTIVITIES

Explore the rest of Scotts Run Nature Preserve (see Hike 30, page 148), Roosevelt Island (see Hike 4, page 27), and also Turkey Run Park. Sample other PHNST segments, especially the new ones as they're opened. Contact the Potomac Heritage Trail Association for updates, and the Metropolitan Washington Regional Outings Program, (202) 547-2326 or **www.mwrop.org,** regarding inaugural segment hikes led by Glenn Gillis and me. When not hiking, consider joining the association.

30 SCOTTS RUN NATURE PRESERVE

KEY AT-A-GLANCE INFORMATION

LENGTH: 4 miles

CONFIGURATION: Modified loop

DIFFICULTY: Easy–moderate

SCENERY: Rolling woodlands, river views

EXPOSURE: Mostly shady; less so in winter

TRAFFIC: Light to moderate on main path to river, especially on warm-weather evenings, weekends, holidays; elsewhere, usually light

TRAIL SURFACE: Mostly dirt or gravel; rocky, rooty near river

HIKING TIME: 2.5–3.5 hours (including dawdle-at-river time)

SEASON: Year-round

ACCESS: Open daily, sunrise–sunset

MAPS: USGS Falls Church; questionably accurate map posted at trailhead and at some trail intersections

FACILITIES: None

FOR MORE INFORMATION: Contact nearby Riverbend Park, (703) 759-9018

SPECIAL COMMENTS: Scott's Run is polluted, so don't touch the water

IN BRIEF

Out-of-sight Scotts Run Nature Preserve, on the Potomac River near the beltway, is well supplied with flora, fauna, river views, and little-used hiking trails.

DESCRIPTION

Hidden away amid upscale subdivisions in Fairfax County, Scotts Run Nature Preserve consists of a hilly, wildflower-riddled tract of riverside woodlands scarcely 4 crow-miles northwest of Washington. For songbirds and other wildlife, it's a sanctuary. For local people, it's a community park. And for hikers, it's one of the metro area's loveliest close-in venues. For many years, owner Edward Burling used the area as a weekend getaway, but also allowed hikers to roam his almost 400 acres. After he died, the tract was sold to a developer. But in 1970, local residents and officials finally managed to fold it into Fairfax County's park system as Dranesville District Park. It was later renamed.

This easy 4-mile hike loops through thickly wooded uplands and reaches the Potomac River in three places. It's hilly enough to provide about 1,900 feet of elevation change. Although there are too few trail signs, you'll see some marginally useful "You Are

Directions

From Capital Beltway (Interstate 495) in McLean, Virginia, take Exit 44 to get onto Georgetown Pike (VA 193) heading roughly west. Proceed for 0.7 miles and then, just after Swinks Mill Road sign on left, and just before Betty Cooke Bridge sign on right, turn right into preserve's main parking lot. If lot is full, go back up pike to small satellite lot, and start hike there.

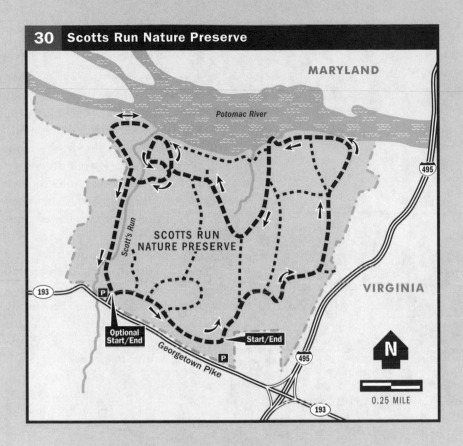

Here" trailside maps, so follow my directions carefully. And do watch for the evolving and signposted Potomac Heritage National Scenic Trail, which is scheduled to pass through the preserve (see Hike 29, page 143). But stay out of the polluted stream and abundant poison ivy, and remember that, when wet or icy, the riverside trails can be tricky or even hazardous.

To get started from the parking lot, head up a flight of wooden steps and into the woods. Proceed along a winding and undulating dirt trail that roughly parallels Georgetown Pike. After passing two side trails on the left, bear right at a fork and cross an eroded gully. Then, at the next fork, turn left and uphill (near the satellite parking lot, off to the right). At a broad unpaved road, turn left and continue gently uphill. Next, at an intersection marked by an unreliable "You Are Here" map, turn right onto a narrow curving trail.

After crossing a bridge spanning a little gully, continue gently uphill. At a T-junction and another suspect trailside map near the preserve's eastern boundary, turn left and keep going. At the next intersection, turn right and head downhill to the river. There, beneath a great arc of open sky, you'll find a stretch of unspoiled Potomac shoreline. Over on the Maryland shore, in the Carderock

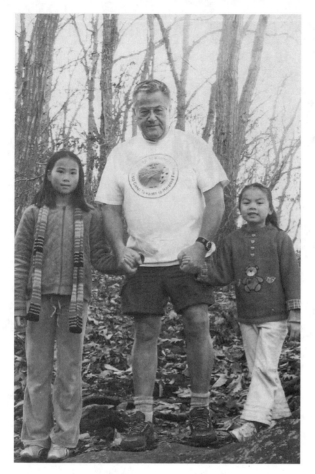

area, lurks part of the Billy Goat Trail. In the river are the shoals known as Stubblefield Falls. In the moist ground at your feet, hunt for the tracks of deer and other creatures. Admire but don't touch the biggest nearby tree, a huge, poison ivy–entwined maple. Then head upriver on a narrow trail that's somewhat overgrown. The trail soon becomes a rocky and rooty path that angles uphill, crosses a rock-slab streambed, and skirts the base of a huge rock. About 60 yards beyond the rock, stop at the first of several spots that offer gorgeous views. It's a one-person, fern-fringed overlook just a few steps off the trail. Note the mysterious stone walls in the water below.

You'll find another rewarding overlook just after the main trail is crossed by another trail that sweeps straight downhill. To get there, turn right at the next intersection onto a rocky ledge. Be doubly careful in that the rock can be slippery and is rimmed by poison ivy. Retrace your steps from the ledge, cross the main trail, and continue uphill. The trail is steep at first and then flattens out and curves through the woods. At an intersection near a concrete-embedded pipe called the Flag Pole, go straight through on a broad trail. At the next intersection and trail-side map, take the right-hand trail. At the fork after that, the hike's halfway point, detour to the right to see what's left of Burling's fire-destroyed cabin.

Return to the main trail and follow it downhill to some wooden stairs. Step down and turn right to take a broad gravel path down to the Potomac. There, enjoy additional fine river views and reach a lovely, waterfall-fed, and rock-enclosed pool at the mouth of Scott's Run. But resist the temptation to swim or wade. Start to retrace your route uphill on the gravel path. Then keep going, past the wooden stairs, until you reach Scott's Run. Cross the stream on the concrete stepping posts, and turn right onto a fairly flat trail. Continue, staying to the right wherever the trail forks. At a steep slope, ascend it to reach the top of a ridge. Pause to view the river off to your left (great views in leafless winter), and then follow the trail down to the mouth of Scott's Run. Be careful because the trail is steep, rocky, and rooty—and hemmed in by poison ivy. Enjoy the pool and waterfall and then head back. At the stream in the stepping-posts area, don't step across. Rather, turn right onto the broad gravel trail that goes gently uphill for half a mile to the trailhead.

NEARBY/RELATED ACTIVITIES

Explore nearby Great Falls Park and Riverbend Park, farther west along Georgetown Pike (see Hike 32, page 157).

31 FRASER PRESERVE

KEY AT-A-GLANCE INFORMATION

LENGTH: 6 miles

CONFIGURATION: Modified loop

DIFFICULTY: Easy–moderate

SCENERY: Woodlands, river views, remnants of 200-year-old canal

EXPOSURE: Mostly shady; less so in winter

TRAFFIC: Very light to light; occasionally heavier when summer camp is in session

TRAIL SURFACE: Chiefly dirt, some gravel; rooty, muddy in places

HIKING TIME: 2.5–3.5 hours (including dawdling at old canal)

SEASON: Year-round

ACCESS: No restrictions, but call preserve manager before visiting

MAPS: USGS Seneca; sketch map posted at kiosk

FACILITIES: None

FOR MORE INFORMATION: Visit National Conservancy's Web site, www.nature.org; call Virginia chapter, in Charlottesville, (804) 295-6106; call preserve manager Joe Keiger, in Arlington, (703) 528-4952; call on-site caretaker John Thayer, (703) 757-0288

SPECIAL COMMENTS: Observe posted regulations; don't drive into preserve, even if gate is open

IN BRIEF

Fraser Preserve is a private nature sanctuary in the northwestern corner of Fairfax County close to the Potomac River. It's open to the public and a delightful and secluded place to hike.

DESCRIPTION

Fraser Preserve is a 220-acre tract of rolling woodlands and floodplain some 14 miles northwest of Washington. Formerly a Washington family's summer refuge, the property was bequeathed to the Nature Conservancy in 1975. A Washington church uses a small inholding as a children's summer camp and church retreat A single-lane paved road links the preserve's gated entrance to a cleared area containing the camp's lodge and a caretaker's cottage.

The preserve is slowly reverting to an untamed woodland state, in keeping with the

----

Directions ⟶

From Capital Beltway (Interstate 495) in McLean, Virginia, take Exit 44 to get onto Georgetown Pike (VA 193) heading roughly west. Proceed for 7.7 miles, passing through community of Great Falls at 6.3-mile mark. Then turn right at traffic light onto Springvale Road (VA 674) and proceed for 2 miles. Then, just after Beach Mill Road comes in from right, follow road as it makes sharp left turn at yellow arrow, continue for about 25 yards, and take first right to get back on Springvale (which cleverly becomes VA 755). Continue for about 0.5 miles and turn left onto Allenwood Lane. Park on shoulder close to Springvale.

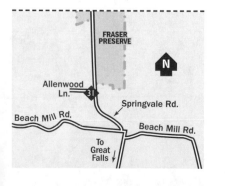

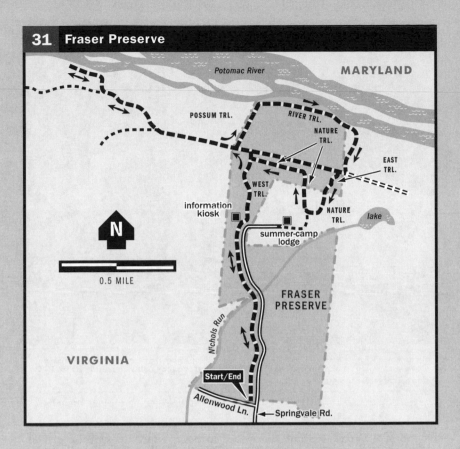

conservancy's emphasis on eco-preservation. Mature deciduous trees dominate the hillsides, with a sprinkling of pines, hollies, and spicebushes that provide wintertime color. Alder thickets thrive on the floodplain, and come alive with birds—and bugs—during the warm-weather months. Maples and sycamores lean out over the river. Wildflowers flourish, and resident animals range from deer to salamanders.

This hike is a 6-mile modified loop on well-maintained trails, with about 1,200 feet of elevation change. It's "modified" to include an out-and-back, history-oriented excursion into undeveloped land owned by the Northern Virginia Regional Park Authority.

To get started from the roadside trailhead, return to Springvale Road, turn left, and walk down a narrow paved road about 100 yards to the preserve's entrance. Head north into the preserve on a gravel road that gently descends for about half a mile before crossing a stream (Nichols Run) and then gently climbs.

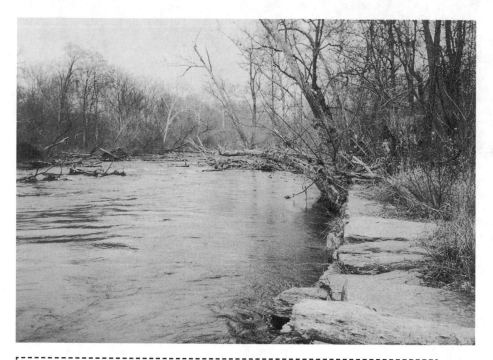

This stone wall was part of a bypass canal built by the Potowmack Company under its first president, George Washington.

At the end of the road (0.8 miles from the entrance gate), turn left onto the blue-blazed West Trail. Pause first at a kiosk, and then head downhill for about a third of a mile. At the bottom of the hill, turn left onto a level, unpaved road that follows a sewer-line right-of-way. Stay on the road as it crosses a grassy expanse marking another right-of-way (a buried oil pipeline, at right angles to the sewer line). Continue along the gravelly road, which gradually becomes more of a woodland trail, and be sure to stay to the right whenever a side trail tempts you to veer left (no, I'm not being political).

After about a mile on the road/trail, you will see the Potomac River on the right. Turn onto a short side trail leading down to the water. At the riverbank, pick up a narrow angler's trail that wriggles upstream for about 100 yards, roughly paralleling a narrow channel between the bank and a small island. Don't stray off the trail; poison ivy thrives in this area (see page 7 for more on avoiding it). Watch for the remains of stone walls on both sides of the channel.

A little farther on, past the island, you will find yourself atop a massive piece of old wall that ends at an inlet (see photo above). The stone work is a remnant of one of several short 18th-century canals built by the Potowmack Company as part of its fitful effort to make the Potomac commercially navigable (the small island is still called Potowmack Island). In the 1820s the insolvent company handed over its remaining assets to the Chesapeake and Ohio Company.

Retrace your steps to the main road/trail, and head back to the preserve. At the pipeline right-of-way, turn left onto a dirt trail leading down to the river. The river's edge marks the hike's halfway point, 3 miles from the trailhead. If the Potomac seems narrow, remember that you're looking at wooded islands, not the far shore. In leafless winter, though, you'll get more open views of the river.

Now turn right onto the River Trail and head downstream for about half a mile on a dirt trail. Rain makes the trail muddy; horses' hooves make it even muddier. Also watch out for stinging nettles and poison ivy close by the trail. Follow the trail inland, go right at a fork, and then head upstream alongside Nichols Run.

Turn right onto the sewer-line road, go about 15 yards past a gate, and then turn left and head uphill on the blue-blazed East Trail. Note that the sewer-line road and River Trail are scheduled to become part of a wonderfully ambitious project called the Potomac Heritage National Scenic Trail, which is being developed along the Potomac (see Hike 29, page 143, for more information).

From the East Trail, you will be able to see the only private dwellings that are visible beyond the preserve. Some of these homes are perched above a dam-impounded lake that interrupts Nichols Run on its way to the Potomac. Puff up the trail for several hundred yards and watch for a short metal post splashed with vivid red paint. There, turn right onto the red-blazed Nature Trail, which snakes across the preserve to the West Trail. The trail itself is faint (and invisible when the leaves are down), so be sure to follow the blazes.

On reaching the West Trail, turn left and uphill to return to the kiosk. From there, head back to the trailhead.

NEARBY/RELATED ACTIVITIES

After doing the hike once (so you know the route), do it again as a moonlight hike. Return on the same day to try for birdsong at morning and starshine at night. Pick a clear-sky evening when the moon is full. Take along good company, a flashlight, and insect repellent if necessary. Listen for owls, too. Skip the Nature Trail, which is difficult to follow at night. Instead, after hiking the River Trail, take the sewer-line road over to the West Trail and return that way to the trailhead.

Explore the network of informal trails that crisscross the undeveloped Northern Virginia Park Authority lands located upriver from the preserve. You can do that by heading away from the river and uphill on one of the side trails near the ruined canal. You will be on low bluffs bordering the Potomac, which will be visible occasionally through the trees. Also watch for the turquoise blazes marking the route of the Potomac Heritage National Scenic Trail.

Also consider becoming a preserve volunteer. Contact the conservancy's Virginia chapter or call preserve manager Joe Keiger (see contact information on page 152).

RIVERBEND PARK AND GREAT FALLS PARK 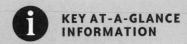 32

IN BRIEF

Riverbend Park and Great Falls Park in Fairfax County, offer hikers Great Falls, great vistas, and a great time in a magnificent Potomac River setting.

DESCRIPTION

Only about 15 miles from the White House, the Great Falls area is probably the metro area's finest close-in natural attraction. There, the broad and smooth Potomac River suddenly tumbles almost 80 feet in a series of rapids, and then squeezes through narrow, mile-long, and sheer-walled Mather Gorge. National Park Service (NPS) lands protect both banks and provide riveting views of nature at work. On the Virginia side, Great Falls Park stretches the length of the gorge and beyond, and inland, too, to cover 805 acres of rocky shoreline and wooded uplands laced with hiking trails. Adjoining the park to the north is Fairfax County's 409-acre Riverbend Park, which has wooded uplands, hiking trails, and a pretty floodplain shoreline.

This hike is a two-park, 9.8-mile loop leading through the uplands, to the falls, along

KEY AT-A-GLANCE INFORMATION

LENGTH: 9.8 miles (with shorter options)

CONFIGURATION: Modified loop

DIFFICULTY: Moderate–hard

SCENERY: Uplands, river vistas

EXPOSURE: Shady; less so in winter

TRAFFIC: Usually light, but heavy–crowded in falls area on warm-weather weekends, holidays

TRAIL SURFACE: Mostly dirt; some pavement, gravel; rocky in places

HIKING TIME: 5–6 hours

SEASON: Year-round

ACCESS: Riverbend open daily at 7 a.m.; closes 5–8:30 p.m.; Great Falls open daily, sunrise–sunset (closed December 25)

MAPS: USGS Rockville, Seneca, Vienna, Falls Church; PATC Map D; ADC Northern Virginia; so-so sketch maps in free park brochures

FACILITIES: Toilets, water, phones at visitor centers; snack bar at Great Falls center; toilets at Georgetown Pike parking lot; toilets, water at Matildaville

FOR MORE INFORMATION: Contact Riverbend Park, (703) 759-9018 or www.co.fairfax.va.us/parks/river bend, and Great Falls Park, (703) 285-2966 or www.nps.gov/gwmp/grfa

Directions

From Capital Beltway (Interstate 495) in McLean, Virginia, take Exit 44 to get onto Georgetown Pike (VA 193) heading roughly west. Stay on pike for 4.7 miles. Then turn right onto River Bend Road (VA 603). Drive 2.2 miles and turn right onto Jeffery Road (VA 1268). Proceed for 1.3 miles, past Riverbend Park's main entrance, to parking lot at end of gated road, next to park's former nature center. *Note:* Nearing gated road's end, note posted closing time—to avoid staying overnight in park.

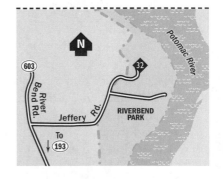

32 Riverbend Park and Great Falls Park

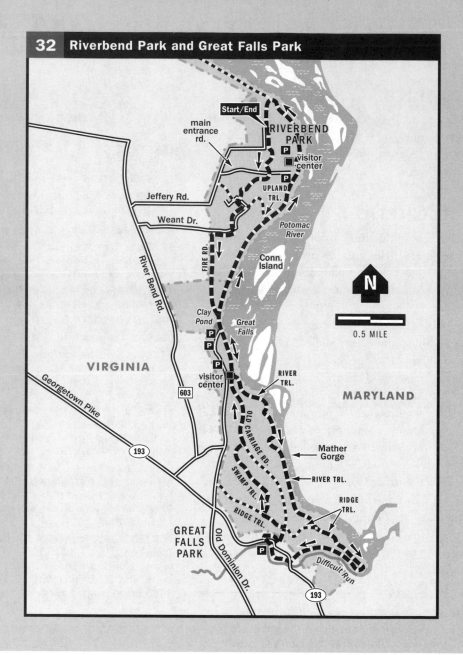

the gorge, and onto the floodplain. You'll experience assorted scenery, impressive vistas, and about 2,200 feet of elevation change. The route has limited blazes and signposts, so follow my directions closely—and avoid the poison ivy. To get started from the trailhead, walk back along the entrance road for 200 yards, turn left, and head downhill on a paved one-lane road. Go 200 yards, and turn right at a signpost onto the red-blazed Upland Trail. The undulating dirt trail will take you through the heavily wooded hills and stream valleys common to both parks.

On the Upland Trail, you'll cross the park's entrance road and then encounter a series of signposted trail junctions. Stay on the Upland Trail until you reach a junction where there's a post promising that it's 0.75 miles back to the visitor center (Riverbend's) and 0.2 miles to the river. There, turn right to leave the Upland Trail and head uphill.

Avoiding several side trails, follow the unmarked trail as it levels off and goes mostly and gently downhill. It emerges from the woods at the intersection of two gravel roads, one L-shaped, the other gated. Turn right onto the L-shaped road and head uphill to where it becomes a paved road (Weant Drive) and forms a junction with a two-sign gravel road ("Fire Road" and "Private Drive"). There, turn left onto the signed road. Follow it mostly downhill to the Great Falls visitor center's vast parking area and Clay Pond (read the explanatory label). Cross the lot to take a short path leading toward the river. At the end of the path, turn right onto the broad and gravelly Potowmack Canal Trail, which parallels the ruined canal.

The canal was one of five built by the Potowmack Company, starting in 1785, to make the Potomac navigable and open up waterborne trade with the interior. The company's first president was an ardent advocate named George Washington. After four years, though, he left to become the first president of a larger entity. The Great Falls canal was opened in 1802. For two decades, it had enough boat traffic to support the adjoining town of Matildaville, started by Henry "Light-Horse Harry" Lee (Matilda was his first wife; Robert E. was his son). But the company, canal, and town foundered. In 1828 the company's property and rights passed to the Chesapeake and Ohio Canal Company, which tried again on the Maryland side of the river (see Hike 15, page 81). Although ultimately it failed, it left behind what are now some fine hiking venues.

Stay on the gravelly path until you reach the large and exhibit-loaded Great Falls visitor center, at the hike's 2.7-mile mark. There, do what you must, and then continue on the same path into a grassy open area that was the site of an amusement park a century ago and is now a picnicking area that's thronged with visitors in warm weather. On your left you'll find short paths leading to three cliff-top overlooks, where you'll get superb views of the river, falls, and gorge—and maybe see kayakers braving the churning waters and onlookers watching safely from the overlook on the Maryland side (within the C&O Canal National Historical Park). On the way to the third overlook, note the post on which record flood levels are marked—and look skyward to see the 1936 and 1972 marks.

Returning from the third overlook, turn left as soon as possible and walk about 30 yards to swing left onto a twisty cliff-top path. Follow it for 200 yards, and then swing left to get onto the blue-blazed and rather rocky River Trail, which you'll be on for 1.3 miles. En route, read the information boards and explore some of the unmarked short side trails on the left to peer down into

Mather Gorge. The 200-foot-wide gorge is a 2-million-year work in progress, being created by the ever-erosive river cutting down through bedrock. At a signage-free intersection, go straight through to cross a stream valley on steep wooden steps. Continuing, you'll pass several trailside overlooks, and then turn right and inland to cross the old canal bed and reach a T-junction. There, turn left and proceed, first passing ruined Lock 2 and then passing a deep, man-made rock cleft where Locks 3, 4, and 5 once stepped the canal down to the river. Continuing along the gorge, you'll find that the scenery gets wilder, the trail rockier, and the going slower—partly because the moody river requires watching. When unruffled, it glitters harmlessly. But when turbulent, it resembles a strong brown god—sullen, untamed, and intractable.

From the semi-overgrown Cow Hoof Rock overlook, near the end of the gorge, the trail angles inland and climbs uphill steeply, as you should. Then turn left onto the Ridge Trail, at the hike's 4.3-mile mark. Continue for about half a mile along that woodland trail, and then swing right to descend to the Difficult Run Trail. At the bottom, turn left and proceed to a lovely off-the-beaten trail place—Difficult Run's mouth on the Potomac. Then follow the streambank inland and mostly uphill on the fire road alongside the picturesque stream. Where the road levels off, bear left at a trail sign onto a muddy-when-wet dirt trail that follows the stream under trestled Georgetown Pike (VA 193). At a roadside parking lot next to Difficult Run, you'll be at the hike's 6.1-mile mark—and also on the Cross County Trail (see facing page).

Next, cross the pike very carefully (blind curves hide speeding cars) to get onto a woodland dirt trail that leads 200 yards gently uphill. At the trail's end, turn left onto and up the Ridge Trail. Go about 200 yards and then turn right to walk past a no-horses–no bikes barrier to get onto the Swamp-Ridge Connector Trail. It undulates for 0.4 miles through deep woods and then plunges downhill to a junction, where you should turn left onto the level Swamp Trail. Go 0.4 miles and then turn left onto the broad and level Old Carriage Road near what's left of Matildaville. Continuing, pass the visitor center again. Then swing right to the trail along the canal, and head upriver. Beyond the canal, jog left onto a gravel path, and proceed to leave one park and reenter the other. When passing the park boundary, note and listen to the low 19th-century dam that spans the river just below Conn Island to feed Washington's major water-supply intake.

For the next 2 miles, you'll experience some of the best riverside hiking I know. You'll be on the floodplain where the Potomac makes the big bend for which the park is named. You'll also be on a section of the evolving Potomac Heritage National Scenic Trail (see Hike 29, page 143) and simultaneously on the new-as-of-late-2005 Potomac Gorge Interpretive Trail.The mostly smooth but sometimes muddy trail is flanked by mature sycamores, cottonwoods, and maples, as well as pawpaws, bushes, and wildflowers. And watch for springtime songbirds, summertime butterflies, wintertime water birds, and anytime bald eagles (they live on Conn Island—and unusually far inland for eagles).

About a mile past the dam, you'll reach the Riverbend visitor center. Then continue on the riverbank trail. Where the trail doglegs and a sign points across a small footbridge and toward the nature center, resist temptation and stay on the main trail. Keep going on the heavily pawpaw-lined trail (help yourself in September), and then, after crossing a wooden footbridge, turn left at the next fork to start the hike's final half mile. Walk uphill on a gravel road, pass a pond, and, at a signpost symbolically banning horses and bikes, turn left onto a narrow dirt trail leading to the parking-lot trailhead.

For a 5.3-mile sampler of this hike, just do the first part from Riverbend to the Great Falls visitor center and its overlooks, and then go back along the river-side trail. When doing the full hike in the fall or winter, reverse the route so you'll be doing the riverside trail in the morning sunshine.

NEARBY/RELATED ACTIVITIES

Explore other trails, such as Riverbend's Meadow Trail and Great Falls's Matilda-ville Trail. Linger at both visitor centers to see the nature exhibits and confer with eager-to-help staffers. Try some of the many year-round programs offered by the parks.

33 CROSS COUNTY TRAIL:
Colvin Run Mill to Potomac River

KEY AT-A-GLANCE INFORMATION

LENGTH: 8.7 miles (with shorter options)

CONFIGURATION: Out-and-back

DIFFICULTY: Easy–moderate

SCENERY: Stream valley, woodlands, river views

EXPOSURE: Mostly shady; less so in winter

TRAFFIC: Generally very light–light; heavier north of Georgetown Pike

TRAIL SURFACE: Dirt or dirt and gravel, with some muddy stretches; short stretch of pavement near mill; gravelly old road north of pike

HIKING TIME: 3.5–4.5 hours

SEASON: Year-round

ACCESS: Open daily sunrise–sunset

MAPS: USGS Falls Church; PATC Map D; ADC Northern Virginia: FCPA CCT maps #9 and #10 (also available on FCPA Web site)

FACILITIES: Toilets, water, phone at mill; toilet at Georgetown Pike parking lot

FOR MORE INFORMATION: Contact Fairfax County Park Authority, (703) 289-2500 or www.fairfaxcounty.gov/parks/cct; Fairfax Trails and Streams, www.fairfaxtrails.org; Colvin Run Mill, (703) 759-2771 or www.fairfaxcounty.gov/parks/crm

IN BRIEF

The northernmost section of the Cross County Trail (CCT) in Fairfax County follows a lovely and leafy stream valley through upscale suburbia from a historic mill to the Potomac River.

DESCRIPTION

The Cross County Trail is the only trail I know that essentially was constructed beneath the hikers' feet. In the mid-1990s, Bill Niedringhaus blithely envisioned a trail spanning heavily built-up Fairfax County between the Potomac River and the Occoquan River. He reasoned that the existing stream valleys—already protected parkland—could be linked to create such a trail. In 1999, with other pioneers, he started leading hikes along the route, even though that meant using sidewalks and shoulders and sometimes going astray. But they persevered, both in hiking the right way and pitching the concept. The eventual result was a coalition of public officials, trail-user groups, and other organizations and individuals that finally put a mostly off-road trail under the hikers' feet in 2006.

Directions

From intersection of Capital Beltway (Interstate 495) and Leesburg Pike (VA 7) near Tysons Corner, Virginia, take Exit 47A onto Leesburg Pike (VA 7) heading roughly west. Keep going for about 5 miles, and then turn right onto Colvin Run Road. Proceed for 0.2 miles, past gravel driveway leading to mill on left, and then go 0.1 mile and turn left into large paved parking lot.

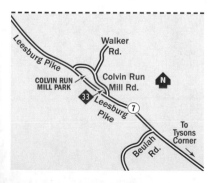

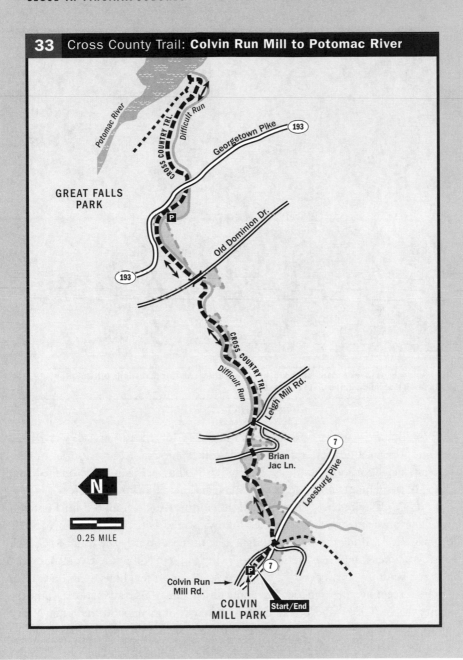

33 Cross County Trail: **Colvin Run Mill to Potomac River**

The CCT is evolving as a key part of the county's network of trails. It stretches from Great Falls Park in the north, where it connects with the Potomac Heritage National Scenic Trail (see Hike 29, page 143) to Occoquan Regional Park in the south, where it will eventually connect with the Bull Run–Occoquan Trail (see Hike 49, page 239). In between, it crosses the multicounty W&OD

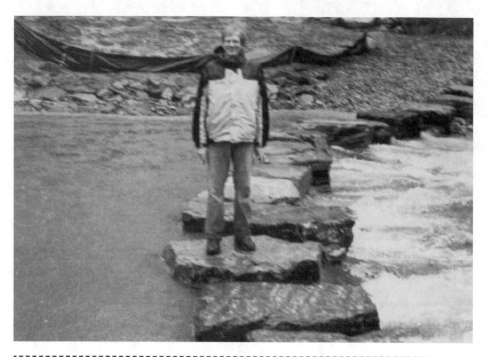

Bill Niedringhaus takes a stand on the rocky fair-weather crossing that spans Difficult Run on the trail that he dreamed up in the 1990s.

Trail (see Hike 34, page 167) and has links with local trail networks in Fairfax City and Reston. In effect, it's the 41-mile-long spine connecting a series of what are really neighborhood parks, as reflected in it's having been built for the use of hikers, bikers, equestrians, joggers, runners, and neighborhood strollers.

For a CCT sampler, I have selected the northern end for an 8.7-mile out-and-back hike on a mostly dirt trail that follows scenic Difficult Run down to the Potomac River. Along the way, you'll see a lot of trees (mostly the usual oaks, hickories, sycamores, tulip trees, and beeches, many of them still in their youth), myriad birds and wildflowers (depending on the season), only a few houses, and few or no vehicles (except in a parking lot). But you will see numerous trail markers, some displaying the CCT logo and others bearing different numbers and the letter N or S (signifying that you're so many miles from the trail's north or south terminus). Remember to stay on the trail and let the poison ivy and other plants grow in peace.

To get started from Colvin Run Mill's parking lot, take the short path over to the general store and barn, and then walk downhill past the miller's house and alongside the old millrace to reach the grandly restored two-centuries-old mill, which is the only operating gristmill from the 19th century left in the county. Note the fine old millstones standing guard near the mill, and then swing around the building to the left and head across the grass to where Colvin Run Road approaches Leesburg Pike. Cross carefully and continue on an old paved road that

heads roughly eastward. After going about 200 yards and passing some maintenance buildings, you'll slide into the woods on a gravelly and level dirt trail
alongside a little stream. In about 0.6 miles, you'll cross a stream at the first of the
fair-weather crossings, consisting of cylindrical concrete stepping-stones. (*Note:*
Heavy rain can make both crossings unusable; ice can make them slippery.)

Continuing, you'll come to an area where the trail starts to undulate a bit
and crosses a quiet cul-de-sac (Brian Jac Lane) in a parklike area between upscale
houses. It then reaches an open area of parkland, where it turns right and follows
the edge of a grassy hill up and then down before crossing Leigh Mill Road and
ducking back into the woods and onto the Difficult Run floodplain. Watch for a
signposted side trail on the right. There, either continue on the main trail or,
especially if it's muddy, get onto the side trail, which will take you dryly above
the floodplain and then reunite you with the main trail.

Next, you'll get to the second fair-weather crossing, this time across Difficult
Run, and you'll find yourself leaping across on huge rocks that have been posi-
tioned in the stream. On the far side, you'll pass a large stand of bamboo and a
dilapidated old wooden building that is the hike's only direct evidence (aside
from the mill) that the area has a history. In an open area, look high above you to
see the underside of Old Dominion Drive. Next, after crossing a small stream on
a metal bridge (note the little wooden one nearby, if it's still there, provided
informally by a local equestrian), you'll reach the rebuilt parking lot at Georgetown Pike.

Go to the far end of the lot to get on the CCT-designated 1.3-mile trail segment that lies within Great Falls Park and follows the tumbling stream down to the
Potomac at the southern end of the Mather Gorge. You'll start by passing safely
under the busy pike, and then you'll follow a braided, eroded, and muddy path
along the stream until you jog upward for a few feet and get on an old gravel road
(now a fire road) that will take you down to the river. You'll probably find that the
riverbank, thoughtfully equipped with rocks for sitting on, is a wonderful spot for
lingering, having a picnic, contemplating being in nature's realm, and looking far
across the water for tiny people scrambling on the Billy Goat Trail on Bear Island.
When ready, make your way back to Colvin Mill the way you came (except that at
the hillside detour, you should just stay on the main trail if it's dry).

Your options for a shorter CCT hike include doing a 6-mile out-and-back to
the Georgetown Pike parking lot, but you'd miss the best part of the CCT's Difficult Run stretch. Alternatively, you could avoid missing it by driving to the pike
parking lot and doing an out-and-back 2.6-miler to the Potomac, staying close to
the stream the whole way. Yet another choice would be to spot a car at the same
parking lot and hike from the mill all the way to the river and then back to the
car, for a scenic outing of 5.7 miles. And if you're feeling ambitiously eager for
something longer, try one of CCT specialist Henri Comeau's outings by spotting
a car at Riverbend Park and doing a one-way trek of almost 10 miles from the
mill to and through Great Falls Park.

NEARBY/RELATED ACTIVITIES

Explore Colvin Run Mill and its companion structures. Ask about its numerous programs and other events for both children and adults, especially the mill tour, which is a revelation of early 19th-century mechanical ingenuity and a chance to see grain being milled—and to buy some at the mill's general store. Special summer events include the hands-on churning of ice cream, which sweetly toothed hiker Carol Ivory recommends (as, at other times, she favors a posthike trip along nearby Walker Road to Thelma's, renowned for decades for its home-made ice cream).

Consider becoming a volunteer at the mill or joining the Friends of Colvin Mill; call the mill for details. Also consider joining Fairfax Trails and Streams, **www.fairfaxtrails.org**, the grassroots trail and environmental-advocacy group founded by Bill Niedringhaus.

Explore other sections of the CCT, taking advantage of the convenient access points where you can spot a car and do a one-way hike.

W&OD RAILROAD REGIONAL PARK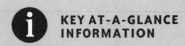

IN BRIEF

This ribbony park trail enables hikers to get lots of exercise, scenery, and fresh air in the Vienna/Reston portion of Fairfax County.

DESCRIPTION

Much as a dachshund is three dogs long and half a dog high, so the Washington & Old Dominion Railroad Regional Park is several parks long and a tiny decimal fraction of one park wide. More precisely, it's 45 miles long and 0.0189 mile wide—as can happen when an abandoned railroad right-of-way becomes a park. The park extends across northern Virginia between urban Alexandria and exurban Purcellville. Its chief attraction is an end-to-end, multiuse, and gently sloping paved path known as the W&OD Trail.

This hike uses the close-in and scenic trail section between Vienna and Reston. About

---

Directions ———————➤

From Capital Beltway (Interstate 495) in Merrifield, Virginia, take Exit 49 onto I-66 heading west. Drive less than 2 miles and take first exit (Exit 62). After 0.8 miles on exit ramp, get onto Nutley Street heading north toward Vienna. Drive 0.7 miles and turn right onto Courthouse Road. Drive 0.75 miles and turn right onto Maple Avenue (Vienna's portion of Chain Bridge Road or VA 123). Drive 0.4 miles and turn right onto Park Street. Drive 0.2 miles and turn right into Vienna Community Center parking lot.

Or use Metro to get to trailhead: Take Orange Line train to Dunn Loring–Merrifield Metro station, take Metrobus 2C to Maple Avenue and Park Street, and then take to sidewalk for 0.2 miles to trailhead. Contact Metro, (202) 637-7000 or www.wmata.com.

KEY AT-A-GLANCE INFORMATION

LENGTH: 13 miles

CONFIGURATION: Out-and-back

DIFFICULTY: Moderate

SCENERY: Woodlands, parklands, hedgerows, creeping-closer suburbia

EXPOSURE: Mostly open; even more so in winter

TRAFFIC: Generally light; light–moderate on warm-weather evenings, weekends, holidays

TRAIL SURFACE: Almost all pavement, with crushed-gravel option

HIKING TIME: 5–6 hours

SEASON: Year-round, but best from fall through spring

ACCESS: Open daily until dark

MAPS: USGS Vienna; map in official W&OD trail guide (revised edition)

FACILITIES: Toilets, water, phones at, near trailhead, off-trail near half-mile posts 17, 18; toilet near post 15; water near post 16.5

FOR MORE INFORMATION: Contact W&OD Trail office in Ashburn, (703) 729-0596; NVRPA, (703) 352-5900; or the Friends of the W&OD (FOWOD), www.wodfriends.org

SPECIAL COMMENTS: On warm-weather weekends and holidays, stay to right on paved trail to avoid speeding cyclists and in-line skaters

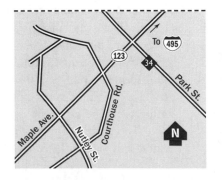

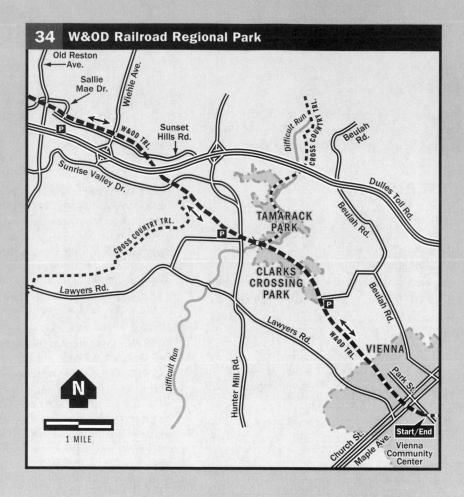

34 W&OD Railroad Regional Park

6.5 miles long, it's flanked by other parklands that make the 100-foot-wide former right-of-way seem broader and greener. West of Vienna, the paved trail is paralleled by a crushed-gravel horse trail. The paved trail is the most popular, largely with cyclists and in-line skaters. Signs identify the major thoroughfares along the trail. Brown signposts and white numerals painted on the trail every half mile measure the cumulative distance from Alexandria. By contrast, the gravel trail has little signage, some hills, and sparse traffic (mostly a few joggers and strollers, and an occasional biker or equestrian). It also has thicker hedgerows, where wildflowers burst into scented bloom and the birds warble sweet in the spring. Consider using both trails to provide diversity on your out-and-back outing. And be sure to watch for other users and be attentive when crossing streets and roads.

To get started from the parking lot, head for the adjoining paved trail, turn right, and proceed. After about 0.2 miles, pass W&OD half-mile post 11.5 and then quickly reach Maple Avenue, Vienna's store-and-eatery–lined and traffic-clogged main street. Cross carefully at the traffic light (note the athletic figure on the crosswalk sign). Continuing, cross less-busy Church Street and reach the Vienna railroad station, one of six surviving W&OD stations. A modest wooden structure dating from around 1860, it's now leased by a model-railroading group, but may eventually become a W&OD museum.

Then slip out of Vienna and into a landscape of hedgerows, parklands, woodlands, and sky. After passing W&OD post 13, enjoy the first installment of Clarks Crossing Park. If it's spring, pause to take in the hike's lone and dazzling forsythia forest, next to a small parking lot. If it's summer, admire the hike's lone, gorgeous, and tree-sized hydrangea bush nearby. And (for contrast) note, on a treeless hill, what may still be the hike's lone mansion. Then press on, past a mile of the park's bottomlands.

After W&OD post 14, cross Difficult Run by bridge. It's the hike's lone significant stream, snaking northward across Fairfax County to the Potomac River. Half a mile later, in spring, listen for the choral shrilling of spring peepers. Also watch for signs that you're also on a stretch of Fairfax County's Cross County Trail (see Hike 33, page 162). Then, just past the hike's lone trailside outhouse, cross a paved road again for the first time in 3 miles. It's Hunter Mill Road, where the trail starts going uphill, mostly very gently, for nearly 2 miles. After crossing Sunrise Valley Drive, duck under the Dulles Toll Road, just before W&OD post 16. Scan the open embankments for wildflowers, which help to visually offset the commercial buildings rising along the toll road. About half a mile later, on the far side of Sunset Hills Road, note the hike's lone water fountain, complete with a bowl for pets (it was donated by the nearby plumbing firm). The trail then levels off, having accumulated most of the hike's 500 feet of elevation gain.

Just after passing the hike's lone array of trailside fast-food outlets, you'll reach and cross busy Wiehle Avenue and start to see more of Reston's buildings. After going by a trail shelter and bulletin board, cross Old Reston Avenue. On the far side, head for a small, white-painted wooden hut. Just short of W&OD post 18, it's the hike's halfway mark and the former Wiehle railroad station. Peering inside, note the half-door ticket counter, where the last ticket was sold in 1951. Note the hike's lone convenience store nearby. Then recross Old Reston Avenue and return to the trailhead.

NEARBY/RELATED ACTIVITIES

If hit by posthike hunger, head for the Sunflower Vegetarian Restaurant, (703) 319-3888, a pan-Asian eatery on Chain Bridge Road a mile southwest of the trailhead. On Saturday mornings from June to October, forage at the Vienna Farmers Market, (703) 281-3530, three blocks from the trailhead. Visit the FOWOD Web site, www.wodfriends.org, to learn about the fight to keep threatened sections of the trail from becoming a treeless right-of-way for new transmission lines. Also, at any time of year, consider joining FOWOD.

35 MASON NECK STATE PARK AND MASON NECK NATIONAL WILDLIFE REFUGE

KEY AT-A-GLANCE INFORMATION

LENGTH: 12.9 miles (with shorter options)

CONFIGURATION: Modified loop

DIFFICULTY: Moderate–hard

SCENERY: Bay views, marshlands

EXPOSURE: Mostly shady; less so in winter

TRAFFIC: Usually very light–light; moderate in and near state-park picnic area on warm-weather weekends, holidays

TRAIL SURFACE: About 75% dirt, 25% pavement

HIKING TIME: 4.5–6 hours (including beach pauses and marsh gazing)

SEASON: Year-round, but best from fall through spring

ACCESS: State park: open daily, 8 a.m.–dusk, entrance fee; wildlife refuge: open daily sunrise-sunset

MAPS: USGS Fort Belvoir, Indian Head; sketch map in free NWR brochure and posted at trailhead

FACILITIES: Toilets, water at state-park picnic area; water, phone at state-park visitor center; toilet at wildlife-refuge trailhead

FOR MORE INFORMATION: See Description

SPECIAL COMMENTS: Wildlife-refuge trails closed December–June

IN BRIEF

A state park and adjoining national wildlife refuge, both on a secluded peninsula in the southeastern corner of Fairfax County, provide a protected habitat for wildlife and some fine woodland and shoreline trails for hikers.

DESCRIPTION

For more than three decades, Mason Neck State Park and Mason Neck National Wildlife Refuge have played a vital role in keeping much of the Mason Neck peninsula green and in helping to restore the area's once-imperiled bald-eagle population. The park and refuge, together with other public lands, now cover most of the 9,000-acre peninsula, which juts

----

Directions ⟶

From Capital Beltway (Interstate 495) in Springfield, Virginia, take Exit 57A onto I-95 heading southwest, toward Richmond. If you start from Washington, head southwest on Shirley Memorial Highway (I-395) to automatically be on I-95 when you cross beltway. From beltway, drive about 6.5 miles south on I-95 and take Exit 163 to Lorton Road (VA 642). Go left onto Lorton Road and head east for 1.3 miles. Turn right onto Armistead Road, drive several hundred yards, and then turn right onto Richmond Highway (US 1). Drive 0.8 miles and turn left onto Gunston Road. Proceed generally southeast for 4.6 miles. Turn right onto High Point Road and go 1 mile to contact station (en route, after 0.7 miles; note refuge trailhead parking lot on left). Then continue for 2 miles to parking lot at state-park visitor center. *Note:* Arrive early on warm-weather weekends and holidays; if main lot and nearby picnic-area lot are full, walk back along entrance road to Wilson Spring Trail parking lot, and start hiking there.

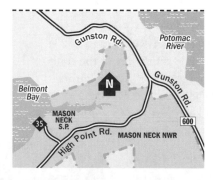

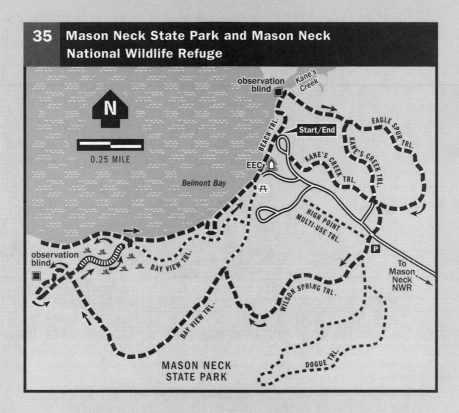

into the Potomac River roughly 25 miles of Washington. They are managed cooperatively as a huge nature preserve that also provides humans with various recreation opportunities.

The 1,813-acre park and 2,227-acre refuge are largely an area of rolling woodlands. Although most of their acreage is closed to the public, each of them has a modest trail system that enables hikers to sample the local scenery. However, now that the two systems have been linked by a paved path, I have replaced my original two short and separate hikes with a grand tour of 12.9 miles, with only about 650 feet of elevation change, although shorter options are available.

The trails are generally well marked and well maintained, with those in the park also having color-coded trail names (but few blazes). They are only lightly used, in that nearly all visitors head for the park's waterfront visitor center and nearby picnic area. Be sure to stay on the trails and off the poison ivy. Take along field glasses and a bird book, and remember that winter is the best time to spot waterbirds and eagles. Also remember that the refuge is very buggy in summer.

To get started from the park's parking lot, walk back along the entrance road for just a few yards to turn left onto the Kane's Creek Trail (blue) and into the oak,

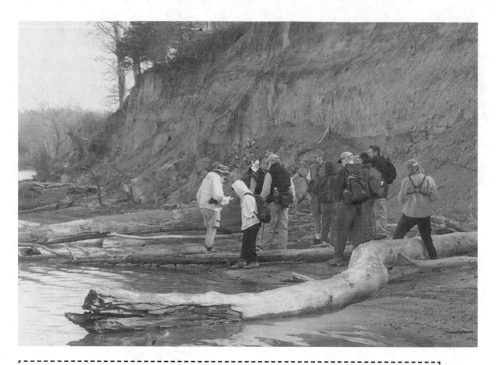

Fallen trees and crumbling cliffs give hikers sad pause along the park's shoreline, which is beset by wave erosion and water pollution.

hickory, and beech woods and southward. At the first intersection, about 0.6 miles later, turn sharply left to stay on the trail, which makes a clockwise 0.8-mile half loop to a T-junction, where it meets the Eagle Spur Trail (silver). Turn left and take the undulating 1.25-mile-long trail mostly northward to an observation blind over-looking Kane's Creek. (It replaces the excellent blind at the creek's mouth that was closed for environmental reasons.) Step inside. Scan the skies and the creek, and watch for such rewarding sights as eagles, ospreys, and (in summer) water lilies.

Leaving the blind, return to the T-junction and turn left to do the last 0.25-mile piece of the Kane's Creek Trail to reach a familiar intersection. There, turn left onto the Wilson Spring Trail (yellow) and proceed for 0.2 miles, carefully crossing the entrance road, to reach a parking lot and the paved High Point Multi-Use Trail, about 3.2 miles into the hike. Turn left and follow the trail south and east for 1.75 miles, mostly alongside the entrance road, until you reach the refuge's parking lot on the right on High Point Road. There, about 5 miles into the hike, pause to read the information boards and prepare for a 3.25-mile round-trip excursion through the refuge (not shown on the map).

The refuge was established in 1969 as the country's first federal sanctuary for bald eagles. The impetus came from the alarming fact that the local eagles (like those elsewhere in the lower 48 states) seemed headed for extinction thanks to habitat loss and pesticide use, and the peninsula seemed headed for suburban development. However, with significant help from the Nature Conservancy, a public–private coalition was launched successfully in the mid-1960s to help reverse the situation and preserve what is now the heart of the refuge—the 250-acre Great Marsh. It also contributed to the eagles' comeback (just as nationally the species is no longer listed as endangered). The species' recovery has been remarkable along Virginia's lower Chesapeake Bay and its tidal tributaries, including the Mason Neck area. In 1977 the region had only 33 pairs of eagles (they mate for life), whereas, by the spring of 2006, the total had risen to 485 pairs.

The marsh is a year-round faunal delight where you'll have a chance to benefit from what Thoreau called "the tonic of wilderness." Ducks, geese, and swans pass through in the spring and fall, with some wintering there. In summer, swallows and other insect eaters cruise the wetland, and herons and egrets dot the marsh like blossoms. The woods shelter migratory songbirds as well as resident birds, deer, and other creatures. The eagles number about 60 in winter, including both migrants (from the far north) and residents, and roughly 20 in summer. They nest and roost in tall trees, and roam the local waterways. Starting in November or December, they take six months or more to raise their young.

To get started from the parking lot, take the gravel road leading deeper into the refuge. After about 50 yards, turn right onto the blue-blazed and dirt-surfaced Wood-marsh Trail, which undulates gently through the woods. At about 0.8 miles, you'll reach a signposted T-junction. There, turn right to begin a loop segment that passes a display shelter (the left-hand trail goes to Eagle Point). The trail swings generally to the left. After several hundred yards, pause at another T-junction and a fence across the main trail. If the fence is open, continue on the trail; if it's closed because eagles are nesting nearby (as a large sign will explain), pause for one paragraph.

Continuing on the main trail, stop at the display shelter, where you can learn about eagles. After that, follow the trail as its swings left and down to the edge of the marsh. There, about halfway into the hike, linger at an observation platform. After that, swing left and take the marsh-edge trail to Eagle Point. After passing Hickory Pass coming in from the left, you'll reach a semi-marshy area spanned by a bridge.

But if you've been stopped by the closed fence at the T-junction, turn left there and take Hickory Pass downhill on what is, in effect, a shorter-by-0.8-miles alternative route to the bridge area. Along the way, if you know your hickories, watch for four different species. Cross the bridge, and then cross a second one, which is rickety but safe. If it's winter, pause on the bridge to look up for an active eagle's nest. After the bridge, turn right and proceed to the trail's end at Eagle Point. There, look again for the treetop nest. Also scan the endless marsh for a chance to see the way of an eagle in the air.

Leaving Eagle Point, retrace your steps to the second bridge. Don't turn left to cross it; rather, just continue up the trail, which leads to the signposted T-junction where the loop started. There, turn right and head back to the parking-lot trailhead. Then take the paved path back to state park and the Wilson Spring Trail parking lot—at the hike's 10-mile mark. Then head west on the winding Wilson Spring Trail (yellow) for about 0.8 miles and into a hillier and more open area.

Staying on the main trail, you'll pass an information board and the new Dogue Trail (on the left), and then swing north to a T-junction, where you'll turn left onto the Bay View Trail (red). Proceed for 1 mile, heading west and then northwest and pausing to peruse several information boards that explain the local ecosystem, to reach a four-way intersection. Next, perform an 0.8-mile maneuver consisting of crossing the intersection and doing a counterclockwise mini-loop that goes back through the intersection and down a short flight of steps to reach a wooden board-walk. Along the loop, between intersection crossings, pause at an overlook and then an observation blind, both to your right, to look out at a marshy inlet. Also pause on the boardwalk to scan a woodsy marsh area where beavers have left their marks.

At the end of the boardwalk, leave the trail and walk a few yards to the beach to start an out-and-back detour. Turn left and get onto a dirt bluff trail that leads along the edge of the beach. Go as far as you can, and then descend to the beach (you may have to hop over a small tidal channel) to continue on the sand as far as a tangle of dead trees. Stay on the sand for the return leg. Scan Belmont Bay, watch for birds, avoid the washed-up debris, read the unsafe-for-swimming signs, and contemplate the park's shoreline plight. Note the exposed tree roots, as well as the trees that have already bitten the sand. The park loses one to two feet of shoreline each year to erosion. Water pollution has killed the aquatic plants that would otherwise reduce the erosive action of waves.

Back at the boardwalk, continue roughly eastward and close to the curving shoreline for the hike's final 0.8 miles. You'll be on a mixture of dirt trail and board-walk sections that follow the bluffs and offer inviting overlooks. At the edge of the picnic area, follow the fence line across the grass. Just past bluebird box number 1, turn left onto a narrow downhill trail with steps. At the bottom, turn sharply left to follow the trail clockwise around a tidal pond. Then cross the boat launch's parking area and ascend the steps to reach the bluff top near the visitor center and trailhead. Use my description and map to plan shorter outings for yourself. Also consider using a car shuttle to avoid walking the 3.4 miles total between the park and refuge.

For more information on the park and refuge, contact the park, (703) 339-2385 or **www.dcr.state.va.us/parks/masonnec.htm;** call or visit the visitor center, (703) 339-2380; and call the refuge office in Woodbridge, (703) 490-4979.

NEARBY/RELATED ACTIVITIES

The park's visitor center has informative brochures, exhibits, and staffers. Ask about events and programs, such as the guided canoe trips, both by day and moonlight. (Hours: weekdays, 10 a.m. to 6 p.m., April through October; week-ends, 10 a.m. to 5 p.m., November through January; closed in February.)

Explore Pohick Bay Regional Park, Gunston Hall Plantation, and Mead-owood Special Recreational Management Area, all of which you'll pass on your drive back along Gunston Road.

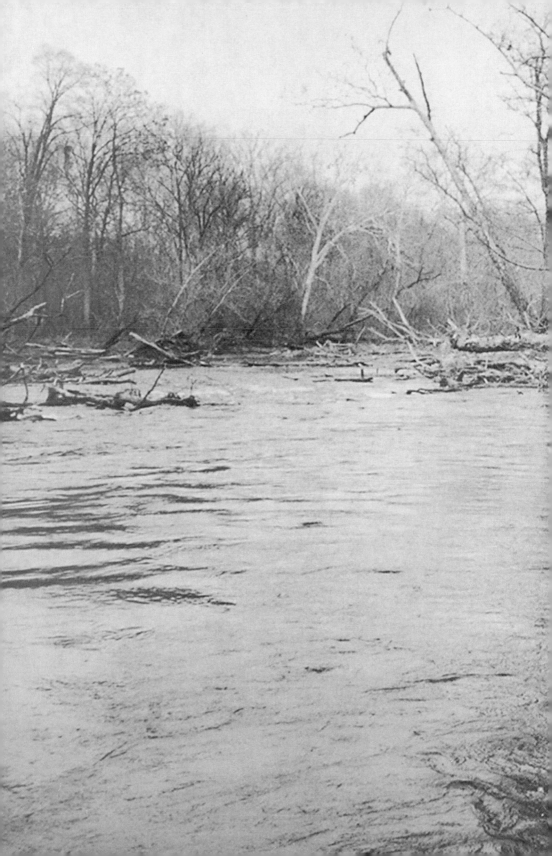

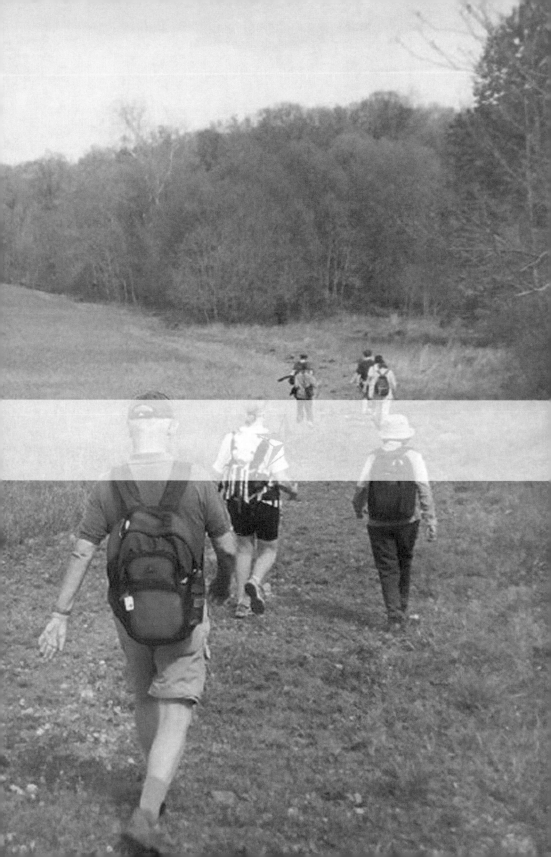

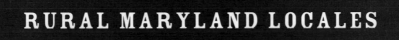

RURAL MARYLAND LOCALES

36 C&O CANAL TOWPATH:
Washington to Harpers Ferry

KEY AT-A-GLANCE INFORMATION

LENGTH: 62.1 miles (with 2 shorter options)

CONFIGURATION: One-way

DIFFICULTY: Extremely hard

SCENERY: Woodlands; river and tow-path views; glimpses of communities, farmlands, and suffering hikers

EXPOSURE: Partly open, partly shady; dark at night

TRAFFIC: Generally light, especially before sunrise and after sunset

TRAIL SURFACE: Mostly dirt, with sandy, pebbly, rocky, grassy patches; pavement stretches at start and end

HIKING TIME: 17–21 hours

SEASON: Spring, but only on last Saturday in April

ACCESS: Advance registration (including fee) required

MAPS: USGS Washington West, Falls Church, Seneca, Vienna, Waterford, Poolesville, Point of Rocks, Harpers Ferry; sectional sketch maps in BSA booklet "184 Miles of Adventure: Hiker's Guide to the C&O Canal"

FACILITIES: Toilets at trailhead, 16+ towpath locations; phones at 6 locations; food/drink stops at 7 trailside locations and Highacre; toilets, water at Highacre; bike patrols on hike route, medical teams at food/drink stops

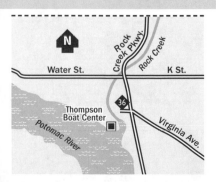

IN BRIEF

This hike answers the question, "Can I experience the glorious C&O Canal National Historical Park in springtime by taking one long hike instead of several short ones?"

DESCRIPTION

This hike is unlike any other in this book. It's much longer and much more difficult, even grueling. It's actually an organized event held only once a year. It features manned food-and-drink stops, medical teams, and bike patrols. It requires participants to register in advance. And I include it here because it's a great way for hikers to challenge themselves, to savor the glories of spring along the Potomac River, and to experience the camaraderie of the hiking trail.

The full hike is 62.1 miles, or 100 kilometers, in length (but comes with two shorter options). It's a one-way hike along the Potomac from Washington, D.C., to Harpers Ferry, West Virginia. It's also a one-day hike, the particular day being the last Saturday in April. And that day starts at 3 a.m. and, for most participants, lasts well into the evening.

Directions

From Washington's Mall area, drive west on Constitution Avenue and turn right (north) onto 23rd Street NW. Go several blocks and then turn left onto Virginia Avenue. Go several more blocks and cross Rock Creek Parkway to enter Thompson Boat Center parking lot, catty-corner from Watergate. *Note:* Parking at Thompson's is metered during day and forbidden overnight, but parking on nearby streets is permitted without fee or time limit on weekends. It's best, though, to get a ride to the trailhead for this one-way hike.

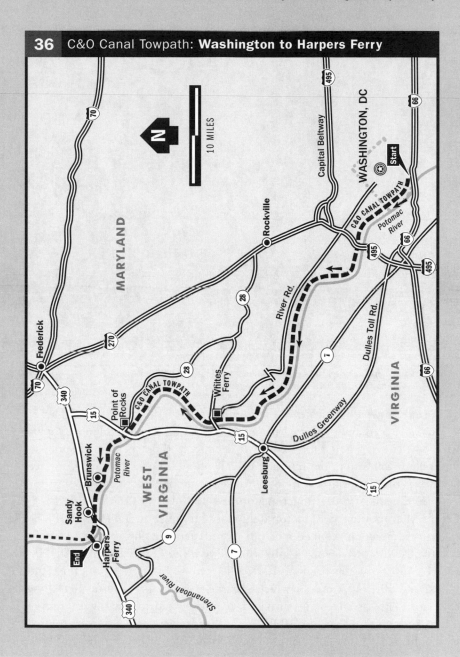

36 C&O Canal Towpath: **Washington to Harpers Ferry**

The 100K, as it has long been called, was started in 1974 by Ray Martin and Loren Friesen. They were inspired by a 50-mile outing on the C&O Canal towpath organized in the 1960s by Bobby Kennedy, who, in turn, had been motivated by his brother Jack's presidential concern about the American people's physical fitness. As Ray remembers, he and Loren decided to "ratchet up the challenge"

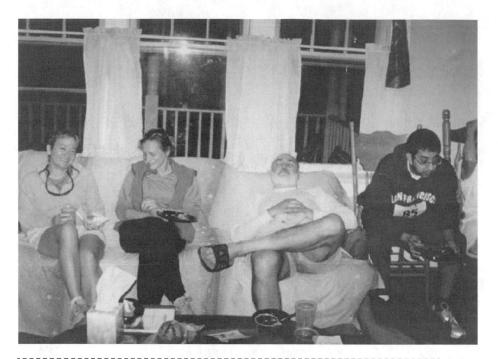

The 2006 finishers included 100K veteran Mike Darzi (center), 50K first-timer
Shaleen Khurana, and 50K/80K veteran Pat Hopson.

and use the towpath to achieve "the round figure of 100 kilometers." Thereafter, a core of rugged and dedicated (if not obsessed) hikers and volunteers managed to keep the event going for some two decades without benefit of sponsorship, umbrella organization, the Internet, or cell phones. For a long time, in fact, the event was run out of the back pocket of coordinator Roger Clark.

In the mid-1990s, Roger negotiated to fold the 100K into the Sierra Club's Metropolitan Washington Regional Outings Program (MWROP). Subsequently, although it retained much of its independent and idiosyncratic character, the 100K slowly evolved into what is now the One Day Hike (ODH). The ODH consists of the original 100K plus two shorter versions, the 50K (31 miles) and 80K (49.7 miles), which start later in the day and farther along the towpath. This arrangement provides would-be participants with reasonable alternatives to the do-or-die 100K. And all three versions end in Harpers Ferry at Highacre, a cozy old house rented for the event from the Potomac Appalachian Trail Club.

Currently, between 150 and 200 people from a dozen states and several foreign countries sign up to do the ODH. They're wonderfully diverse, varying considerably in size, shape, sex, age (teens to 70s), ethnicity, hair color, clothing choices, and hiking style. Nearly all of the 50K and 80K starters make it all the way to Highacre, as do half or more of the 100Kers. The causes of nonsuccess are exhaustion, dehydration, foot problems, or weather conditions (but all dropouts are well taken care of). The causes of success are individual preparedness, motivation, and determination, plus the active presence of some 60 volunteers.

In the following brief account, I focus on the 100K, but encourage novices to start by trying the 50K. For more details on all three versions, as well as photographs, advice on where to stay after the hike and how to get back from Harpers Ferry, and the ODH results since 1997, visit the event Web site, **www.oneday hike.org**.

Preparation is the key to success in the 100K. As the Web site says, "Hiking 62.14 miles in a single day is a challenge, even for people in good physical condition. It means having to cover a distance that's 10 miles longer than two back-to-back marathons. It means having to average 3 miles an hour (including rest stops) just to finish by midnight (having started at 3 a.m.) [and thereby meet the checkpoint cutoff times]." That's why MWROP's ODH planning committee (of which I am a longtime member) organizes local training hikes over the four months before the big day. Such hikes are essential for building stamina, toughening the feet, accustoming the leg muscles and mind to long-distance flatland hiking, and learning to drink while walking fast.

To get started on the hike (assuming you're registered), proceed to the trail-head, in the Thompson Boat Center parking lot. Then, promptly at 3 a.m., leave with the other hikers and do a half-mile out-and-back along the Potomac (that segment helps keep the 100K kilometrically exact). Then get onto the milepost-studded restored towpath near milepost zero and head out of the District and into Maryland. You'll stay close to the Potomac forever. You'll also have recurrent views of the river, farmlands, and wildflower-dotted woodlands, as well as the ruined canal's old locks and lock houses.

You'll find that the dirt-surfaced towpath is mostly level and smooth, with some grassy stretches. But it can be hard when dry, and soft and muddy when wet. It's also dark for the hike's first few hours—and again in the evening, when most participants are still out there, under the wide and starry sky. On the way to Harpers Ferry, you'll encounter volunteer bike patrols and discover that hikers tackle the 100K in different ways. Some buddy up, some don't. Some talk, some don't. Some zone out, some use the mileposts to pull themselves along. And you'll pass through—and doubtless pause at—several combination checkpoints, food and drink stops, and first-aid stations.

After about 61 miles, watch on your left for a footbridge spanning the Potomac. There, cross over into Harpers Ferry, and follow the signs for just over a mile uphill to Highacre. There you'll be welcomed with applause, camaraderie, drink, food, and a place to sit down or collapse. Perhaps you'll congratulate yourself. Perhaps you'll wonder why you did such a crazy thing. And perhaps you'll find it useful to reflect on Mike Ambrose's views of the event. He first did the 100K in 1988—"for entirely noble and sane reasons"—as a fund-raiser in support of a District soup kitchen, but then wound up doing it over the many ensuing years "for the exercise and the chance to walk in the rain with friends whose mental health was not entirely certain."

Each year, during training hikes for the event, says Mike, "a few conversational themes occur with predictability. One is that our bodies were not designed for this, and there's something foolish or even perverse in the undertaking. Another is that we must be insane to do such a thing. Then, during the event itself, the insanity theme becomes more urgent and more frequent as the evidence accumulates. There's a new bodily ache every mile, we have blisters in improbable places, and there's no relief in sight. By this time, it's obvious that we are nuts. And just to prove the point, we continue. Then, when we reach the end of the 100K, there's a wonderful relief and a profound sense of accomplishment, followed by the instant clarity of full-on sanity: we never have to do *that* again!"

NEARBY/RELATED ACTIVITIES

Be sure to train hard and well, and get to know the towpath by trying other towpath hikes in this book, by going on organized hikes, or by exploring on your own. And if you stay over after the hike, explore historic Harpers Ferry (see Hike 59, page 285).

C&O CANAL TOWPATH:
Monocacy River Aqueduct to Calico Rocks

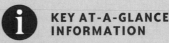 37

IN BRIEF

On this C&O Canal towpath hike, there's more scenery and less trail traffic than on the others in this book. After crossing a massive and historic stone aqueduct, hikers can savor the pleasures of a tranquil riverside trek in rural Maryland.

DESCRIPTION

This 10.8-mile C&O Canal towpath hike in southern Frederick County closely follows the gloriously unspoiled Potomac River upriver from a point a couple of hundred yards past towpath milepost 42 to half a mile beyond milepost 47—and back. It also follows the old canal, of course, but in this area the former waterway is just a dry and overgrown trough. As part of the C&O Canal National Historical Park, the hike route is rich in woodlands year-round. It displays tree leaves and blossoms and wildflowers galore during the warm-weather months and plays host to migratory birds in spring and fall. Its winter glory consists of almost constant views of the nearby river, plus towering riverbank sycamores with their stark white upper trunks and branches. What's delightfully lacking year-round in this area some 50 miles northwest of Washington is a lot of human foot traffic. At times in the fall, I've encountered more deer than people.

KEY AT-A-GLANCE INFORMATION

LENGTH: 10.8 miles

CONFIGURATION: Out-and-back

DIFFICULTY: Easy–moderate

SCENERY: Woodlands, river views, colorful rocks

EXPOSURE: Mostly shady; less so in winter

TRAFFIC: Very light; slightly heavier on warm-weather weekends, holidays in trailhead, Nolands Ferry areas

TRAIL SURFACE: Chiefly hard-packed dirt (muddy when wet); 560 feet of stone

HIKING TIME: 3.5–5 hours

SEASON: Year-round, but especially lovely in late fall, early winter

ACCESS: Open daily, dawn–dusk

MAPS: USGS Poolesville, Point of Rocks; map on board at trailhead

FACILITIES: Toilet at trailhead; toilets, water at pumps (if working) at Indian Flats, Nolands Ferry, Calico Rocks

FOR MORE INFORMATION: Call Great Falls visitor center, (301) 299-3613; visit park's Web site, www.nps.gov/choh; call park's headquarters office in Sharpsburg, (301) 739-4200; read canal history in Hike 15, page 81

Directions →

From junction of Capital Beltway (Interstate 495) and I-270 in Maryland, head northwest on I-270 for about 6 miles. Get off at Exit 6B in Rockville onto MD 28, heading generally northwest. Stay on MD 28 for about 30 miles as it undergoes several name changes. About 0.4 miles past Dickerson (still on MD 28), turn left onto Mouth of Monocacy Road. Go 1.3 miles to parking lot at end, turning left at fork en route.

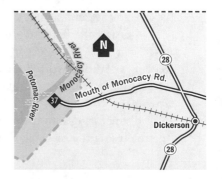

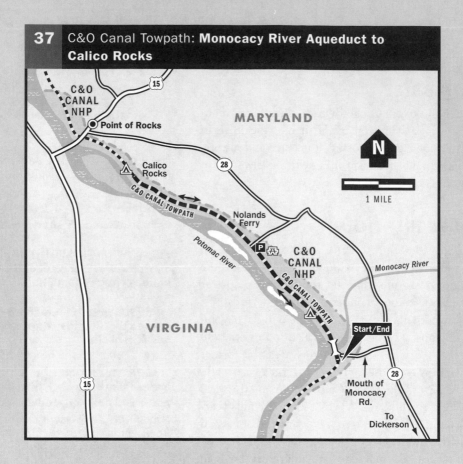

37 C&O Canal Towpath: **Monocacy River Aqueduct to Calico Rocks**

At the trailhead, the most conspicuous sight is the huge aqueduct that carried the canal and its towpath across the Monocacy River. Built of pinkish quartzite quarried at the base of nearby Sugarloaf Mountain, the seven-arched, 560-foot-long aqueduct was an engineering marvel when completed in 1833. It's still impressive, even though it's been battered by Confederates (who tried to demolish it), storms, and age; it's now held together by metal supports.

To start the hike, step onto the towpath, turn right, and head for the aqueduct, with the Potomac on your left. Crossing the aqueduct, be thankful that recent renovation work has included the addition of a smooth-surfaced walkway. Halfway across, pause to take in the views up and down the Monocacy. Downstream, on your left, it joins the Potomac. Upstream, you'll see the shallow waterway disappearing into the woods. On the aqueduct itself, look for a faded stone plaque listing the original contractors.

Stepping off the structure onto the familiar dirt-surfaced towpath, head into the woods and upriver. You'll pass the Indian Flats camping area (an old fording place) and then milepost 43. Go another mile or so along the towpath and you'll find more river views and fewer trees, along with (if it isn't winter) myriad wild-flowers in the canal bed. Then you'll get to Nolands Ferry, with its large picnic area and parking lot served by an access road that crosses the canal bed.

Like other Potomac riverbank locations surnamed "Ferry," Nolands had a long history as a crossing place. The ford there was used as part of a traditional Native American pathway between what came to be Maryland and the Carolinas— a route later adopted by colonists. Ferry service was started in the 1750s, and a small trading settlement developed. However, the building of the C&O Canal and of a bridge across the Potomac at Point of Rocks, a few miles upstream, led to the isolation and decline of Nolands. A bridge across the canal there in the 1850s proved economically futile. Today, all you'll see of the old community are the bridge's stone abutments on each side of the canal. Just beyond those relics, watch for a mysterious stone building on the riverbank. It's actually a water intake and treatment facility that serves Frederick County communities.

Beyond milepost 46, you'll be on one of the most scenic stretches of the hike. There, it's tempting to linger and watch the play of sunlight on the nearby river set against the looming backdrop framed by Catoctin Mountain. And if the season is right, the old canal to the right will look less like a canal bed than a wildflower gar-den. The color scheme is enhanced by multihued rock outcroppings along the canal's far side. The rock is variously referred to as Potomac marble, calico marble, or Potomac breccia. It's actually a conglomerate, or pudding stone, consisting of multicolored pebbles embedded in a limestone matrix. It looks its colorful best just after a light rain.

About half a mile beyond milepost 47 is the hike's halfway mark (5.4 miles) and your turnaround spot, the Calico Rocks camping area, on the outskirts of Point of Rocks. The camping area sports none of the colorful rocks, but it does have an unusual maple with a hollowed-out trunk and an overcoat of fungi. Walk down to the riverbank and linger awhile, especially if you brought lunch. If you're feeling peppy, continue along the towpath for about a mile to see the little com-munity of Point of Rocks, with its ugly but essential bridge across the Potomac. If not, just return directly to the Monocacy trailhead.

NEARBY/RELATED ACTIVITIES

On driving back from Monocacy in the warm-weather season, stop at one of the produce stands on MD 28 to buy fruits and vegetables. Or, if you have time, detour to visit family-run Homestead Farm, which has an unusually large variety of fruit, including gooseberries (a rarity in the metro area), for both picking and buying. The farm is on Sugarland Road, off MD 28; call (301) 977-3761 or visit **www.homestead-farm.net**.

38 LOWER MAGRUDER TRAIL AND MAGRUDER BRANCH TRAIL

KEY AT-A-GLANCE INFORMATION

LENGTH: 9.7 miles (with shorter options)

CONFIGURATION: Modified out-and-back

DIFFICULTY: Moderate

SCENERY: Parklands, woodlands, stream valleys

EXPOSURE: Mostly shady; less so in winter

TRAFFIC: Very light–light; heaviest in vicinity of recreational park's sports facilities on warm-weather weekends, holidays

TRAIL SURFACE: Mostly dirt with some muddy stretches; some pavement, grass

HIKING TIME: 4.5–5.5 hours

SEASON: Year-round

ACCESS: Open daily, sunrise–sunset

MAPS: USGS Damascus; ADC Montgomery County; sketch map on Web site below

FACILITIES: Toilets, water at shelter close to trailhead

FOR MORE INFORMATION: Contact Montgomery County Departments of Park and Planning, www.mc-mncppc.org

SPECIAL COMMENTS: Watch for poison ivy

IN BRIEF

An out-of-the-way stream valley in northernmost Montgomery County now has a modest trail system that enables hikers to enjoy a restful woodland setting where plants and animals thrive.

DESCRIPTION

This hike is a mostly out-and-back outing of 9.7 miles and only 650 feet of elevation change. It starts with part of a paved trail that extends north to Damascus. It then continues on a dirt-surfaced trail that extends south to Seneca Creek. And it ends with a loopy coda that's a mix of park and nonpark trails and road shoulders. Both main trails are well maintained and well marked, but use my directions for the coda.

To get started from the parking-lot trailhead, head downhill for 0.1 mile to the paved Magruder Branch Trail. Turn left and follow it for about 1 mile as it curves and undulates north and east through an open area. It then enters the woods and curves gently downhill into Magruder Branch Stream Valley Park. The mostly deciduous trees are the usual local mix of oaks, hickories, and beeches, plus some conifers. Stay on the main trail until you reach a signposted dirt trail heading gently uphill to your

----

Directions ⟶

From junction of Capital Beltway (Interstate 495) and I-270 spur in Maryland, head northwest on I-270 (toward Frederick) for about 15 miles. Get off at Exit 16, and proceed on exit ramp for 0.5 miles, staying to right at fork (marked Exit 16A, to Damascus). Merge onto Ridge Road, and proceed for 4.3 miles (crossing MD 355 en route). Then turn right onto Kings Valley Road, proceed for 0.6 miles, turn left into park's first entrance, and go about 100 yards to parking lot near playing field.

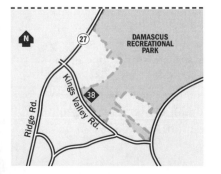

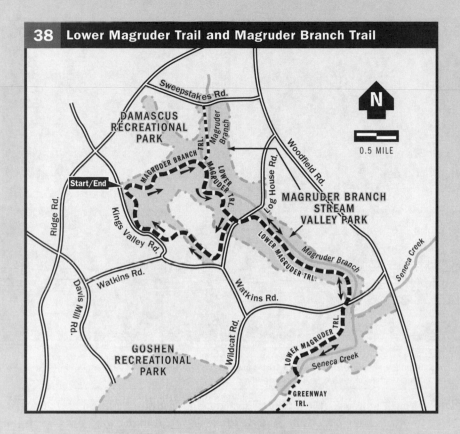

right. That's the blue-blazed Lower Magruder Trail, which was finished in 2003. But before taking it, continue for 80 yards to peruse Magruder Branch, and then return.

Heading south on the blue-blazed dirt trail for the next 0.9 miles, you'll go gently up and down through the woods to reach Log House Road. Cross the road carefully, go eight yards to a trail T-junction, turn left, and keep going. For the next 1.7 miles, you'll be mostly on or near the stream's right bank and on a wooded floodplain that sprouts wildflowers in the spring. Ignore the side trails, and contemplate the mysterious 90-degree turn made by the main stream.

On reaching Watkins Road, cross carefully, turn right, and walk uphill for 80 yards to find more blue blazes on the left. Over the next 1.1 miles, you'll first be in an open area of fields and then in open woods on a level trail until you finally reach Seneca Creek at the hike's 4.9-mile mark and your turnaround spot. However, before leaving, take the stepping-stones across the creek to reach the Greenway Trail (see Hike 23, page 114).

When you're ready, follow the blue blazes back to the trail's T-junction just before Log House Road, at the hike's 7.7-mile mark. Then, start the hike's final and

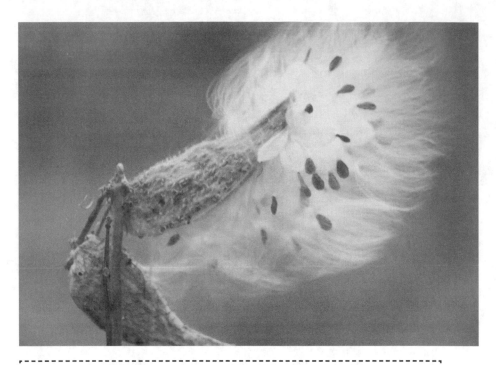

Look for milkweed plants near Seneca Creek; monarch butterflies depend on them, and shutterbugs watch for the exploding seedpods.

new-to-you 2-mile leg by continuing straight and slightly uphill on the dirt trail. Next, after traversing a gravelly parking lot, swing right to get onto the Log House Road shoulder. Keep going for about 0.25 miles, past large and tidy houses, to the road's T-junction with Watkins Road. Then turn right to continue down the right side of Watkins for 40 yards, and then angle downhill into the woods to pick up a faint and unmarked trail that levels off on the floodplain. Ease to the left to get close to a small stream (Wildcat Branch), and follow it to a short embankment. Ascend to a road (Founders Way) amid large houses, turn left, and follow it to Kings Valley Road. Turn right and walk uphill. Turn right into an entrance to Damascus Recreational Park, pass a basketball court on the left, and then swing left to get onto the paved Magruder Branch Trail. Follow it to the shelter near the trailhead.

For an easier full-length hike, do a straight out-and-back, without the loopy coda. For a shorter hike, just turn around sooner. For a 4.2-mile loop, skip the Lower Magruder Trail south of Log House Road. For an 8-mile hike in wet or icy weather, stay on the mostly paved Magruder Branch Trail (see the map).

NEARBY/RELATED ACTIVITIES

After the hike, detour to family-owned Butler's Orchard, (301) 972-3299 or www.butlersorchard.com, which has the best strawberries I've picked so far in the metro area.

LITTLE BENNETT REGIONAL PARK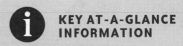

IN BRIEF

This northern Montgomery County park is a hiker's delight, with a magnificent upland meadow, a lovely grove of tulip trees, and other treats.

DESCRIPTION

Located about 23 miles northwest of Washington, Little Bennett Regional Park is Montgomery County's largest park, covering almost 3,650 acres (a small piece lies in Frederick County). It affords much splendid scenery, birds and other wildlife, a trail network, and few human trail users other than occasional equestrians. This hike is a challenging 12.6-mile grand tour, with about 4,000 feet of elevation change. The mostly dirt trails are unblazed, but the major intersections are signposted. The trails west of Little Bennett Creek are in good shape, but off-limits to bikers and equestrians. Those in the more rugged eastern area are twice as hilly (says my altimeter) and rather muddy, thanks to equine hooves. But don't be deterred. Mud washes off, and my irreverent eye sees a purpose in liquidity: fewer whizzing bikers. Yes, good can come of brook water and mud. The major meadow trails are mowed periodically in summer, but the grass grows rapidly and ticks

KEY AT-A-GLANCE INFORMATION

LENGTH: 12.6 miles (with shorter options)

CONFIGURATION: Modified loop

DIFFICULTY: Quite hard

SCENERY: Wooded hills, meadow vistas, stream valleys

EXPOSURE: Shady; less so in winter

TRAFFIC: Usually very light; light at its heaviest

TRAIL SURFACE: Mostly dirt, plus some gravel, grass, pine needles; rocky, rooty, muddy in places

HIKING TIME: 7–8 hours

SEASON: Year-round

ACCESS: Open daily sunrise–sunset

MAPS: USGS Germantown, Urbana; sketch map on free park pamphlet

FACILITIES: None at trailhead; phone at Hawks Reach Activity Center; roadside toilets, water, phone near campground's loop C; toilets on Purdum Trail

FOR MORE INFORMATION: Contact park manager, (301) 972-6581; visit Montgomery County Departments of Parks and Planning Web site, www.mc-mncppc.org

SPECIAL COMMENTS: Watch for posted signs about staying away when park has one of its occasional "managed deer hunts"

Directions

From junction of Capital Beltway (Interstate 495) and I-270 spur in Maryland, head northwest on I-270 (toward Frederick) for about 18 miles. Get off at Exit 18 and turn right onto Clarksburg Road (MD 121). Drive east on Clarksburg for 2.3 miles (go straight through intersection with MD 355, ignoring park sign there that points left to park's campground office). Then, after reaching bottom of hill on straight road, take first right—at gravel-road intersection—into small parking lot.

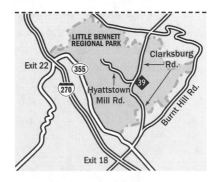

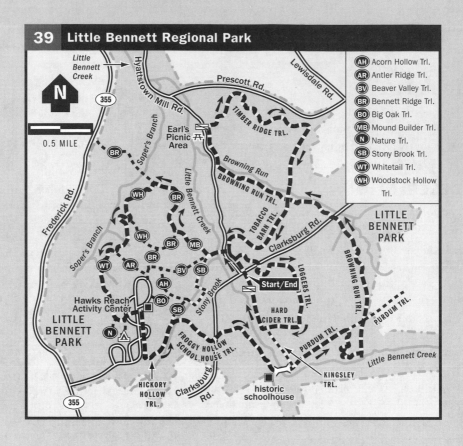

39 Little Bennett Regional Park

Little Bennett Creek

N

0.5 MILE

Hyattstown Mill Rd.

Prescott Rd.

Lewisdale Rd.

355

Earl's Picnic Area

TIMBER RIDGE TRL.

Browning Run

BROWNING RUN TRL.

Soper's Branch

Little Bennett Creek

Frederick Rd.

Soper's Branch

TOBACCO BARN TRL.

Clarksburg Rd.

LITTLE BENNETT PARK

BROWNING RUN TRL.

PURDUM TRL.

LOGGERS TRL.

Start/End

HARD CIDER TRL.

PURDUM TRL.

Little Bennett Creek

KINGSLEY TRL.

Stony Brook

Hawks Reach Activity Center

LITTLE BENNETT PARK

N

FROGGY HOLLOW SCHOOL HOUSE TRL.

HICKORY HOLLOW TRL.

Clarksburg Rd.

historic schoolhouse

355

AH Acorn Hollow Trl.
AR Antler Ridge Trl.
BV Beaver Valley Trl.
BR Bennett Ridge Trl.
BO Big Oak Trl.
MB Mound Builder Trl.
N Nature Trl.
SB Stony Brook Trl.
WT Whitetail Trl.
WH Woodstock Hollow Trl.

BR WH BR BR WH BR MB WT AR BR BV SB AH BO SB

abound. So, use common sense plus long pants or insect repellent. Stick to the trail anyway, in that poison ivy lurks.

The hike starts with a counterclockwise loop of 5 miles through the area west of Little Bennett Creek. To get started from the parking lot, return to and cross Clarksburg Road. Follow gravelly Hyattstown Mill Road for about 300 yards. Then turn sharp left onto the Beaver Valley Trail. After crossing Little Bennett Creek, turn left, and follow the trail as it swings right and away from the stream, and heads gently uphill. At the next major intersection, turn right onto the Mound Builder Trail—named for the local Allegheny mound-building ants. Watch for trail-side mounds, but avoid the ants, which bite. Continuing, turn right at a T-junction onto the Bennett Ridge Trail. At an open hilltop meadow, turn left onto the Woodcock Hollow Trail and enjoy a scenic half mile of hiking. Ease on uphill a bit, and then turn right at the next junction onto the undulating Whitetail Trail. Over the next mile and a half, be sure to ignore the Antler Ridge Trail, cross two small streams, and then follow a lovely fern-lined third stream uphill.

At the next junction, ignore the "Nature Trail" sign and turn left; also stay left at the next "Nature Trail" sign. Reach and carefully cross a road, one of several in the park's campground area. Keep going up the trail to emerge from the woods at another road—the area's main access road. Cross it alertly to reach Hawks Reach Activity Center, 3 miles into the hike.

Continuing, follow the paved road very gently uphill for almost half a mile. Where it curves right, watch on your left for the aptly named Hickory Hollow Trail. Take it, and head downhill on a steep and rocky path. Then turn left onto the Stony Brook Trail. After about 300 yards, turn right onto the Froggy Hollow School House Trail, cross the brook, and start climbing.

Emerging from the woods onto a level, grassy trail, stay to the right as you pass a white house. At a road (Clarksburg Road again), cross watchfully, jog left, and return to the trail. For the next half mile, you'll follow a woodland trail, and then reach a one-room schoolhouse, well preserved, boarded up, and fenced in. It served the local community—known as Kingsley and named for the local King family—from the 1890s until the 1930s, when the Great Depression finished off the area's already meager economy. Then turn left and take the nearby bridge over Little Bennett Creek. Cross a grassy area, which has a convenient picnic table if you want to linger. Birds and butterflies also favor this spot (the park is one of the metro area's butterfly hot spots).

Then head for the nearby gravel road to march uphill and embark on the hike's second, longer, and tougher segment—a 7.6-mile embellished figure eight through the eastern part of the park. Alternatively, to shorten the full hike to 5.6 miles, just turn left and follow the level gravel road (the Kingsley Trail) back to the trailhead for 0.6 miles (see below for two other shorter-hike options).

The mostly open road is part of the Purdum Trail (but ignore the trail sign pointing to an off-road trail). It provides the hike's steepest uphill stretch before leveling off, crossing a primitive campground, and becoming a dirt trail in the woods. At a four-way intersection, turn right onto an unnamed trail (opposite what the signpost calls the Loggers Trail). However, if there's snow on the ground, stay on the Purdum Trail (see below). Revealed to me by a passing equestrian and only faintly marked, the unnamed trail wriggles downhill to a small and sometimes muddy floodplain, and then glides left to follow a small creek upstream (Little Bennett Creek again). At a white pole—the hike's halfway mark—turn right and walk about 50 yards to look at the quite lovely creek. Then turn around and follow the white poles uphill on a gas-pipeline right-of-way, which crosses the Purdum Trail to become the Browning Run Trail.

At the next fork, bear left into the woods, staying on the Browning Run Trail. Proceed gently downhill on the horse-churned trail. Emerging in a meadow, cross a small stream, pass through a T-junction (Pine Knob Trail goes to the left), and then carefully cross an active road (Clarksburg yet again). Back in the woods, go either way at a trail fork. Where the trails reunite, cross a small stream and continue to another meadow, and then walk straight through the trail's intersection with the

Tobacco Barn Trail. Then return to the woods, dodge the mud, and reach a gravel road (Hyattstown Mill Road again). Turn right and follow it to Earl's Picnic Area. There, head for a nearby vehicle barrier and turn right onto the Pine Grove Trail.

For half a mile, you'll ascend through the pines on a winding trail that's needle-soft underfoot. At a T-junction in a clearing, turn right onto the Timber Ridge Trail. Stay on it for half a mile as it snakes through the woods. At an unmarked fork, go either way; both paths veer left and reunite. Soon after passing a sign warning of a private residence that you'll never see, pitch downhill into a serene and majestic grove of tulip trees. The only such grove I know, it's stunning, both for its expanse and for the towering trees with their tulip-shaped leaves and yellow-green-orange flowers. After crossing a small stream and starting to climb out of the grove, turn right at a junction and head uphill to break out of the woods.

Then step onto the Tobacco Barn Trail—and into an area of rolling grassy slopes fringed with woods beneath the open sky. Pause to look at the ruined tobacco-drying barn nearby and then head downhill on a curving, mowed path. At the bottom, follow the trail into the woods and across Browning Run, and then cross the Browning Run Trail to stay on the Tobacco Barn Trail as it skirts a meadow where butterflies, bluebirds, and dragonflies sometimes put on aerial displays.

Reenter the woods for a mostly downhill trek on a narrow, rocky, rooty, and muddy trail section. Go right at the first fork to stay on the Tobacco Barn Trail (never mind the "Loggers Trail" sign). When you reach a road (Hyattstown Mill Road), turn left and proceed for a few hundred yards. Then turn left onto the Loggers Trail, just past where the Beaver Valley Trail goes right. Do another hill climb, contend with a bit more mud, bear right at the first fork, and continue until a road appears (Clarksburg Road again). Cross carefully at an uphill angle of 45 degrees to find the trail. Ascend to reach an unmarked T-junction, turn right, and proceed downhill. At the next junction, turn left onto the Loggers Trail.

After more climbing, turn right at a T-junction onto a sometimes mucky but level old farm road—the Loggers Trail continued. Finally, reach a fork and swing right onto the Hard Cider Trail. It's the hike's longest downhill stretch, extending more than half a mile. It's also rocky and muddy. On reaching a level gravel road (the Kingsley Trail), turn right and walk a third of a mile to the trailhead.

You don't have to do the full 12.6-mile hike. For an 8.2-mile hike, just do the second segment by using the Kingsley Trail to get to the Purdum Trail. For a 3-mile sampler, drive along Hyattstown Mill Road to Earl's Picnic Area and do a loop using the Pine Grove, Timber Ridge, and Tobacco Barn Trails, and then the road.

NEARBY/RELATED ACTIVITIES

After the hike, detour to visit a nearby cluster of historic sites, including Hyattstown Mill, the miller's house, and the Ziegler Log House. To get there from Clarksburg Road, turn right onto MD 355, go about 3 miles, turn right onto Hyattstown Mill Road, and proceed for about 0.5 miles.

SUGARLOAF MOUNTAIN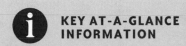

IN BRIEF

Washington's nearest mountain is vista-rich Sugarloaf Mountain, located in southern Frederick County. One can hike up, around, and down it in half a day.

DESCRIPTION

Sugarloaf Mountain looms above rolling farmlands about 30 crow-miles northwest of Washington. Privately owned, it is managed as both a nature preserve and public recreation area. Although it attracts many visitors, they're mostly sightseers and picnickers who prefer the roadside overlooks and the summit. For hikers, the 3,300-acre property offers good trails, a lungs-and-muscles workout, and a beguiling natural setting. At its best, it's wildflower-pretty in spring, green-bower scenic in summer, turning-leaf colorful in autumn, and snow-dusted ethereal in winter. Birds, deer, and other four-footed creatures are plentiful, as are copperheads and rattlers. Coyotes are sometimes seen.

The now heavily wooded preserve exists because Sugarloaf intrigued vacationing Chicagoan and cyclist Gordon Strong when he pedaled by in 1902. He acquired

KEY AT-A-GLANCE INFORMATION

LENGTH: 8.1 miles (with shorter options)

CONFIGURATION: Loop

DIFFICULTY: Moderate–hard

SCENERY: Upland woodlands, sweeping vistas

EXPOSURE: Mostly shady; less so in winter

TRAFFIC: Usually light; heavier on warm-weather weekends, holidays, especially on and near summit

TRAIL SURFACE: Roughly half hard-packed dirt, half rocky and rooty

HIKING TIME: 3.5–4.5 hours

SEASON: Year-round

ACCESS: Open daily, sunrise–sunset; road within park opens 8 a.m., closes 1 hour before sunset

MAPS: USGS Urbana, Buckeystown, Poolesville; map on free flyer available at preserve (also on Stronghold Web site)

FACILITIES: Water, phone at trailhead, with toilet nearby; toilet at East View parking lot; summer snack bar near West View lot (weekends, holidays)

FOR MORE INFORMATION: Contact Stronghold Inc., (301) 869-7846 or www.sugarloafmd.com

Directions

From junction of Capital Beltway (Interstate 495) and I-270 spur in Maryland, head northwest on I-270 (toward Frederick) for 22 miles. Get off at Exit 22, turn right onto MD 109, and head west for about 3 miles. Then turn right onto MD 95 (Comus Road) and proceed for 2.5 miles to small parking area at base of mountain, just outside entrance gate. If lot is full, drive to one of upper lots and start hike there (see map). *Note:* Gated entrance road closes 1 hour before sunset.

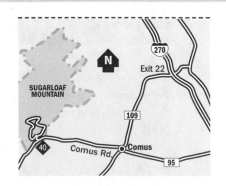

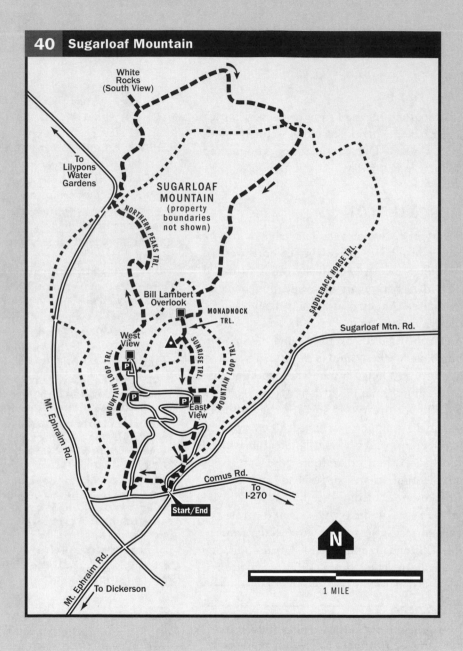

40 Sugarloaf Mountain

White Rocks (South View)

To Lilypons Water Gardens

SUGARLOAF MOUNTAIN (property boundaries not shown)

NORTHERN PEAKS TRL.

SADDLEBACK HORSE TRL.

Bill Lambert Overlook

MONADNOCK TRL.

Sugarloaf Mtn. Rd.

West View

SUNRISE TRL.

MOUNTAIN LOOP TRL.

MOUNTAIN LOOP TRL.

East View

Mt. Ephraim Rd.

Comus Rd.

To I-270

Start/End

Mt. Ephraim Rd.

To Dickerson

N

1 MILE

the mountain piecemeal, and turned it into a private preserve, complete with a vacation mansion. He opened the grounds to the walking public on weekends. He retired there in 1936. When he died in 1954, the estate was already in the hands of the present owner—his nonprofit foundation called Stronghold Inc.

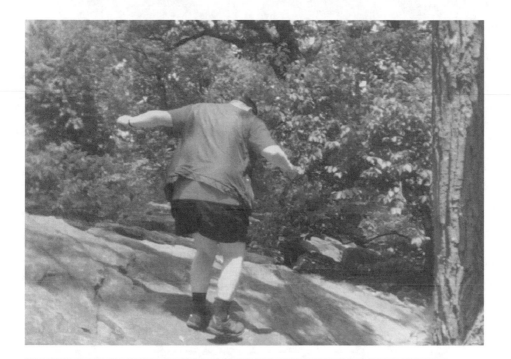

On visiting Sugarloaf, "DK," a German film director, broke into a jig (much as Jacques d'Amboise honored the Appalachian Trail).

This 8.1-mile woodland hike—essentially the same one that has long been promoted by the Potomac Appalachian Trail Club (PATC)—is a clockwise loop featuring 3,500 feet of elevation change and several superb overlooks, including the summit. The PATC-maintained trails are named, blazed, color coded, and signposted. To get started from the parking-lot trailhead, walk up the paved entrance road, pass between two small buildings, and turn left onto a paved path. Proceed past a "Smokey Says" sign, toilet, and shed. Detour to the left to see the remains of Strong's original cabin and his and his wife's simple crypt. Continuing, at the next paved road, turn left and follow it downhill for about 50 yards. Then turn right onto the combined white-blazed Mountain Loop Trail and yellow-blazed Saddleback Horse Trail. The two-in-one trail will take you into the oak-dominated woods typical of the hike route. At the next junction, go straight, staying on the gently climbing white-blazed trail. At the following junction, turn left onto the combined white-blazed trail and blue-blazed Northern Peaks Trail.

At the junction after that, stay to the left, on the blue-blazed trail, and follow it through the backcountry. Then head downhill to reach a short stretch of level and blue-blazed gravel road. Next, turn right onto a dirt trail and follow the blazes steeply uphill. At the next signposted junction, go straight (on what is actually a side trail), and proceed to White Rocks (South View); 3.3 miles into the hike, it's a superb place to linger and from which to admire the Frederick Valley. From there, return to the main, blue-blazed trail. Swing left and follow its undulating

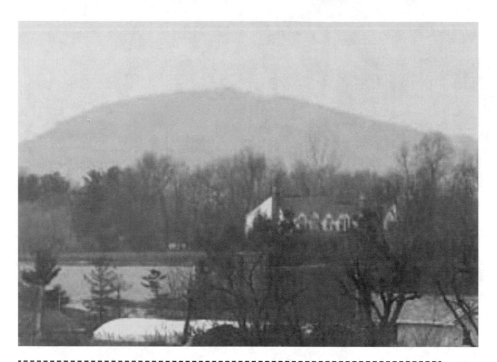

An outlier of the Blue Ridge, Sugarloaf is a huge and wooded slab of mostly quartzite that rises very distinctively above the plain.

course for about 2.5 miles. En route, you'll cross the yellow-blazed horse trail and encounter a large pile of rocks that gets reworked, sometimes creatively, by passing hikers. Later, after skirting or crossing several rocky outcrops, you'll traverse a dark grove of conifers.

At the next junction, stay left on what is again the combined blue- and white-blazed trail. Then, at the junction after that, turn right and head steeply uphill on the blue-blazed trail. At an intersection, turn right and head for the nearby Bill Lambert Overlook. Look around, and retrace your steps to cross the blue-blazed trail and head uphill on the red-blazed Monadnock Trail (geologically, Sugarloaf is a monadnock—an outlier of the Blue Ridge). Walk sharply uphill for several hundred yards to the summit, a flat and massive rock slab covering about an acre. Head for the tree- and bush-rimmed edge in search of viewing spots. Also, climb the highest nearby rock; at 1,282 feet above sea level, you'll be some 800 feet above the surrounding farmlands.

From the summit, head back down the red-blazed trail to the first junction, turn right onto the orange-blazed Sunrise Trail, and then walk down a steep hill. At East View, a popular picnicking area more than 400 feet lower than the summit, pause to take in more fine views. Then, turn left (eastward) onto a short connecting trail, and then turn right onto the white-blazed Mountain Loop Trail. Follow the white blazes downhill, carefully crossing a paved road twice (that's the road leading to the upper parking lots and areas of the mountain). On the way down, watch on your left for a glimpse of Gordon Strong's mansion, which is off-limits to scruffy hikers but can be rented for weddings and other events.

Use the map to devise shorter options for yourself. For instance, start at West View and do the Northern Peaks Trail in either direction for a 5.5-mile loop, or take the steep, green-blazed trail to the summit and return on the red-blazed and blue-blazed trails for a 1.5-mile loop.

NEARBY/RELATED ACTIVITIES

Consider supporting Stronghold Inc., the foundation that keeps Sugarloaf going (without benefit of government funding), by becoming a member or on-site volunteer; for details, contact the foundation (see page 193). Also ask about the status of the preserve's long-term research project to develop a blight-resistant American chestnut tree.

Detour to visit the Lilypons Water Gardens, which covers more than 300 seasonally colorful acres, sells aquatic plants and ornamental fish, and also mounts public events. Still owned by the same family, the business was started as a goldfish farm in 1917 by an opera buff who later named it for renowned coloratura Lily Pons. For driving directions and the events schedule, call (800) 999-5459 or visit the Web site, **www.lilypons.com.**

41 WOODSTOCK EQUESTRIAN PARK

KEY AT-A-GLANCE INFORMATION

LENGTH: 9.5 miles (with shorter options)

CONFIGURATION: Modified loop

DIFFICULTY: Moderate

SCENERY: Fields, woodlands

EXPOSURE: Mostly open; even more so in winter

TRAFFIC: Very light to light; relatively heavier in terms of four-footed traffic than two-footed traffic, especially on weekends, holidays

TRAIL SURFACE: Mostly grass, grass and dirt, or dirt, with some muddy stretches; some gravel stretches

HIKING TIME: 4.5–5.5 hours

SEASON: Year-round

ACCESS: Open daily, sunrise–sunset

MAPS: USGS Poolesville; ADC Montgomery County; sketch map posted at Web site below (but differs somewhat from trails on ground)

FACILITIES: Toilets, water at Owens Park recreation center (but access may be iffy); none at trailhead but likely to be built eventually

FOR MORE INFORMATION: Contact Montgomery County Departments of Park and Planning, www.mc-mnc ppc.org; call Friends of Woodstock, through Montgomery Parks Foundation, (301) 767-0002

IN BRIEF

A new equestrian park in western Montgomery County gives hikers free rein to roam serenely through woodland-fringed farmlands under open skies.

DESCRIPTION

From a hiker's perspective, Woodstock Equestrian Park is a lovely work in progress. The work consists of transforming two donated tracts of private farmland into an 824-acre Montgomery County park with two equestrian centers and some 15 miles of trails. Most of the trails have now been laid out, named, and signposted, and although the park won't open officially until late 2006 or 2007, hikers, equestrians, birders, and strollers (but not bikers) are already and equally welcome to use them. However more horsey the park may become in the future, it's presently one of the metro area's best farmland-hiking venues. And that's why I have devised a 9.5-mile hike, with about 1,350 feet of elevation change, to cover much of it. Follow my directions carefully, but be open to improvise on the trail as the park

----

Directions ——————————————————→

From junction of Capital Beltway (Interstate 495) and I-270 spur in Maryland, head northwest on I-270 (toward Frederick) for about 6 miles. Get off at Exit 6B in Rockville to get onto MD 28. Stay on MD 28 for about 17 miles as it successively becomes West Montgomery Avenue, Key West Avenue, and then Darnestown Road; then (0.8 miles after crossing Beallsville Road, or VA 109) turn right at signposted gates onto gravel entrance road of Dr. William Rickman Equestrian Center. Proceed for 0.2 miles to parking lot.

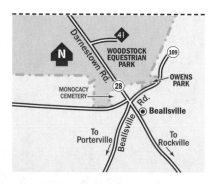

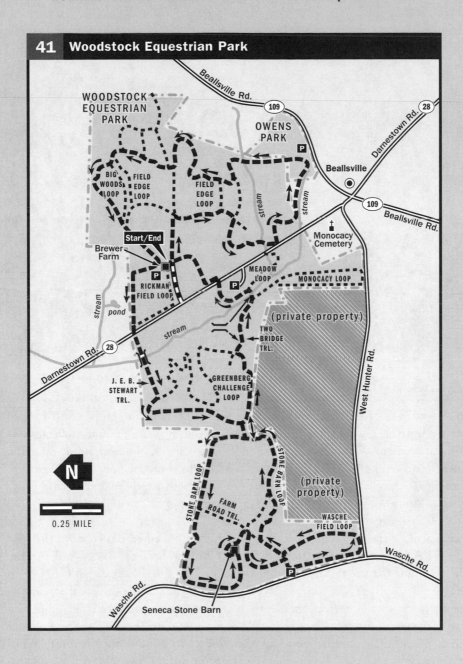

41 Woodstock Equestrian Park

evolves. And use my words and map to create shorter hike options. (*Note:* In warm weather, check for ticks after hiking.)

Just north of Poolesville and roughly 25 miles northwest of Washington, the park lies in the county's vaunted agricultural reserve—and also in horse country

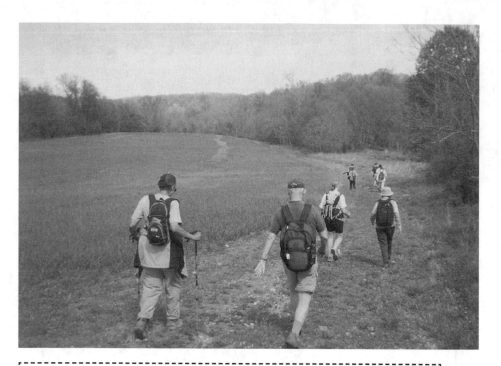

Hikers on the Greenberg Challenge Loop follow the edge of the woods that border open areas farmed under a lease arrangement.

(more than 10,000 horses live in the county). Most of the land is still farmed under lease arrangements with local farmers, and much of the trail mileage consists of broad mowed strips along the edges of the fields. Nonfarm flora and fauna also flourish in the park. The woods and hedgerows include oaks, hickories, beeches, dogwoods, maples, and some conifers, with a rich understory of bushes and wildflowers. The park also has a great variety of birds and butterflies.

I have organized the hike as five short legs starting at the parking lot for what will be the Dr. William Rickman Equestrian Center. To start on the first leg—1.6 miles to Owens Park—head east on the Straight Shot Trail. At the first signpost, turn right and follow the Field's Edge Loop uphill and then downhill to go straight onto a woodland trail that crosses a small stream to reach a four-way intersection. There, turn right and continue to the edge of a field, turn left onto the Potomac Hunt Loop, and follow the field edge uphill and then downhill. Near the bottom, turn left onto a faint trail leading uphill through open woods. When the trail disappears, bushwhack to the right to reach a grassy trail overlooking Darnestown Road. Swing left and take the trail down to a small clearing. Then turn left and head uphill to a T-junction. There, turn right and follow an old road downhill and then gently uphill alongside a small stream. At the top of the hill, swing left into Owens Park.

For the hike's second leg—a 2-miler back to the trailhead area—head north from the recreation center alongside a playing field. Then either take the new trail (if built) or bushwhack northward through the young woods, following the ribbon route markers. After crossing a stream, head uphill to reach a power-line right-of-way. There, turn left, walk 50 yards, and then turn left onto a trail that undulates through the woods to eventually reach a fork. There, turn right, march downhill to a T-junction, turn right, and keep going until you get to a large field and the Field's Edge Loop again. Proceed uphill, staying to the right, and cross the power-line right-of-way. Pause to take in the sweeping views.

Continue along the field edge, and go straight at the next two signposts to stay on the Field's Edge Loop. At the third one, bear left to stay on it. Then pass to the left of a line of young trees, and follow the field edge as it swings to the left. Next, at a Big Woods Loop signpost, take the dirt trail into the woods, turn right at the next T-junction, and press on. After passing a bullet-riddled old car, swing left at a signposted fork, and go straight through at the next T-junction (where the Big Woods Loop turns left). Stay on the unnamed main trail, cross the right-of-way again, and reach the edge of a field. Stay to the right along the field edge to reach the next signpost, where you'll see the trailhead parking lot on your left.

There, turn right to slip into the next field and begin the hike's third leg, which spans 1.3 miles. Follow the Rickman Field Loop to Darnestown Road, and cross carefully to get onto the undulating, gravel-surfaced J. E. B. Stewart Trail (surely the park planners meant "Stuart"). At the next signpost, turn left and then right to get onto the Greenberg Challenge Trail. Follow the field edge, and then swing left across a piece of the field to continue along the edge, keeping the woods on your right.

At the next signpost, start the hike's fourth leg, of 1.1 miles, by turning right and walking through the woods to reach yet another huge field, and turn right onto the Stone Barn Loop. Follow the field edge counterclockwise in a semicircle along the park's property line. En route, you'll cross the Farm Road Trail. Finally, you'll reach the Seneca Stone Barn, perched grandly on an open hillside. Built of local sandstone in the English style, it dates from around 1800 and remained in use until the 1950s.

Next, continue past the barn and downhill to start the hike's fifth leg, a wiggly 2-mile circuit. Stay on the Stone Barn Loop, but bear right to reach and turn right onto the Farm Road Trail. Proceed uphill and then swing right onto the Old Orchard Trail, which arcs through the woods and rejoins the old farm road. Turn right and then left to get to the Wasche Field Loop. Follow the field's perimeter counterclockwise, and then turn right onto the old farm road. Take it downhill until you get to a clearing on the right. There, take an unnamed trail into the woods, staying right at a fork, to rejoin the Stone Barn Loop. Turn right and proceed to where you started that loop. Turn right, go back through the woods, and return to the Greenberg Challenge Loop.

This time, go straight and downhill along a fence to start the hike's final, 1.5-mile leg. On reaching some woods, turn right onto the Two Bridges Trail, and follow it across a bridge to eventually reach the lobe of a large field. Cross the lobe, and follow its edge to the field. Staying to the left, walk uphill until you reach a signpost. There, turn left and cross the second bridge to reach a gravel path—the Meadow Loop—near a paved parking lot that will serve the future Moritz Greenberg Equestrian Center.

Turn left and follow the curving path until you get close to Darnestown Road; then cut across to the road, cross it carefully, and turn left. Then, just before a narrow bridge, veer right to bushwhack for about 40 yards across some rough and a small stream. Next, swing right and follow the edge of this final field to see what's left of the 19th-century Brewer Farm outbuildings. Finally, swing right to get onto the gravel road that leads about 100 yards to the trailhead parking lot.

NEARBY/RELATED ACTIVITIES

Return to further explore the evolving park. Visit historic Monocacy Cemetery (see the map). Consider joining the Friends of Woodstock; call (301) 767-0002 for more information.

CATOCTIN MOUNTAIN PARK AND CUNNINGHAM FALLS STATE PARK

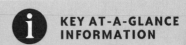

IN BRIEF

These two parks north of Frederick in Maryland's Blue Ridge region are endowed with a touch of wilderness, a sense of history, and exceptional vistas. They also enable hikers to practice three of Hugh Macintosh's four principles of optimal day hiking.

DESCRIPTION

Located scarcely 60 miles northwest of Washington, Catoctin Mountain Park and Cunningham Falls State Park let arriving visitors know immediately that they're far removed from the urban plains. The air is fresher and cooler, the sky is bigger, trees are everywhere, and the endless ridges rolling softly to the horizon evoke a sense of being in a mountain fastness. Such a place can be restorative, as I learned on a 1991 fall hike led by Louise Snell. Later, I expanded her route and also applied three of the four principles of optimal day hiking I deduced from hiking with Hugh Macintosh. They are 1) enjoy mountain vistas, 2) sustain a good pace but break for a leisurely lunch and short siesta, and 3) end a summer hike at or in water.

Directions ⟶

From junction of Capital Beltway (Interstate 495) and I-270 spur in Maryland, drive northwest on I-270 for about 32 miles to Frederick. There, turn right onto US 15 (Catoctin Mountain Highway) heading north and proceed for about 17 miles to Thurmont. There, take MD 77 exit ramp (on right), turn right at bottom of ramp, and proceed westward on MD 77 (Foxville Road) for about 3 miles. Turn right onto Park Central Road and into Catoctin Mountain Park. Then immediately turn right into visitor-center parking lot—or use overflow parking lot on left.

KEY AT-A-GLANCE INFORMATION

LENGTH: 11 miles (with shorter option)

CONFIGURATION: Loop

DIFFICULTY: Moderate

SCENERY: Wooded uplands, waterfall, sweeping vistas from overlooks

EXPOSURE: Mostly shady; less so in winter

TRAFFIC: Very light–light; heavier on warm-weather weekends, holidays; heaviest near falls, lake

TRAIL SURFACE: Mostly rocky or sandy; some boardwalk, pavement, grass; quite rooty

HIKING TIME: 6–8 hours (including vista, siesta, and lake time)

SEASON: Year-round, but best in fair fall weather on hunter-free Sundays

ACCESS: Open daily sunrise–sunset

MAPS: USGS Blue Ridge Summit, Catoctin Furnace; PATC Map 5; ADC Frederick Co.; sketch maps in free park brochure

FACILITIES: Toilets, water, phone at visitor center, park headquarters; toilets, water near Hog Rock

FOR MORE INFORMATION: Contact Catoctin Mountain Park, (301) 663-9388 or www.nps.gov/cato; and Cunningham Falls State Park, (301) 271-7574

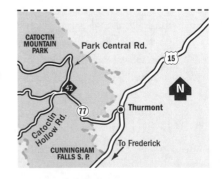

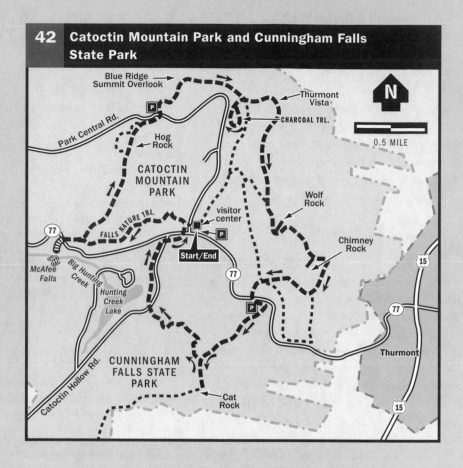

42 Catoctin Mountain Park and Cunningham Falls State Park

As alluring as it is, the Catoctin-Cunningham area is still recovering from severe despoliation. During the 19th century, Catoctin Mountain—an outlier in the eastern part of the Blue Ridge region—was stripped of timber chiefly for making charcoal for local iron-smelting furnaces, for which iron was mined nearby. Huge amounts of wood were needed. For instance, the amount of wood needed to make charcoal for 25 years for just the Catoctin Furnace (now a ruin in the state park) equaled all of the timber on an area much larger than that now covered by the two present parks combined. By 1900, much of the Thurmont area had been reduced to logged-over woodlots and submarginal farmlands. Three decades later, the federal government assembled more than 10,500 acres of land as a demonstration project—one of about 50 nationally—for restoring the environment and creating recreation facilities. In 1945 the demo area was transferred to the National Park Service (NPS). Nine years later, it was divided very roughly in half, with Maryland getting the southern portion for a state park and NPS retaining the rest as Catoctin National Park.

This 11-mile clockwise circuit loops through both parks and has a cumulative elevation change of about 2,100 feet. Try the hike in any season, but remember that hunting is allowed in Cunningham in the fall (except on Sundays), and that Catoctin's Park Central Road is closed in winter. That road is also closed at times because the park contains the out-of-sight presidential retreat known as Camp David (which began as Franklin D. Roosevelt's Shangri-La). And while hiking, stay out of the poison ivy, watch for snakes, and pay attention to the trail signposts and my directions. You'll find that the trails are generally kept in good working order and are well marked with signposts. Cunningham's trails are also blazed, but Catoctin's are not.

To get started from the visitor center, cross Park Central Road and then cross the overflow parking lot to pick up the Falls Nature Trail, on the right, and to disappear into the woods. After crossing a bridged stream and passing some large boulders, curve to the left and climb a short, rather steep slope. Going moderately uphill for about a mile, you'll traverse an area decorated with huge boulders. Some are as big as a bus, others merely car-sized.

After the trail noses downhill to link to a nameless trail, go left to detour a few hundred yards into the state park. Start by heading downhill to MD 77, turning left, and walking about 70 yards along the road. Then cross carefully into a parking lot. At the lot's far end, proceed on the boardwalk that follows Big Hunting Creek upstream to the base of one of Maryland's highest and loveliest waterfalls, known locally as McAfee Falls. Stay on the boardwalk both to protect the fragile riparian environment and to admire the stepped cascade easing 78 feet down the gorge. Then return along the boardwalk and unnamed trail and slip back into the national park. At the junction of choice, go straight through and uphill, toward Hog Rock.

On a northeasterly course, the trail gains some 600 feet in elevation while passing through areas of moss, grass, and rockiness. En route, watch on the right for a landmark tree—a tall and splendid sassafras. Note the species' odd habit of displaying three shapes of leaves, sometimes on the same branch. As Frederick Law Olmsted commented, sassafras is "very sportive in its form of foliage." In leafless winter, you'll know it by its much-furrowed, old-looking, red-brown bark. The trail then passes by a large rock formation on the right, descends, crosses a small streambed by bridge, and nips uphill to Hog Rock. There, on the hike's highest promontory (1,671 feet above sea level), take in the views. Then resume your journey and swing left. On reaching a fork, jog right and continue past a small boulder field.

Eventually, the trail smooths out into level grassiness. At Park Central Road, cross carefully and head for a well-appointed parking area (about 3 miles into the hike), complete with picnic tables, trash cans, water, and toilets. From there, follow the trail as it descends through maples and oaks, and rises toward the next viewpoint, the Blue Ridge Summit Overlook. As the trail turns left and runs along a squat rock ridge, you'll reach a plateau. Shortly thereafter, turn left onto a short side trail and see what the overlook looks over, including Pennsylvania.

Back on the main trail, turn left, and press on through the woods for about a mile as the path undulates and starts curving to the right, or south. At a four-way intersection, turn right to take a side trip on the Charcoal Trail. It's a self-guiding half-mile loop trail that explains the area's ruinous former industry. To get there from the main trail, head for a nearby parking area and, just past an interpretive sign, turn left onto the Charcoal Trail. Then return to the intersection, and go straight, heading east and south toward the next overlook, Thurmont Vista. At a fork, bear right to reach the vista and perch at the hike's 5-mile mark. Consider taking a Hugh Macintosh–style lunch break.

Continuing south for about three-quarters of a mile, follow a wooded ridgeline that's initially level but then descends. At a junction, stay to the left. At the next junction, turn left onto a short side trail leading to Wolf Rock. There, be careful about your footing, in that there are many deep crevices. And don't expect much of a view, because it has been greatly reduced by healthy tree growth. Back on the main trail, head for the next overlook, Chimney Rock, a half mile to the southeast. A right turn onto a short and rocky side trail leads to Chimney Rock along with its big boulders, deep crevices, and glorious views.

Returning to the main trail, stay and curve to the right and west as the trail pitches sharply downhill through an understory of mountain laurel. At a four-way intersection, go straight, continuing to descend, and reach MD 77 near the park headquarters, 7 miles into the hike. Cross the road to return again to the state park and to pick up the trail leading to the sixth and final overlook, Cat Rock. Alternatively, you can shorten the hike by 2.3 miles, down to 8.7 miles, by avoiding that trail and instead turning right to walk along the MD 77 shoulder to the visitor center.

The trek to Cat Rock is a somewhat strenuous haul of about a mile horizontally and about 600 feet vertically, on a yellow-blazed trail that swings west and south. Halfway up, notice but don't take an orange-blazed trail on the right. At the top, head for the main overlook, a noble rock formation to the right of the trail— and also where Hugh first showed me his technique for a postlunch catnap. Take in the view, but don't take the trail past Cat Rock. Instead, head back down the way you came. Then go left onto the orange-blazed trail. Follow it across the wooded slopes for just over a mile and steeply downhill to the Hunting Creek Lake area. If it's summer, note the inviting 43-acre lake and its sandy beach. At Catoctin Hollow Road, cross carefully, turn right, and proceed for just over half a mile to MD 77, staying on the left shoulder. Cross MD 77 even more carefully. Then turn right, and walk along the shoulder for a few hundred yards to the trailhead.

NEARBY/RELATED ACTIVITIES

After the hike, if it's summer and you've taken a long lunch and short nap at an overlook, abide by Hugh's third principle by cooling off in the lake. Then, when passing through Frederick, honor his fourth principle by having a microbrew at ambience-rich Jennifer's Restaurant, (301) 662-0373, located at 207 West Patrick Street, or at upscale-ish Zest, (301) 662-8171, located at 201 South Market Street. Then shop for used books at Wonder Book & Video, (301) 694-5955, located at 1306 West Patrick Street and open until 10 p.m. (but closed on Saturdays).

Contact both parks (see page 203) to learn about their various programs, which are conducted both outdoors and indoors.

In the summer or fall, stop in Thurmont to buy peaches and apples at Pryor's Orchard, (301) 271-2693; to get there from the trailhead, go back 2 miles on MD 77, turn left onto Pryor Road, go 0.5 miles, and turn left into the orchard.

In mid-October, linger in Thurmont to attend the Catoctin Colorfest, an annual arts-and-crafts show, **www.colorfest.org**.

43 PATUXENT RIVER PARK:
Jug Bay Natural Area

KEY AT-A-GLANCE INFORMATION

LENGTH: 7.5 miles (with shorter option)

CONFIGURATION: Modified loop

DIFFICULTY: Easy–moderate

SCENERY: Wooded hills, meadows, tidal marshes, river views

EXPOSURE: Shady; less so in winter

TRAFFIC: Usually very light to light; heavier on warm-weather weekends, holidays, near visitor center, in nature study area

TRAIL SURFACE: Mostly hard-packed sand; some pavement; short stretches of boardwalk, wood chips, mud

HIKING TIME: 3–4 hours

ACCESS: Open daily, 8 a.m.–posted closing time; day-use fee

MAPS: USGS Bristol, Lower Marlboro, free sketch map of Jug Bay available at visitor center

FACILITIES: Water, toilets, phone at visitor center

FOR MORE INFORMATION: Call Jug Bay park office, (301) 627-6074; visit www.pgparks.com/places/parks/jugbay.html

SPECIAL COMMENTS: Hunting is allowed, so call Jug Bay park office to ask where and when—but remember that Maryland has no-hunting-on-Sundays law

IN BRIEF

Plants and wildlife thrive in the scenic Jug Bay portion of Patuxent River Park, in Prince George's County, Maryland. Another life-form that does well in that setting is the visiting hiker.

DESCRIPTION

The Patuxent River, Maryland's longest in-state waterway, wriggles south for more than 100 miles through woodlands, wetlands, and farmlands—and urbanized areas—to reach Chesapeake Bay. Like the rest of the bay's watershed, it suffers from poor water quality and other environmental ills. Even so, under a program launched in the early 1960s, much of its river valley is protected as publicly owned and limited-use open space.

The program has also resulted in some fine hiking venues, such as Patuxent River Park. The park consists of several areas of great natural beauty dotted along the lower Patuxent. Of those, my choice is the delightful 2,000-acre Jug Bay Natural Area, some 20 miles southeast of Washington.

Directions

From Capital Beltway (Interstate 495 and I-95) near Forestville, Maryland, take Exit 11 and head southeast on MD 4 for 7.8 miles to Upper Marlboro. There, turn right onto MD 301 and head roughly south for 1.7 miles. Then turn left onto Croom Station Road and go 1.6 miles. Next, turn left onto Croom Road and go 1.5 miles. Then, at Patuxent River Park sign, turn left onto Croom Airport Road and drive east for 2.1 miles, passing Duvall Road (on left). At next park sign, turn left onto park entrance road. Drive 1.5 miles to parking lot near visitor center and park office.

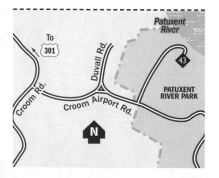

43 Patuxent River Park: **Jug Bay Natural Area**

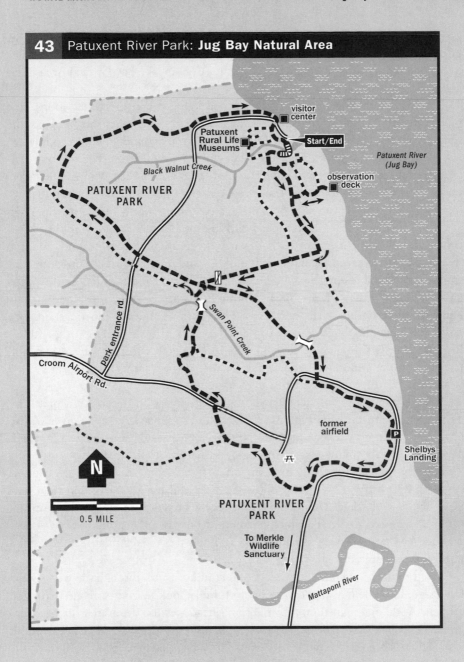

Named for a lakelike stretch of the river, the Jug Bay Natural Area is well equipped with scenery, vistas, trails, and especially birds. Except for birders and hikers, though, most visitors focus on other attractions, such as the visitor center, several buildings known as the Patuxent Rural Life Museums, and a nature study area. Adjoining the area is the Merkle Wildlife Sanctuary, a large state-owned preserve renowned for its bird life. Together, the two areas form one of the finest mid-Atlantic birding spots, so take along field glasses and reference books. The two areas are also linked by the worth-taking Chesapeake Bay Critical Area Driving Tour.

This 7.5-mile hike consists of a modified loop, or pair of stacked loops. The mostly woodland trails wind through rolling hills and wetland marshes, and past the site of a historic airfield. Mud, bugs, and poison ivy are common, but steep hills are not—and the hike's elevation change totals only about 600 feet. The Jug Bay Natural Area's trails are not blazed, but most of them are marked with simple directional signs. However, there are trail stretches, especially at the beginning, that are short on such signage, so you should make attentive use of my directions and map.

To get started from the trailhead parking lot, directly across from the visitor center, head down a gravel path toward the museum complex and into the woods. Pause at or pass the museum buildings, and then turn right onto an inconspicuous dirt trail leading steeply downhill. At the bottom, turn left and proceed along a dirt trail through the Black Walnut Creek Study Area, a lush and marshy tangle of trees, bushes, ferns, and vines. Then turn right at a T-junction and keep going, on a winding boardwalk that spans the creek. Turn right at a fork, and follow the boards through the marsh. When you reach the foot of a steep hill, pause to survey a pond on your right. In the warm-weather months, it's filled with cattails, other aquatic plants, and noisy amphibians.

Next, climb a set of steps on the left, pausing at an observation platform. Then continue to the top of the rise on a rather rooty path that soon gives way to a wide trail of hard-packed sand with large trees overhead. At a junction, turn left and head roughly south, passing through another junction.

At the junction after that, turn left off the main trail to take a detour of about 200 yards round-trip. Follow the side trail for 50 yards, and then turn right to bushwhack downhill next to a gully on your right. At the bottom, turn right onto a dirt trail, which becomes a boardwalk leading to a two-story wooden observation deck overlooking Jug Bay's freshwater tidal marshes and a vista that probably has not changed in a century.

Return to the main trail, turn left, and continue south through the woods on a low ridge. In the fall, as the leaves start to tumble, look for views of the bay off to the left. At the next junction, turn right and head west on a trail that ranges from level to undulating. Arriving at yet another junction, go straight, and be prepared for mud if there's been rain recently. About 80 yards after passing a gate, you'll reach the intersection that serves as the hike's central node—and to which you'll be returning.

Turn left there and go straight at a junction about 50 yards down the trail. About a quarter-mile along, there's an often wet and muddy stretch of trail. Approaching Swan Point Creek, you'll go downhill. Don't take the apparent path to your right, but step carefully along the wider, rooty section on the left. Cross the bridges spanning the creek's two branches, keep going, and then ascend the creek bank to reach level ground.

Continuing through the open woods, you'll reach Croom Airport Road (part of the driving-tour route). Cross the road and then, at a directional sign, turn left onto a wide, grassy path. Keep going, and in a few yards, you'll be out in the open in a huge, pancake-flat field that is currently leased and cultivated by a local farmer. You'll also be walking along the perimeter of what was the country's first black-owned and -operated airfield. Opened as Riverside Field in 1941 by John W. Greene Jr., it was used for wartime flight training until 1944. Later reopened by Greene as the Columbia Air Center, the facility was permanently closed in 1958.

Follow the perimeter hedgerow to the corner of the field, and then turn right at a directional sign. Continuing, you'll have the field on your right (and note the lone tree out there) and the paved road on your left. When you see a Shelbys Landing sign on the left, cross the road to detour about 100 yards down to a small dock to peruse the bay. Then return to continue along the edge of the field. Watch for and take an unpaved old road leading into the woods on the left. Go about 150 yards and turn right onto a narrow dirt trail marked by a directional sign. Proceed on that trail as it snakes through the woods. Go straight through a four-way intersection. Eventually you'll reach Croom Airport Road again, and be at the hike's halfway point.

There, turn left and walk along the shoulder. Watch on the right for a green gate. Cross to walk past the gate and onto yet another muddy stretch of trail. Then, at a T-junction where there's a sign saying that the trail straight ahead is only for hikers, swing left instead. Proceeding, cross entrenched Swan Point Creek again by approaching it on a steep and pebbly trail segment and then leaving it on a rocky and rutted segment. Next, swing right at a fork, and then turn left at the next T-junction. At the T-junction 70 yards after that, turn left and walk another 70 yards to reach the hike's central node again. Go straight through to reach the park entrance road.

Cross the road, walk past a set of posts, and proceed on an old roadway set between steep banks. But then the trail rises and levels off. At the next junction, turn right. The trail leads to a field and a grassy path. There, turn right and continue across the partly open field, and then scoot back under the trees.

As the path curves east, you'll go past several side trails on the left and then get a final go at a very muddy stretch of trail. At the park entrance road, swing left and follow it for about a third of a mile to the trailhead.

To shorten your hike by 2.5 miles, down to 5 miles, you can cut off a portion by turning right on first reaching Croom Airport Road, and then heading west on a 0.6-mile connecting trail (shown on the map) to turn right onto the main trail and continue.

NEARBY/RELATED ACTIVITIES

Explore the Patuxent Rural Life Museums, which are generally open on Sunday afternoons from April through October. They include a tool museum, blacksmith shop, tobacco farming museum, and 1880s log cabin. In the warm-weather months, sign up for a guided birding walk, nature hike, or (best of all) a sunset boat tour. Or take a rental canoe or kayak out on the bay. Call the Jug Bay park office for details (see page 208).

After doing the hike, roam at least some of the adjoining 1,670-acre Merkle Wildlife Sanctuary (entrance fee). Be sure to visit the observation platform, which, I have been assured (by naturalist GB Ludwig), is a fine spot for birding, napping, and cooing. Also stop by at the visitor center. For information and directions, call the sanctuary, (301) 888-1410 or visit **www.dnr.state.md.us/ publiclands/southern/merkle.html.**

Take the 4-mile Chesapeake Bay Critical Area Driving Tour between Jug Bay and Merkle (you can also hike or bike it). Call the Jug Bay office or sanctuary for details.

PISCATAWAY PARK 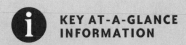 44

IN BRIEF

Piscataway Park, in Prince George's County, preserves the view across the Potomac River from Mount Vernon. But hikers can also use it to trek through both the past and present.

DESCRIPTION

In the late 18th century, the view across the Potomac River from George Washington's Mount Vernon estate was one of woods and cultivated fields. More than two centuries later, it still is.

A mix of private and public actions saved the developmentally challenged shoreline lying only 14 miles south of the White House. In the early 1950s, local groups and citizens launched an effort to protect it. Then, in 1961, Congress authorized Piscataway Park to preserve "the historic and scenic values . . . of lands which provide the principal overview." Using more easements than ownership, the

- -

Directions ———————————➤

From Capital Beltway (Interstate 495 and I-95) in Oxon Hill, take Exit 2 or Exit 3 and long exit ramp to get onto southbound MD 210 (Indian Head Highway). Proceed about 8.3 miles, and then turn right onto exit ramp leading to Bryan Point Road. Follow service road, and turn right onto Bryan Point Road. If you miss exit ramp, turn right at next traffic light onto Livingston Road; then turn right onto Biddle Road and left onto Bryan Point Road. Proceed 3.5 miles. After passing Cactus Hill Road on left, continue for about 200 yards. At "All Visitors" sign, turn right onto gravel road and proceed 100 yards to parking lot near visitor center (pay entrance fee there). On leaving park, use Biddle and Livingston to get back onto MD 210.

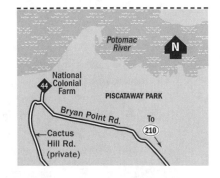

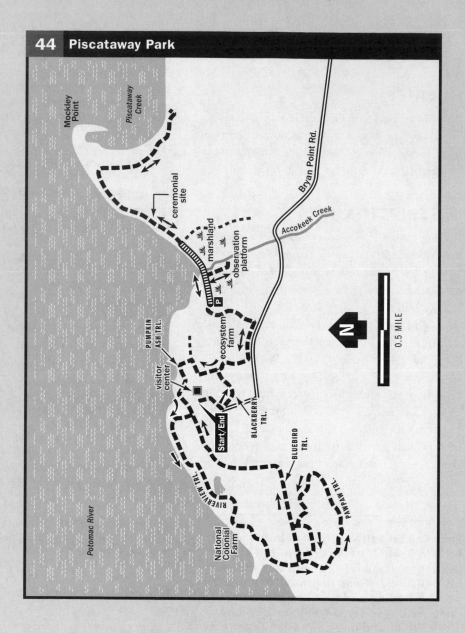

44 Piscataway Park

Mockley Point

Piscataway Creek

Bryan Point Rd.

Accokeek Creek

ceremonial site

marshland

observation platform

P

PUMPKIN ASH TRL.

ecosystem farm

visitor center

BLACKBERRY TRL.

Start/End

BLUEBIRD TRL.

RIVERVIEW TRL.

PAWPAW TRL.

National Colonial Farm

Potomac River

N

0.5 MILE

present-day park extends along the riverbank for about 6 miles and covers about 5,000 acres.

This hike is a country ramble in an area where past and present mingle. It includes a reconstructed colonial-era farm featuring now-rare crops and livestock breeds, as well as a modern organic farm. Among its other attractions are views of Mount Vernon, a Native American ceremonial site, an arboretum, and a marsh. The mostly level, 8.5-mile hike is only partially blazed and signposted, so follow my directions closely, especially on the segment after the colonial farm. Also, expect little shade and a bit of mud.

To get started from the trailhead parking lot, walk back to the paved road. Turn left onto the grassy shoulder and walk along the edge of the woods for about 50 yards. Turn left onto the Blackberry Trail at a half-hidden trail sign. Follow the purple blazes through the woods.

At the far side, you'll reach the fenced-in, eight-acre Robert Ware Straus Ecosystem Farm. It develops improved methods of intensive and sustainable organic farming. Like the colonial farm, it's run by the Accokeek Foundation at Piscataway Park, which also manages the park's trails and visitor center for the National Park Service.

Touch not the electrified antideer fence. Turn right to walk along it. At the end, turn right onto an open gravel road. At a paved road (Bryan Point Road), turn left, and follow the shoulder for 200 yards, staying left. Then, at the "Tayac" sign, turn left onto a dirt road and follow it through fields going wild. Cross a parking lot onto a woodland path, then settle in for a scenic hike of just over a mile along the river. The hike begins with a boardwalk jaunt across a large freshwater tidal marsh fed by Accokeek Creek.

In the warm-weather months, the marsh is a green carpet dotted with color, mostly the red, pink, or white blooms of flowering plants and the wing patches of red-winged blackbirds. Water birds ply the shore. Insects create a sonic background for the boom of a bullfrog or the whistle of an osprey. In winter, you'll mostly experience browns, grays, and silence. The browns may well include bald eagles.

After the marsh, you'll pass through a small wooded swamp and then step off the planks and onto a paved woodland path. About 20 yards later, step into the open at a junction with an unpaved farm road. Turn left and follow the road along the riverbank to the site of a large, precolonial Piscataway village. The area remains sacred to the villagers' descendants, who gather there each spring for a ceremony. Pause to view the ceremonial wigwam, other artifacts, and the plaque honoring Chief Turkey Tayac (1895–1978).

Continuing, stay near the river, which is shielded by thickets. The passing fields are part of a special farm where schoolchildren learn about farming and ecology. Eventually, you'll enter some woods and leave the river as the road swings right. When you next reach the water, it'll be at Piscataway Creek's estuary—also the turnaround spot, 2.25 miles into the hike. Look around, and note the bushes brightened in summer by honeysuckle flowers, butterflies, and dragonflies (and poetically remember the dragonfly hanging like a blue thread loosed from the sky). On the estuary's far side, look for mammoth Fort Washington, built in 1824 to guard the river approach to the capital. Then begin your return to the ecosystem farm. En route, just after the end of the boardwalk, detour for a quarter-mile round trip into the marsh on a trail bordering Accokeek Creek. Watch on the left for an observation platform. Use it to marsh gaze, and then walk back.

At the ecosystem farm, again, change course. First, you'll proceed along the fence all the way to the end. Then turn right along a second fence line. Turn left at the second side trail, near bluebird box number 42; and walk to the riverbank. There, at the farm's solar power generator, eyeball Mount Vernon, turn left, and follow the grassy riverbank path.

At a trail junction (that's the Blackberry Trail again, on the left), proceed on the signposted and yellow-blazed Pumpkin Ash Trail, which leads a half mile to the visitor center. From the center, head west on a dirt path. Just before getting to an avenue of cedars, turn right onto the signposted Riverview Trail. It's an open, blue-blazed, mowed-in-season grassy trail that's 0.8 miles long but hidden from the river by thickets. On approaching a fenced enclosure, leave the trail to turn right and then right again to take a stairway to the boat dock. The dock provides a fine view of Mount Vernon year-round.

Back on the main trail, detour to the enclosure known as the Museum Garden. A key part of the National Colonial Farm, it features plants grown and used by the colonists. Later you'll see more of the farm and perhaps some staff members and volunteers, who wear period garb and interact informatively with visitors.

After leaving the garden, turn left, walk to the end of the fence, and turn right onto a gravel road. After passing the caretaker's residence, a driveway, and an old out-kitchen on the right, leave the road and swing right onto a grassy trail (part of the Riverview Trail). Follow it past a pond on the left. Then swing sharply right and head into the woods on a dirt trail. Soon after crossing a stream and out in the open again, turn right at the first of six junctions and walk past overgrown fields. Turn right at the next junction. Turn right at the third junction, along the shore, and swing left along the edge of the woods. Turn right at the fourth junction, out in the open. Turn right at the fifth junction (ignore the trail sign pointing straight ahead to the Bluebird Trail), and walk about 50 yards uphill—to the sixth junction. There, turn right and then left onto the signposted and white-blazed Pawpaw Trail. It's a narrow dirt trail that arcs for half a mile through a hilly and heavily wooded area. Watch for labeled trees, mature trees, baby trees (especially pawpaws), wildflowers, and poison ivy.

The Pawpaw Trail ends at the upper edge of a mowed area dotted with labeled young trees and shrubs representing more than 125 species that grew in southern Maryland in the colonial era. They make up the park's six-acre Native Tree Arboretum, started in the 1980s. Roam among the plants and then follow the edge of the woods westward (away from the Pawpaw Trail). Turn left onto a gravel road (part of the Bluebird Trail), walk ten yards, and turn left again onto a grassy path to semicircle around what park literature alleges is a chestnut grove. Continuing, you'll arrive at the junction of the Pawpaw Trail and the short trail up from the Bluebird Trail. This time, turn right onto the short trail and then right again onto the blue-blazed Bluebird Trail, and head out into the open.

Follow the road east, between a pasture on the left and the lower part of the arboretum on the right. Beyond the pasture, turn sharply left to stay on the gravel road and Bluebird Trail. Heading north, follow the road as it swings right past some stables and reaches a junction. There, turn sharply left and continue, following the blue blazes past the farm's livestock area. Then pass the driveway again. Continue, keeping the Museum Garden on your left, and head down the cedar avenue that leads to the start of the Riverview Trail. At the end of the avenue, detour through a gate on the right to circle past the colonial farm's old farmhouse, out-kitchen, smokehouse, "necessary" (outhouse), and kitchen garden. Then return to the trailhead.

NEARBY/RELATED ACTIVITIES

Tour the colonial farm, attend a special event (such as African-American Heritage Day, in August), or become a volunteer; contact the foundation for details (see page 213).

45 AMERICAN CHESTNUT LAND TRUST LANDS

KEY AT-A-GLANCE INFORMATION

LENGTH: 7.6 miles (with shorter options)

CONFIGURATION: Modified loop

DIFFICULTY: Easy–moderate

SCENERY: Woodlands, wetlands, fields, old farm buildings, historic cemetery

EXPOSURE: Mostly shady; less so in winter

TRAFFIC: Very light to light

TRAIL SURFACE: Chiefly dirt or grass; some pavement, boardwalk

HIKING TIME: 4.5–5.5 hours

SEASON: Year-round but best from fall to spring

ACCESS: Open daily, dawn–dusk

MAPS: USGS Prince Frederick, Broomes Island; sketch map in South Side brochure available at trailhead, on Web site below (trailhead's crude wall map is unreliable)

FACILITIES: None at trailhead; toilet nearby at Gravatt Lane–Swamp Trail junction

FOR MORE INFORMATION: Contact office of American Chestnut Land Trust, (410) 414-3400 or www .acltweb.org; collect trail guides and other printed materials at trailhead and also at North Side Trailhead

IN BRIEF

In Maryland's Calvert County, a beautiful undeveloped stream valley and adjoining lands have been preserved for the benefit of the environment, community, and posterity—and hikers and others who know where to go.

DESCRIPTION

Parkers Creek winds across central Calvert County some 40 crow-miles southeast of Washington as the last remaining undeveloped stream on Chesapeake Bay's western shore. It's the heart of a 2,700-acre protected area of old tobacco farmlands, woodlands, and marshes that's managed by the American Chestnut Land Trust on behalf of the Nature Conservancy, the State of Maryland, and itself (the ACLT owns 810 acres). Created in 1986 by local citizens averse to subdivisional encroachment, the ACLT takes care of the environment and its wealth of plants and animals, runs educational programs, attracts volunteers, leases fields to local farmers, preserves old farm structures, and welcomes visitors.

Although public access is limited, there are modest but separate trail systems both

---

Directions ⟶

From Capital Beltway (Interstate 495) near Forestville, Maryland, take Exit 11 to get onto MD 4 heading roughly south. Proceed for 35.1 miles to Prince Frederick, initially on MD 4 and then on combined MD 2/4. After crossing MD 402, stay on MD 2/4 for 5 miles to turn left onto Parkers Creek Road. Go 0.5 miles (crossing MD 765 en route), and turn right onto Scientists' Cliffs Road. Go 0.8 miles and, at three-way road intersection, turn left at American Chestnut Land Trust signpost into parking lot.

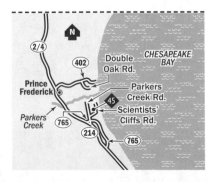

45   American Chestnut Land Trust Lands

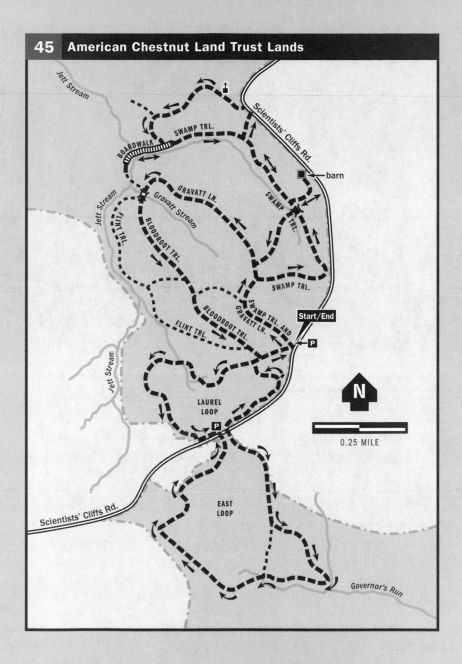

north and south of Parkers Creek. The South Side system is better suited for a longer circuit hike (7.6 miles, with about 1,200 feet of elevation change)—and that's what I present here. The trails are named, mostly color coded, mostly sign-posted, and nicely edged with poison ivy. Follow my directions carefully, and use them and my map to create shorter hikes for yourself. (See my suggestion below

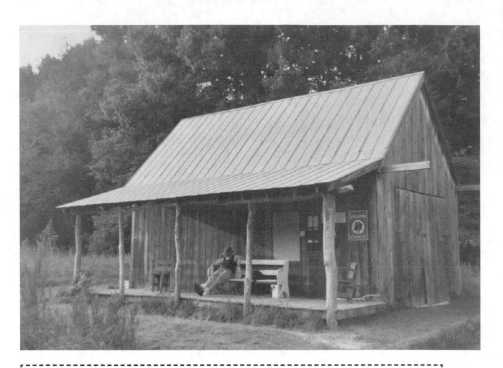

The barn at this hike's trailhead is equipped with trail guides and other materials, and a porch where hikers may safely snooze.

about the North Side.) *Note:* Some hunting is allowed (but never on Sunday), so call ACLT; sign in at both trailhead and East Loop; guard against and check for ticks; and finish hiking by dusk—otherwise, ACLT's posse may come looking for you.

To get started, head for the nearby small barn, sign the register, and take some brochures (including the North Side guide and the bird list). Then get onto the combined Gravatt Lane (red blazes) and Swamp Trail (yellow blazes), which extends perpendicular to the road. After about 300 yards, swing right at a woodland fork to stay on the combined trail. Then pass a fine wood privy, go about 100 yards, and turn right to stay on the Swamp Trail for about 0.6 miles as it winds through a mature woodland area.

Next, at a T-junction where there's a dirt side trail signposted "to the chestnut tree" and a small bridge, be patient and proceed on the main trail for 60 yards. Then, at a "to the Howard Farm site" sign, turn right onto a dirt side trail to do a 0.3-mile out-and-back detour to see a now-dilapidated 19th-century barn. To get there, take the trail uphill to a clearing, turn left, and continue uphill to circle the barn.

Then, on returning to the Swamp Trail, turn right and proceed for about 300 yards to a sign that promises a cemetery and Scientists' Cliff Road. There, turn right onto a dirt trail that goes uphill some 200 yards to the road. Then turn left along the road shoulder, go 20 yards, and turn left onto Cemetery Lane. Follow it uphill about 80 yards to the quaint and restored Hance-Chesley Cemetery. Read the dozen headstones, and use the information board and pamphlet box to put them into historical context.

Then continue into the woods and along a ridgeline on the initially grassy Cemetery Lane. After 0.3 miles, turn left at a T-junction (after noting that the trail you won't be on is, according to a droll trailside sign, "Beyond the graveyard (dead end)." Then head downhill on a dirt trail for about 300 yards to reach the Swamp Trail at a boardwalk T-junction. In a steep section en route, try using the novel rope handrail.

Next, turn right to do a 0.4-mile out-and-back through a heavily wooded and overgrown wetland area where the Swamp Trail lives up to its name, thanks to some energetic beavers. Stay on the long narrow boardwalk and a short piece of dirt trail until your way is blocked by a "the beavers did it" trail sign. Reverse direction and return to the boardwalk T-junction. From there, continue straight on the Swamp Trail for 0.5 miles, passing the side trails to the cemetery and the barn, and then turning right at the "chestnut" bridge to get onto a gently rolling and unnamed dirt trail.

After 220 yards, you'll be in the presence of a rarity—a mature, living American chestnut that's also the largest in Maryland. It's officially 75 feet high but is enveloped by other trees and seems sickly. Even so, it continues to bear burrs (if not viable seeds) and serves as a poignant reminder of the loss of America's great chestnut forests—and, I suspect, as the symbolic root of the land trust's name. Then resume your journey for 180 yards to reach Gravatt Lane. There, turn right to follow that red-blazed trail for about 0.6 miles to Gravatt Stream. En route, pause on the bluff overlooking the swamp, and then descend to the bridge spanning the stream.

Just before the bridge, note on the right the other end of the closed-by-beavers Swamp Trail. On leaving the bridge, you'll be on the Bloodroot Trail (also blazed red) for about 0.6 miles as it passes the Flint Trail (yellow) and ascends gently to reach and follow a wooded ridge. On reaching the Wallace Lane signpost, detour for a 220-yard out-and-back look at the remains of an African American–owned tobacco farm that existed for almost a century, until 2001. Then continue on the main trail as it is rejoined by the Flint Trail and descends gently to reach the Laurel Loop.

Next, turn right to spend about 0.75 miles on the wiggly Laurel Loop—and be sure to follow the white blazes and ribbons. It snakes through an area of scrubby deciduous woodlands with scruffy conifers, crosses what feels like a mountain laurel plantation, drops down to a floodplain, climbs the entire hike's most serious hill, runs behind some backyards, jolts across a couple of deep gullies, and deposits you on Scientists' Cliffs Road. There, turn left and walk along the shoulder for 120 yards to where there's a parking area and, in back, a white blaze and trail sign for your later use.

Cross the road carefully, get onto a grassy avenue next to a large oak tree, and proceed to a pair of signs, one identifying the East Loop and the other asking you to register. Do so, and then embark on a scenic, easy-to-follow, 1.6-mile, clockwise, and green-blazed loop that undulates through hilly woodlands. Eventually you'll reach the road close to where you started. Cross carefully to get onto the last piece of the Laurel Loop, and follow the white blazes through the woods for 0.5 miles to the trailhead by way of the loop's junction with the Bloodroot Trail.

NEARBY/RELATED ACTIVITIES

Do sample the North Side tract and Parkers Creek. To get there from the South Side, return to Prince Frederick, turn right onto MD 402 (Dares Beach Road), go 2.3 miles, turn right onto Double Oak Road, go 0.8 miles, turn left at the "Double Oak farm" sign, and proceed for 0.3 miles to the parking area and trailhead. Sign in and take a North Side brochure.

Following the brochure's map, walk back along the entrance road, turn left onto the main road, and then take the red-blazed Double Oak Road Trail downhill through the woods to the creek. There, launch the waiting guest canoe, and go explore the truly glorious creek. Then either return to the trailhead the way you came (2.6 miles round-trip) or take an alternative route (hint: there's another canoe at the old creek-bridge site).

Consider becoming an ACLT volunteer or member. Participate in the trust's open-to-the-public events, which include guided canoe trips on Parkers Creek and are posted on the ACLT Web site (see page 218).

APPALACHIAN TRAIL:
Weverton to Gathland State Park 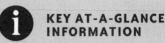 46

IN BRIEF

This outing on South Mountain in western Maryland offers hikers superb views as a reward for a strenuous climb. It also includes an easy ridgetop trail segment, plus an unusual memorial.

DESCRIPTION

South Mountain forms part of the Blue Ridge portion of Maryland and adjoining Pennsylvania. Logged and fought over in the 19th century, much of it is now protected within several Maryland state parks known collectively as the South Mountain Recreation Area. Threading through the area is a 40-mile strip of the Appalachian Trail (AT).

This somewhat challenging out-and-back AT hike features South Mountain's southernmost portion, which rises above the Potomac River in a series of high cliffs. The area, broadly straddling the line between Washington and Frederick counties, lies roughly 60 miles northwest of Washington, D.C. The north-to-south hike is 13.8 miles long (including about a half mile of side trips) and accumulates about 3,000 feet of elevation change between the trailhead at the foot of the mountain and the state-park

KEY AT-A-GLANCE INFORMATION

LENGTH: 13.8 miles

CONFIGURATION: Out-and-back

DIFFICULTY: Quite hard

SCENERY: Mountain woodlands, farmland views, Potomac panorama

EXPOSURE: Mostly shady; less so in winter

TRAFFIC: Usually light; heavier on cliffs and in park on warm-weather weekends, holidays

TRAIL SURFACE: Mostly rocky, with dirt; some rooty, grassy stretches; pavement in park

HIKING TIME: 6.5–8 hours

SEASON: Year-round

ACCESS: No AT restrictions; Gathland State Park open daily, sunrise–sunset

MAPS: USGS Keedysville, Harpers Ferry; PATC Map 6

FACILITIES: None at trailhead; toilet at trail shelter; water, phone, toilets at Gathland

FOR MORE INFORMATION: Contact Appalachian Trail Conservancy, in Harpers Ferry, (304) 535-6331 or www.appalachiantrail.org; and South Mountain Recreation Area, in Boonsboro, (301) 791-4767 (for annual Adventure Guide, send 83¢ SASE to SMRA, 21843 National Pike, Boonsboro, MD 21713)

Directions

From junction of Capital Beltway (Interstate 495) and I-270 spur in Maryland, drive northwest for 31 miles on I-270 to Frederick. At exit 32, swing right to get onto I-70. Proceed for 0.4 miles and, at next fork, stay to left to get onto I-70 heading west. Proceed for 0.9 miles, and then turn right at next fork (I-70 exit 52) to get onto US 340 heading west. Proceed for about 14.5 miles. Then turn right onto MD 67, go 0.1 mile, turn right onto Weverton Road, and go 0.2 miles to gravel parking area on right.

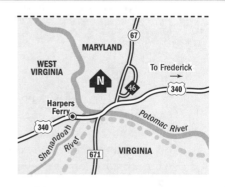

46 Appalachian Trail: **Weverton to Gathland State Park**

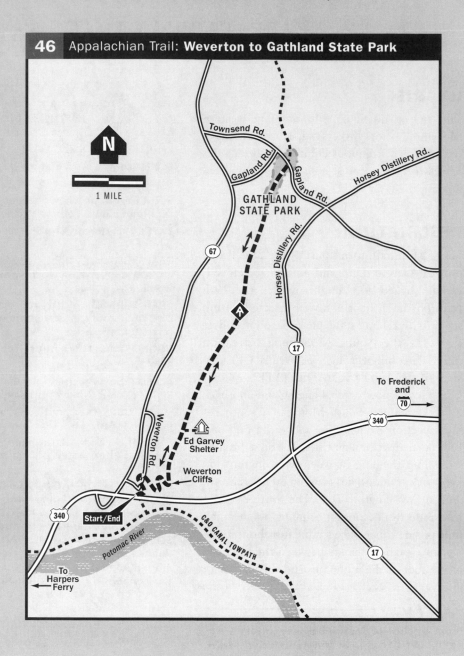

turnaround spot at Crampton Gap. The gap was the site of a September 1862 engagement that was one of several known collectively as the battle of South Mountain. Two decades after the Civil War, the Crampton Gap area was bought by a wealthy writer and ex-war correspondent named George Albert Townsend, who turned it into a mountain retreat of eccentric design. He named it Gathland,

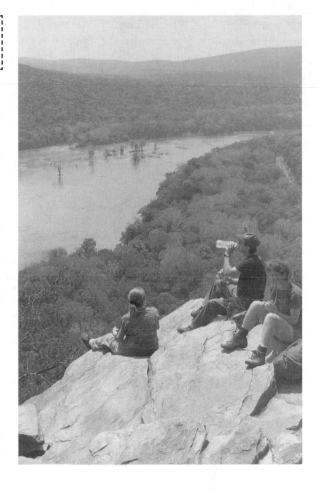

Although you're going to have to chug uphill to reach this spot on Weverton Cliffs, you'll get views that are unrivaled in the metro area.

based on his pseudonym, "Gath" (his initials plus *h*) and the biblical city of Gath. He later spiraled into poverty and died, as did his estate. Eventually acquired by the state, the estate became the 135-acre Gathland State Park in 1958.

The hike route passes through mostly deciduous woodlands that provide shade and greenery during the growing season, later turn beautifully autumnal, and then open up in leafless winter. Flowers, ferns, and wildlife add to the seasonal variety. So does poison ivy, so stay on the trail. My preferred fall clothing color is orange, because the no-hunting-allowed AT right-of-way is narrow.

To get started at Weverton, go to the eastern end of the parking lot and take the path that leads just a few yards to the white-blazed AT. Turn left onto the trail and follow it to Weverton Road. After crossing the road (carefully), head for the utility pole where the AT plunges into the woods and then starts going uphill. The trail gains 500 feet in elevation as a mile-long series of switchbacks. En route, detour onto a rocky, signposted, and blue-blazed side trail on the right. Follow it downhill for about 200 yards to Weverton Cliffs, which has, in the late Ed Garvey's words, "one of the most spectacular views along the entire [AT]." On a clear day, you'll get a panoramic view of the Potomac River Valley and environs, especially if you have field glasses. In the fall, watch for migrating hawks, streaming by on a northwest wind, sometimes at eye-to-eye level. Then retrace your steps to the AT.

Continue up the trail as it rises steadily for several hundred feet over the next mile to reach and follow South Mountain's narrow crest line. After about a half mile more, you'll reach a signpost, which points right, toward one of the overnight shelters that dot the AT. Walk a hundred yards and check out the shelter's construction, views (especially in winter), and colorful logbook (trail register).

Completed in 2001, the Ed Garvey Memorial Shelter honors a man who lived, breathed, through-hiked, and wrote up the AT for decades. Volunteers led by master builder Frank Turk erected the shelter and its matching privy and the Roberto Reyes memorial campfire benches.

Beyond the shelter, the trail pitches up and down a bit as it threads through the ridgetop woods for 3.8 miles to Gathland State Park. Here and there, a fleeting view is to be had, usually in winter, but the basic scenery is of the restful green-tunnel variety. You may see deer and wild turkeys—or evidence of them. Be sure to stay with the white blazes. Eventually, the trail noses gently downhill into the state park. There, follow a paved roadway for a few hundred yards to reach a 50-foot-high structure that marks the hike's turnaround. Townsend (Gath) erected it as a memorial to his fellow war correspondents. Then follow the white blazes for 6.7 miles back to the Weverton trailhead.

NEARBY/RELATED ACTIVITIES

During or after the hike, explore Gathland State Park and its collection of Townsend memorabilia and display boards. To learn more about the Appalachian Trail, see Hike 59, page 285.

APPALACHIAN TRAIL:
Interstate 70 to Turners Gap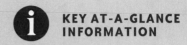

IN BRIEF

This hike, in the central section of South Mountain in western Maryland, provides a ridgetop woodland outing, a short climb in a George Washington monument that doubles as an observation tower, and the chance of having a cooked lunch indoors.

DESCRIPTION

This Appalachian Trail (AT) hike focuses on the part of South Mountain that lies roughly 20 miles north of the Potomac River and some 60 miles northwest of Washington. The hike route extends south from where I-70 and US 40 cross the mountain, winds serenely through the woods, and traverses Washington Monument State Park, where you can practice your vista vision (take along field glasses). What you'll see most on this 10.2-mile, out-and-back hike with 4,000 feet of elevation gain, are deciduous trees, especially oaks and hickories, and rhododendrons and mountain laurels. Also watch for wildflowers, poison ivy, and the autumnal hawk migration. Deer

----

Directions ⟶

From junction of Capital Beltway (Interstate 495) and I-270 spur in Maryland, drive northwest on I-270 for about 32 miles to Frederick. At Exit 32, swing right to get onto 1-70. Proceed for 0.4 miles and, at next fork, stay left to get onto I-70 heading west. Proceed for 11.2 miles. At Exit 42 in Myersville, turn right onto MD 17 (Wolfsville Road). Stay on MD 17 for 1.5 miles (be sure to make sharp right turn in middle of town), and then, at first major intersection, turn left onto US 40 and proceed for 3 miles. Then, going uphill, just past Canada Hill Road sign and graphic hiker sign, pull into roadside parking area on the left.

KEY AT-A-GLANCE INFORMATION

LENGTH: 10.2 miles

CONFIGURATION: Out-and-back

DIFFICULTY: Quite hard

SCENERY:L Mountain woodlands, panoramic farmland vista from tower

EXPOSURE: Shady; less so in winter

TRAFFIC: Mostly light; heavier in state park on warm-weather weekends, holidays

TRAIL SURFACE: Mostly dirt, with rocky, rooty, and paved patches

HIKING TIME: 5.5–6.5 hours (including tower time)

SEASON: Year-round

ACCESS: No restrictions on AT itself; state park open daily, 8 a.m.–sunset

MAPS: USGS Myersville, Middletown; PATC Map 5

FACILITIES: None at trailhead; toilets, water, phone near trail in state park

FOR MORE INFORMATION: Contact Appalachian Trail Conservancy, in Harpers Ferry, (304) 535-6331 or www.appalachiantrail.org; and South Mountain Recreation Area, in Boonsboro, (301) 791-4767 (for annual Adventure Guide, send 83¢ SASE to SMRA, 21843 National Pike, Boonsboro, MD 21713)

SPECIAL COMMENTS: Be careful or stay away during hunting season

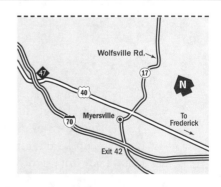

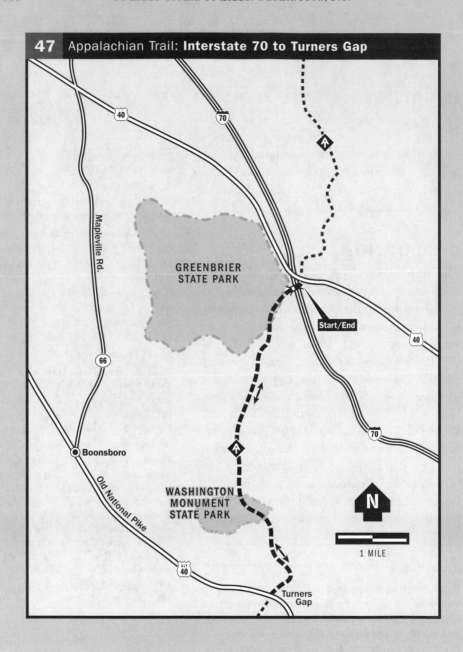

47 Appalachian Trail: **Interstate 70 to Turners Gap**

bound, abound, and are legally protected along the AT, but the right-of-way is narrow, so sport orange during the fall.

To get started from the roadside trailhead, head for a nearby board and go past it to pick up an old asphalt road. After roughly 130 yards, swing left onto a blue-blazed side trail and follow it for 120 yards until you reach a footbridge.

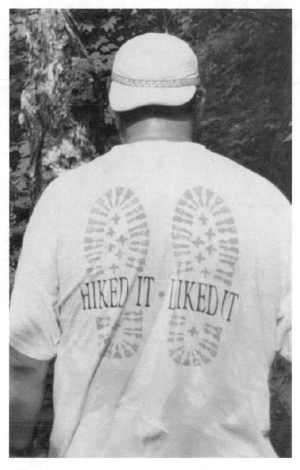

When asked his opinion of this Appalachian Trail section, this hiker said nothing, smiled, removed his backpack, and walked away.

There, the southbound AT comes in from the right to reach the bridge that spans I-70's traffic lanes. Cross the bridge, turn left, ascend some steps, turn right, and proceed along the white-blazed and undulating AT. For the next 2.5 miles, you'll be mostly on old dirt roads. Within the first mile, you'll enter the woods, pass Greenbrier State Park, and twice cross a paved road (Boonsboro Mountain Road). Listen for the lovely sound of silence as you move away from thunderous I-70.

Soon after you cross a power-line right-of-way, head uphill into Washington Monument State Park (like Greenbrier, it's one of South Mountain Recreation Area's several state parks). On reaching a fork, take the rocky and steep side trail leading 0.3 miles to the monument's base, and climb the stairs within the 30-foot-high tower. At the top, on a clear day, revel in one of Maryland's best AT vistas, including the Hagerstown Valley farmlands and ridges beyond to the west. And if it's early fall, watch for migrating hawks riding the northwest winds. From your high perch, you'll see, roughly 2 miles due west, Boonsboro, whose citizens once decided to honor the country's first president. Erected in 1827, their Washington memorial was the country's first. Later, it was used as a Civil War observation post, fell into disrepair, was restored, and then fell down again. The present structure dates from the mid-1930s.

Leaving the tower, descend about 100 yards, and turn right to return to the main trail. Continue downhill half a mile to leave the park. En route, pause at the board at the main parking lot. If you're interested, the park's small museum is nearby. Then turn left, walk 50 yards along the access road, and then cross to turn right onto the signposted AT.

Follow the trail through the woods, uphill at first for half a mile, and then downhill for about a mile, to reach Turners Gap. That's the hike's 5.1-mile mark and turnaround—at US 40A (Old National Pike), and Old South Mountain Inn. Cross the highway (carefully) to learn about the inn's colorful 250-year history, including its years as a National Road stagecoach stop. If it's Sunday, stay for lunch at the otherwise for-dinner-only inn. Or return by road for dinner—by reservation, (301) 432-6155. In either case, you'll find that day hikers are welcome.

Then head back to the trailhead. On the way, consider revisiting the Washington Monument to take a fresh look at the sky and scenery.

NEARBY/RELATED ACTIVITIES

If you do this hike in summer, cool off at nearby Greenbrier State Park, which has beaches, canoe rentals, and a swimming-permitted lake. Also explore nearby Boonsboro (from the trailhead, drive 200 yards up US 40, turn left onto Boonsboro Mountain Road, and go 3 miles to Boonsboro). One unusual attraction is Doug Bast's remarkable history museum (open Sunday afternoons and by appointment); call (301) 432-6969. Or sample the National Pike Festival, held each May; call (301) 733-4876.

To learn more about the AT, see Hike 59, page 285.

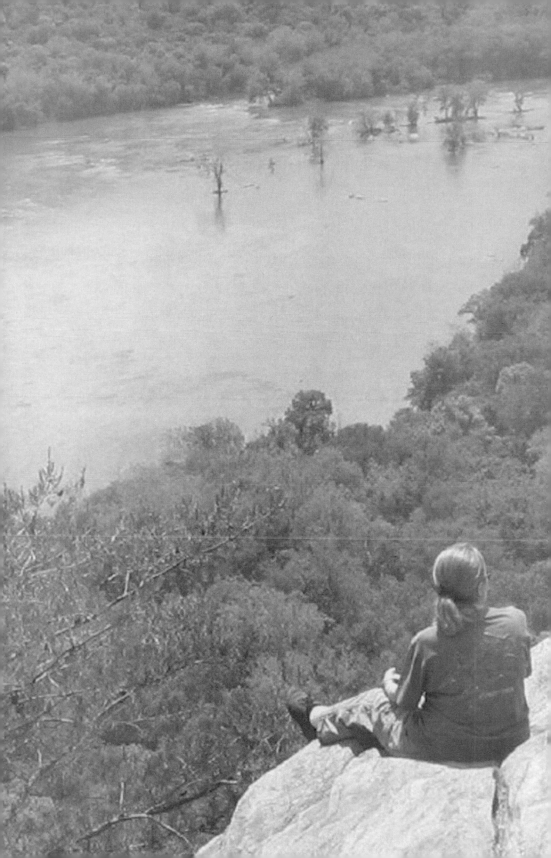

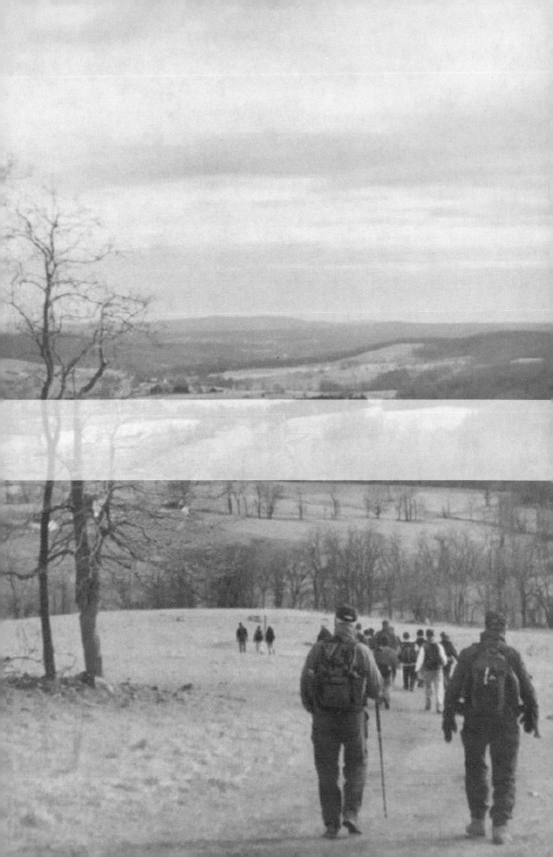

RURAL VIRGINIA AND
WEST VIRGINIA LOCALES

48 BULL RUN MOUNTAINS NATURAL AREA

KEY AT-A-GLANCE INFORMATION

LENGTH: 6.8 miles (with shorter option)

CONFIGURATION: Modified figure 8

DIFFICULTY: Moderate

SCENERY: Hilly woodlands, with sweeping cliff-top vistas of Piedmont farmlands and Blue Ridge

EXPOSURE: Shady; less so in winter

TRAFFIC: Usually light–very light

TRAIL SURFACE: Mostly dirt or grass, with stretches of pavement and gravel; rocky in places

HIKING TIME: 3–4 hours

SEASON: Year-round

ACCESS: Open daily, dawn–dusk; fill out and deposit liability waiver form at trailhead kiosk across from Mountain House

MAPS: USGS Thoroughfare Gap; trail map available on conservancy Web site and also by mail

FACILITIES: None

FOR MORE INFORMATION: Contact Bull Run Mountains Conservancy, (703) 753-2631 or www.brm conservancy.org; visit conservancy office in Mountain House, 8 a.m.– 4 p.m., Monday–Friday

SPECIAL COMMENTS: Comply with use guidelines (available on Web site, by mail, and at trailhead kiosk)

IN BRIEF

In northern Virginia's Haymarket area, about 45 crow-miles west of Washington, lies an out-of-sight nature preserve on an in-sight Blue Ridge outlier, where hikers can find trails, serenity, and a lovely vista-equipped cliff top as the payoff for a moderate climb.

DESCRIPTION

The Bull Run Mountains are both easy to see from a distance and easy to miss close-up. They form a 16-mile-long north–south range that rises hundreds of feet above the gently rolling Piedmont, and their escarpment includes towering white quartzite cliffs compellingly visible from Interstate 66. However, in the few minutes it takes to drive across the narrow range at high speed, one does not encounter any inviting side road or signboard or other inducement to stop and explore (except, maybe, for a fleeting glimpse of a ruined gristmill). Nevertheless, the range, which is an isolated outlier of the Blue Ridge

Directions

From Capital Beltway (Interstate 495) in Merri-field, Virginia, take Exit 49 to get onto I-66 heading west. Proceed for 23.6 miles and then get off at I-66 Exit 40 (Haymarket). Go 0.2 miles to end of exit ramp, and turn left at traffic light onto James Madison Highway (US 15 south). Proceed for 0.5 miles to next traffic light, and turn right onto US 55 west. Proceed for 2.7 miles (crossing railroad tracks at 1.9-mile mark), and then turn right onto Turner Road (also labeled "F289"). Follow Turner Road for 0.1 mile across I-66, and then turn left onto Beverly Mill Drive (F287). Proceed for 0.8 miles to Mountain House, on left and near end of road. Park in gravel area alongside building.

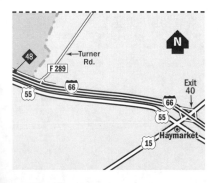

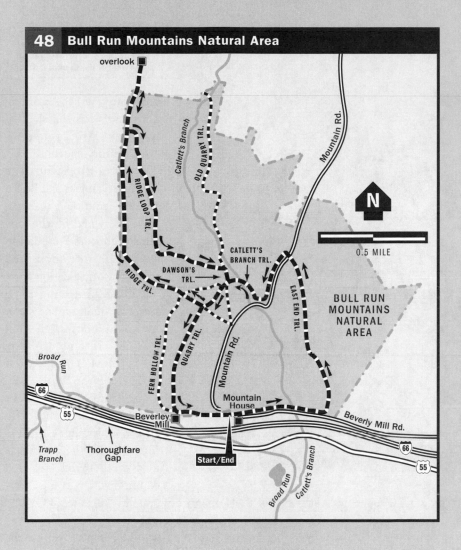

to the west, has a rich and distinctive natural and human history, which makes it wonderfully worth exploring. And an opportunity to do so exists in the form of the Bull Run Mountains Natural Area, established in 2002.

This area, formally known as the Bull Run Mountains State Natural Area Preserve, provides environmental protection for about 2,500 acres of heavily wooded ridges, slopes, and stream valleys. It includes the headwaters of the regionally important Occoquan River and Goose Creek. Its flora include chestnut oaks, hickories, hemlocks, and pines, as well as myriad wildflowers—among them some species rarely found in Virginia. Its fauna include deer, ravens, raptors, and timber rattlesnakes. Its historic sites include old family homesteads and cemeteries and a

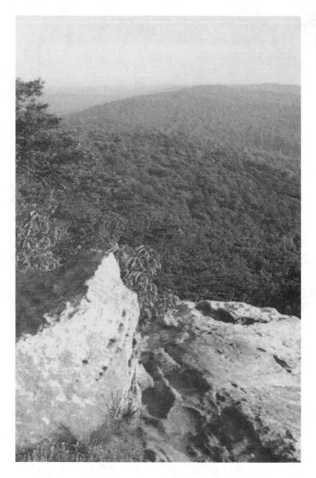

One great charm of the Bull Run Mountains is that such fine overlooks as this one lie less than 30 miles west of the Capital Beltway.

quartzite quarry. Adjoining the preserve is the shell of Beverley Mill, a famous 18th-century gristmill.

Straddling the line between Fauquier and Prince William counties, the preserve is owned by the Virginia Outdoors Foundation (VOF), a state-sponsored nonprofit organization committed to protecting open space throughout the state. Another nonprofit, the Bull Run Mountains Conservancy (BRMC), leases about a third of the VOF land, at the southern end of the range. BRMC uses the leased land and Mountain House (BRMC's on-site headquarters) for both research and educational programs year-round, and it maintains a network of trails open to the public. Together, VOF and BMRC also serve to help keep the metro-area developers at bay.

The preserve's well-maintained trails have names, which mostly reflect the area's history, are color coded, and appear on the preserve's maps. But they're not on the signposts that mark most trail intersections; those carry only the trails' color codes. So be sure to follow the signpost colors (blazes) and my directions and map carefully in doing the following figure-eight hike, which covers 6.8 miles, offers about 2,400 feet of elevation change, and culminates in a vista-rich overlook. To shorten the hike to 5.4 miles, cut off the first part of the hike by first heading north on Mountain Road from Mountain House, then turning left at the first T-junction onto the Ridge Trail, and then following my directions below for the rest of the full hike.

Starting from Mountain House, head east along paved and tree-lined Beverly Mill Drive for roughly 0.5 miles, and then turn left at a roadside marker post to get onto the lime-blazed East End Trail. Proceed gently uphill through the woods on the dirt-and-grass trail for about 0.8 miles. En route, look and listen carefully when you cross a set of active railroad tracks, and ignore a tempting side trail on the right. Then, at a T-junction, turn left onto gravel-surfaced and white-blazed Mountain Road and proceed in a mostly southwesterly direction. At the next T-junction, turn right onto wine-color–blazed Catlett's Branch Trail. Follow it roughly westward across its namesake stream, which may be full enough to induce you to rock-hop.

At the four-way intersection after that, continue straight through, thereby crossing orange-blazed Dawson's Trail, and keep going for some 200 yards on the dark-blue-blazed Old Quarry Trail. At the four-way intersection after that, stay to the right to get onto the blue-blazed Ridge Trail, but note the brown-blazed Quarry Trail (for later use) off to your left. You'll be following the Ridge Trail uphill through the woods—and first west and then north—for about 2 miles to reach and then follow the ridgeline to your cliff-top destination. En route, you'll pass the black-blazed Fern Hollow Trail on the left (after about 0.2 miles) and then the Ridge Loop Trail on the right (after about 1 mile). About 100 yards past that last junction, you'll find a sign marking the BRMC property line. North of that point, you'll be on private property and proceeding at your own risk. However, I think the risk is low because I have heard from reliable sources that the owner is agreeable to letting responsible hikers ascend to the overlook. So keep going for about 0.7 miles on a blaze- and sign-free trail that goes steadily uphill. For the first 0.2 miles yards, you'll be on a narrow woodland dirt trail (be sure to stay to the right at a fork), which then becomes a stony former road. After about 0.3 miles, the road gives way to a narrow dirt trail, which swings left toward the cliff top. Over the next 0.2 miles, you'll be within a few yards of three overlooks to your left.

You'll know the best overlook when you find it. It's a broad rock ledge with magnificent views to the west of Piedmont farmlands with their glinting ponds and isolated hills, and ribbony I-66 with its flyspeck vehicles. And in the western distance you'll see some 75 miles of the great wall of the Blue Ridge proper. You can perch or sprawl on the edge of the ledge and have lots of exposure to sun and verticality (but be careful). Or you can sit safely in the shade and well back from the edge. Looking out across the void, you may well see ravens and various raptors in search of sustenance.

When ready, retrace your steps back to the Ridge Trail and than back to the last junction. There, turn left to get onto the red-blazed Ridge Loop Trail, which roughly parallels the Ridge Trail. You'll be on that steep-and-rocky-in-places downhill trail for about a mile. Then, on reaching a four-way intersection, turn right onto wine-color–blazed Catlett's Branch Trail, and go south on it for about 100 yards. Then, at the next four-way intersection, turn right again to get onto the brown-blazed Quarry Trail and repeat the 200-yard segment of that trail that you walked along earlier.

At the next four-way intersection, cross the Ridge Trail (your previous route) to continue on the Quarry Trail. Follow it south and steeply downhill for 0.2 miles to its junction with the black-blazed Fern Hollow Trail. En route, pause in the quarry area to see the remains of Civil War trenches and read the display boards telling of the area's role in the fight to control Thoroughfare Gap. At the bottom, pause again to look over and read about Beverly Mill (formerly Chapman's Mill), which looms seven stories over its original power source, Broad Run.

Built in 1742, the mill was fought over and damaged during the Thoroughfare Gap action, put back to work and used peacefully until 1951, wantonly destroyed by arson in 1998, and subsequently adopted as a restoration project by the Turn the Mill Around Campaign (to learn more, visit **www.chapmansmill.org**).

Then turn left and head east on the mostly level Fern Hollow Trail. Pause en route to examine several labeled historic sites, including the ruins of the Chapman family house dating from about the 1750s. Also take note of the traffic roar from nearby I-66—a reminder of the importance of Thoroughfare Gap as a road, railroad, and stream route through the Bull Run Mountains. Then after ignoring side trails on the left, turn right at a boardwalked fork to join Mountain Road. Next, follow the road for 100 yards, and then cross the in-use railroad tracks carefully to reach the trailhead at Mountain House.

NEARBY/RELATED ACTIVITIES

Return to the preserve to explore the other trails or to participate in BRMC's various events and other on-site programs. They include hikes and other guided tours, and summer camps for children. For current information, visit **www.chapmans mill.org.** Also consider joining and supporting BRMC (see page 234).

BULL RUN-OCCOQUAN TRAIL 49

IN BRIEF

The Bull Run–Occoquan Trail winds through four adjoining parks in southwestern Fairfax County, Virginia, providing a challenging and picturesque hike.

DESCRIPTION

For a very scenic, long, and rigorous hike within an hour's drive of Washington, D.C., try this one-way, 18-mile trek on the Bull Run–Occoquan Trail (BROT). Located about 25 miles southwest of the city, BROT is the only nearby, lightly used trail on which you can hike in roughly the same direction for 18 miles in a rural setting. That will take you from Bull Run Regional Park to Fountainhead Regional

---

Directions

Car shuttle is required. From intersection of Capital Beltway (Interstate 495) and Braddock Road (VA 620) at beltway Exit 54A in Annandale, Virginia, drive west on Braddock for 1.8 miles. Turn left onto Burke Lake Road (VA 645) and go 4.8 miles. Turn left onto Ox Road (VA 123) and go 1.3 miles. Turn right onto Henderson Road (VA 643) and go 2 miles. Turn left onto Hampton Road (VA 647) and go 1.5 miles. Then turn right into Fountainhead Park and proceed 0.6 miles to car drop-off—parking lot on right. Drive to trailhead (30–40 minutes), as follows. Return 2 miles to junction of Hampton and Henderson. Turn left onto Henderson and go 6.4 miles. Turn left onto Clifton Road (VA 645) and go 2.3 miles, traversing Clifton (where road becomes Main Street). Turn left onto Compton Road (VA 658) and go 6.9 miles (passing under I-66). At "Bull Run Regional Park" sign, turn left onto Bull Run Drive and go 0.9 miles to entrance kiosk. Continue on road for 1.6 miles. Then turn left into parking lot for swimming pool and mini-Frisbee course.

KEY AT-A-GLANCE INFORMATION

LENGTH: 18 miles (with shorter options)

CONFIGURATION: One-way

DIFFICULTY: Extremely hard

SCENERY: Wooded hills, stream valleys, floodplains; fields

EXPOSURE: Shady; less so in winter

TRAFFIC: Mostly very light–light; heavier on warm-weather weekends, holidays, especially near both ends, at Bull Run marina, in Cub Run area (April)

TRAIL SURFACE: Mostly dirt; some grass, gravel, boardwalk, pavement

HIKING TIME: 8.5–10.5 hours

SEASON: Year-round

ACCESS: Open daily, dawn–dusk; entrance fee for nonresidents of NVRPA jurisdictions to enter Bull Run Regional Park

MAPS: USGS Manassas, Independent Hill, Occoquan; trail sketch map in free NVRPA brochure (also available on NVRPA Web site)

FACILITIES: Toilets, water, phones near trailhead, at marina, near Fountainhead

FOR MORE INFORMATION: Contact Northern Virginia Regional Park Authority, (703) 352-5900 or www.nvrpa.org

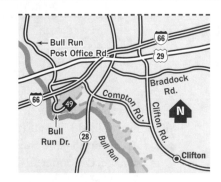

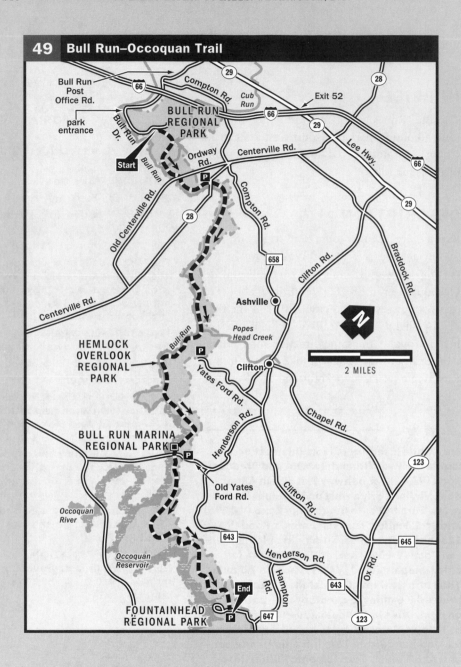

49 Bull Run–Occoquan Trail

Park. For a shorter hike, forgo the car shuttle and do an out-and-back hike from the same trailhead at Bull Run Regional Park; for a 12-mile excursion, for example, turn around at the Bull Run marina. BROT follows the valley carrying Bull Run and the Occoquan River to the Potomac River. It winds through wooded

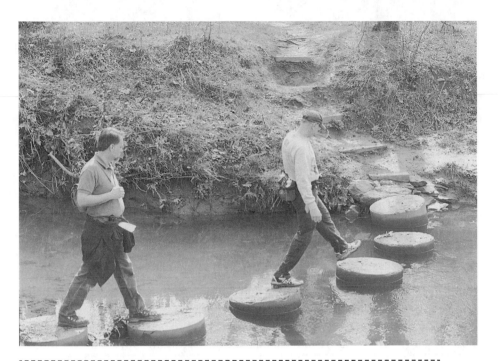

The hiker's way across the mouth of Popes Creek, which is one of Bull Run's major tributaries, remains largely set in concrete.

hills and floodplains, and is marked by a rich assortment of flora and fauna, including large stands of hemlocks and springtime bluebells.

Before setting out, check by phone on trail conditions, (703) 352-5900. Be prepared to turn back if you encounter flooding. Also be prepared for about 3,400 feet of elevation change. Plan to follow the blue-blazed BROT (it's also called the Blue Trail) and its double-sided mileposts giving distances from each end.

To get started from the parking-lot trailhead at Bull Run Regional Park, walk to the entrance road, turn left, and hike along the shoulder toward the warm-season camp store for about 150 yards. Watch and head for a BROT sign on the right. Then cross a small arched bridge onto the blue-blazed trail. The trail curves across a broad and often soggy floodplain under an open tree canopy. On reaching Cub Run, swing right to follow it downstream for more than half a mile.

Continuing, you'll reach Cub Run's mouth on Bull Run and a T-junction. Turn left to stay on BROT and, a mile into the hike, take the bridge across Cub Run. With Bull Run on your right, head downstream. Within the next mile, you'll pass beneath two bridges spanning Bull Run and then be on a hilly woodland trail. After passing under a railroad bridge and through a rocky section (note the stone foundations of a bridge destroyed in the Civil War), you'll reach the mouth of Popes Head Creek, a major Bull Run tributary (about 6.5 miles into the hike). Follow the blue blazes as the trail crosses the steep-banked creek on concrete pillars. Then, step into Hemlock Overlook Regional Park, where you'll be flanked by Bull Run and a hemlock stand for half a mile. Continuing, you'll traverse a picturesque woodland clearing and then pass the ruins of a 19th-century hydroelectric power plant.

For the next mile, you'll stay close to Bull Run as BROT follows the meandering stream across the floodplain. The trail then swings to the left and uphill into the woods. Follow the blue blazes as BROT undulates for a mile on dirt paths and old roads. Follow them out into the open and along the edge of several fields. After passing a Bull Run inlet and stepping across a bridged creek, you'll reach milepost 10/8 and see a broad expanse of playing fields ahead of you.

Head for a blazed post 45 degrees to your right. Then follow more posts—and the marked sidelines—straight across the fields. Turn left at a post topped by an owl, pass two white sideline shelters, and get onto a gravel road, keeping the wooden fence to your left. Near a parking lot, turn right and cross a little creek on a small bridge. Follow the blazes along the edge of a small playing field and then slide under the tree canopy on a dirt trail.

Back in the woods with the blue blazes, watch for a sharp turn to the left and uphill. You'll then pass through Bull Run Marina Regional Park's mature hemlocks and get back close to Bull Run and reach the marina.

From the marina, follow the entrance road out to heavily traveled Old Yates Ford Road (it's the only road spanning the waterway in more than 20 miles). Cross carefully to pick up the trail, which jogs to the right and heads downhill. Then turn left to follow it along Bull Run, which is now part of a huge reservoir.

Stay close to the reservoir for almost half a mile, then follow the blue blazes back into the wooded hills, where you'll zigzag on dirt trails and old roads for the hike's remaining 6 miles. You'll go up and down a lot, cross several small creeks, and catch glimpses of the Occoquan Reservoir.

At milepost 18/0, you'll emerge from the woods at the car drop-off in Fountainhead Regional Park. If you're tempted, turn right and walk 0.4 miles to the marina building, where the observation deck provides nice reservoir views.

NEARBY/RELATED ACTIVITIES

Return to Bull Run Regional Park in April to see the Virginia bluebells in bloom. Take your own walk and time, or go on the annual, ranger-led Bluebell Walk. Call the park for details, (703) 631-0550.

Visit the Manassas Industrial School/Jennie Dean Memorial, in nearby Manassas. The memorial commemorates northern Virginia's first African American school and its remarkable founder, born a slave, who opened it as a private boarding school in 1894. For information and directions, contact the Manassas Museum, (703) 368-1873 or **www.manassasmuseum.org**.

In May and June, visit the garden at Ben Lomond Manor House, in Manassas, to experience the vivid colors and fragrances of 200 old-rose varieties. For information and directions, contact the facility, (703) 368-8784 or **www.ben lomondmanorhouse.org**.

PRINCE WILLIAM FOREST PARK 50

IN BRIEF

Prince William Forest Park, in Prince William County, Virginia, is a huge nature preserve that provides a wonderful habitat for plants, wildlife, and visiting hikers.

DESCRIPTION

Located about 20 miles southwest of the Capital Beltway, Prince William Forest Park ranks as the metro area's largest park. Covering 18,571 acres, it's also the largest woodland expanse within 50 miles of Washington. And I claim that it's the only one worthy of being called a forest, even if it is a young one.

The area was well forested in precolonial times, but over two centuries of farming left the land badly eroded. In 1933 the federal government made it one of the country's 50 or so demonstration projects for restoring the environment and developing inexpensive

- -

Directions

From Capital Beltway (Interstate 495 and I-95), take Exit 57A onto I-95 heading southwest, toward Richmond. If you start from Washington, head southwest on Shirley Memorial Highway (I-395) to automatically be on I-95 when you cross beltway. From beltway, go almost 20 miles on I-95, watch for road sign announcing park, and take Exit 150B to VA 619. Head west on VA 619 (Joplin Road) for 0.4 miles. Then turn right onto park entrance road. Stop at contact station to pay your way. Continue for 0.5 miles, and then turn left onto Scenic Drive. Proceed for 2 miles, and turn left, at sign for Turkey Run campground, onto loop part of Scenic Drive. Go 0.3 miles and turn right onto Turkey Run Road. Continue for 0.3 miles, past campground, to parking lot at Turkey Run Educational Center.

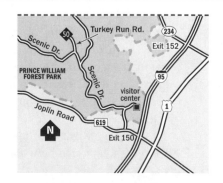

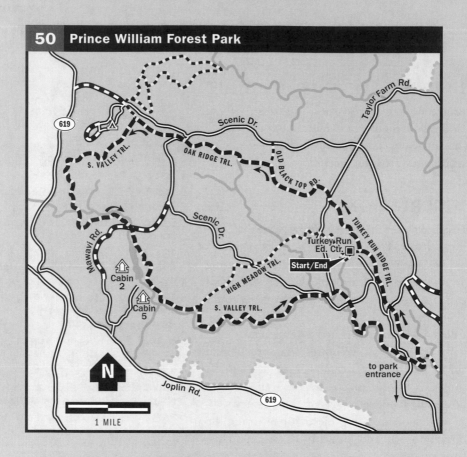

50 Prince William Forest Park

recreation facilities. The Civilian Conservation Corps (CCC) seeded slopes, created trails, and built facilities.

Eventually, in 1948, the area became a national park. Decades of recovery have transformed the depleted farmland. Trees, bushes, wildflowers, and ferns flourish, making springtime treks along the stream valleys a particular delight. Deer, beavers, squirrels, and other wildlife are plentiful. Their habitat extends into the adjoining Quantico Marine Corps Base, much of which is managed as a natural preserve.

This hike is a 12.3-mile counterclockwise loop with about 1,800 feet of elevation change, but only one steep hill. The trails are blazed and signposted (and do stay on them to avoid the poison ivy). You'll get scenic views rather than vistas; there are open areas but no high overlooks. Trail traffic is usually light; most visitors seem to be there to camp, picnic, fish, or take short strolls.

The hike works best in the spring and fall. Summer can be muggy and buggy. Winter, though, can be wonderful. My best time there was a cold but sunny day

Fishing on the park's two lakes is a popular pastime for campers in summer and for great blue herons during most of the year.

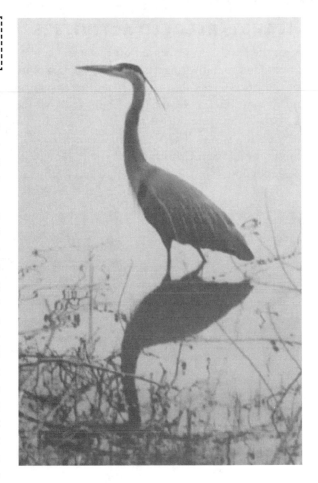

with snow on the ground, deer on the move, and the pileated woodpecker's "great god-call" (to use nature writers Bill and Phyllis Thomas's lovely phrase) echoing through the forest.

To get started from the trailhead, step onto the undulating, dirt-and-gravel–surfaced Old Black Top Road (opposite the parking lot's entrance). Head northwest for 1.8 miles in open country. After crossing Taylor Farm Road and a small stream, watch on the left for the hike's first concrete signpost. There, turn left onto the yellow-blazed Oak Ridge Trail. Follow it for 1.6 miles through the open forest (take care when crossing Scenic Drive).

At a junction, turn left onto the white-blazed South Valley Trail, which will be your path for the next 7.5 miles. First, head roughly south through a fairly open area for almost 2 miles until you reach the South Fork of Quantico Creek. From there, follow the trail as it wiggles southeast close to the tree-lined stream. Cross Mawavi Road (a fire road near the hike's halfway point) and watch for a large beaver lodge in a broad, swampy area. Then, pass two man-made lakes used for canoeing and fishing by summertime campers staying in the nearby CCC-built cabins. Below the second lake, the stream valley is postcard-pretty and one of the park's most attractive trail segments.

Continuing, cross Scenic Drive for the second and third times, hike up and over the hike's only significant hill, and pass side trails leading off to parking lots C, B, and A. Then, cross Scenic Drive again and take the first left onto the 1.4-mile Turkey Run Ridge Trail. Follow the dark-blue-blazed trail uphill, heading northwest. Cross Scenic Drive one last time. Then traverse a hilly and forested area to reach the trailhead at the Turkey Run Educational Center.

NEARBY/RELATED ACTIVITIES

Visit the park's visitor center, off the entrance road. It has nature exhibits, maps, books, and friendly rangers. After the hike, explore historic Dumfries, at the head of Quantico Creek's estuary. To get there, stay on VA 619, cross I-95, and turn north onto US 1 at Triangle. In Dumfries, visit the Weems-Botts Museum, (703) 221-3346. In winter, drive along the estuary on Possum Point Road to see migratory tundra swans. They leave on about March 19 (oddly, that's when the swallows return to San Capistrano). If you're hungry, try Tim's Rivershore Restaurant & Crabhouse (703) 441-1375, on Cherry Hill Road (see note on page 250).

LEESYLVANIA STATE PARK 51

IN BRIEF

While locomoting at the right time through Lee-sylvania State Park, in southeastern Prince William County, hikers can commune with nature, admire the Potomac River, and visit sites associated with Virginia's celebrated Lee family.

DESCRIPTION

Leesylvania State Park lies on a peninsula poking into the Potomac River in the Cherry Hill area, about 25 miles southwest of Washington. Its landscape features wooded uplands, wetlands, coastal bluffs, a sandy beach, and hiking trails. Trees and wildflowers flourish there, as do deer, beavers, and other four-footed creatures. Fauna watchers, though, mostly prize the eagles, ospreys, ducks, cormorants, and herons.

The park's origins date to the 1750s, when Henry Lee II developed a plantation called

Directions

From Capital Beltway (Interstate 495 and I-95) in Springfield, Virginia, take Exit 57A onto I-95 heading southwest toward Richmond. If you start from Washington, head southwest on Shirley Memorial Highway (I-395) to automatically be on I-95 when you cross beltway. After going about 13 miles on I-95 from beltway, watch for "Leesylvania State Park" sign and take Exit 156. Follow exit ramp for 0.8 miles, and then curve right for 0.3 miles to get onto VA 784 (Dale Boulevard). Go 0.7 miles and turn right onto Neabsco Mills Road, and proceed for 1.1 miles. Turn right onto US 1, get in left lane and go south for 0.3 miles, and turn left onto Neabsco Road. Go east for 1.5 miles, turn right onto park's access road, and go 0.6 miles to contact station and then to gravel parking lot on right—the trailhead. If it's full, go on to next lot.

KEY AT-A-GLANCE INFORMATION

LENGTH: 7.5 miles

CONFIGURATION: Modified out-and-back

DIFFICULTY: Easy–moderate

SCENERY: Wooded uplands, wetlands, river and beach views

EXPOSURE: Shady; less so in winter

TRAFFIC: On riverfront, mostly heavy on warm-weather weekends, holidays, much lighter at other times; elsewhere, very light–light

TRAIL SURFACE: Mostly dirt; also some boardwalk, pavement, gravel, pebbles, sand

HIKING TIME: 3–4 hours

SEASON: Year-round, but best from late fall until early spring

ACCESS: Open daily, sunrise–dusk; entrance fee

MAPS: USGS Quantico, Indian Head; sketch map in free park flyer; posted park map

FACILITIES: Toilets, water at park office (near trailhead); toilets, water, phone, warm-season food store on riverfront; water at Freestone Point

FOR MORE INFORMATION: Contact the park, (703) 670-0372 or www.dcr.state.va.us/parks/leesylva.htm

SPECIAL COMMENTS: Vroom, vroom (oh, those summer boats)!

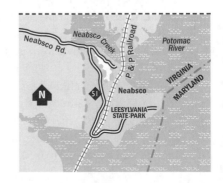

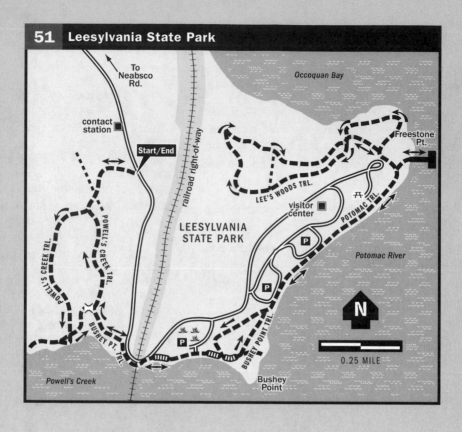

Leesylvania. One of the children born and reared there was Henry Lee III, the Light-Horse Harry of American Revolution fame. The property stayed in the family's hands until 1825. But the Lee link was revived during the Civil War, when a son of Light-Horse Harry's, General Robert E. Lee, had a gun battery installed to help blockade Washington. For a century thereafter, the area was variously used by tobacco farmers, loggers, fishermen, traders, squatters, hunters, and gambling-ship operators. In the late 1970s, philanthropist and playwright Daniel Ludwig acquired much of the area and donated it to the state of Virginia. The park was opened in 1992.

The 542-acre park is a very popular warm-season destination for boaters and beachgoers. The riverfront gets crowded, and the boat engines roar. As hike scouter Bud Zehmer advises, "This bedlam mars the middle section of the hike, so schedule your visit carefully." Of course, the park's at its colorful best in the spring and fall, and some winter days there can be starkly beautiful. This 7.5-mile hike, with only about 1,000 feet of elevation change, includes several short trails and other paths. The major trails are named and signposted, and some trails—but not all—are color coded and blazed, so follow my directions carefully.

To get started from the parking-lot trailhead, head for an interpretive kiosk to pick up a self-guiding booklet keyed to numbered trailside posts. Then hike south on a wide, gently rising trail. The trail levels off and passes a fire road on the right. At an information kiosk where several trails intersect, go right and follow the "Powell's Creek Trail" sign. At a trail fork, turn right to follow the western side of the nominally blue-blazed Powell's Creek Trail loop. You'll quickly lose some elevation and tree cover as you near Powell's Creek. At a set of stairs, detour some 50 feet to view the creek, and then descend the stairs. The trail curves left at the bottom as it follows a gully filled with various aquatic plants. Stay with the trail as it takes you up a moderately steep hill to another set of stairs. At the top, just over a mile into the hike, you'll find a bench and trail junction. Continue straight on the green-blazed Bushey Point Trail (to the left is the Powell's Creek Trail's return loop).

As the trail descends, you'll enter a ravine, pass a marshy area, and cross a bridge. Then, walk up a short incline and some steps to reach the park's access road. Turn right to walk alongside the road. When an obvious path appears on the right, hop aboard to continue along the shore and beneath a railroad trestle (it's the Washington–Richmond main line). The path soon leaves the road, crosses, and traverses some marshy areas. There, in summer, watch for lizard's tail, a tall herb bearing tiny white flowers on drooping spikes. In winter, watch for eagle groupies and their prey, which roost around Bushey Point. At the next trail junction, go straight on the tree-shaded narrow path that runs along the water. Cross a bridge and parking lot, pass a maintenance building on the left, and cross another bridge to reach a trail junction. There, go straight, but note the left-hand trail, which is the one you'll return on.

At the next junction, stay to the left and pass through a tunnel of pawpaws beneath towering tulip trees. Soon after the trail merges with another (on the left), it ends, about 2.5 miles into the hike. Then you'll need to negotiate a trailless area to reach the Potomac Trail. To do so, leave the trees, head slightly to the right, and follow a parking lot to a boardwalk just past the first boat ramp (the well-stocked park store will be off to your left). Stay on the boardwalk until it ends at a second boat ramp. Then walk straight ahead to where the trees resume and the Potomac Trail begins. The half-mile-long, yellow-blazed trail consists of a wide and flat gravel path running between the river on the right and the beach and picnic area. Toward the trail's end, as it begins curving left, you'll reach Freestone Point and draw abreast of a fishing pier to the right. Detour to visit the pier, which provides fine river views.

Return to the main path and turn right, pass through a gate, and continue to a "Lee's Woods Trail" sign and an interpretive kiosk featuring a park map. From the kiosk, get started on the 2-mile-long, red-blazed trail by walking straight and taking a pebbled pathway that curves to the right and uphill. Note the amphitheater on your right, built on the ruins of a 1920s hunting club. Continue up the hill until it flattens out at the Civil War fortification. The path winds around it, passes a replica cannon, and continues straight, affording views of Occoquan Bay to the right. Go through a fence into an open glade and then turn right, following a sign that points to stops #3 and #4 (consult your booklet). Just past #3, go straight on a short spur leading to a fenced area offering more views of the bay. If it's winter, watch for eagles, which roost in that area.

Return to the main trail and swing right and downhill. At the junction at the bottom, turn right onto a wider and stonier trail and immediately begin to ascend. As the trail curves to the right and levels out, look for the ruins of the house built in 1825 by Henry Fairfax, Leesylvania's first post-Lee owner. The building burned down a century later. Ascending again, stay on the main trail and ignore the side roads as you proceed toward stop #8, the site of the original Lee mansion, which was destroyed by fire in the 1790s. There, take a sharp turn to the right and continue upward to an open glade. Then it'll be more downhill, initially on stairs. Reaching a trail fork, turn right and keep going. At the next junction, just continue (don't bother with the signposted Escaped Gardens detour, advises Bud Zehmer).

The trail climbs another hill, and at the top is a gated enclosure around the Lee-Fairfax family cemetery (Henry Lee II is there). Follow the trail to the right, toward stop #11. It meanders through the woods, past a fire road and an above-ground sewer pipe, to reach an intersection where you should turn left and initially head downhill. Stay on the main trail as it curves to the right and undulates back to the kiosk near the amphitheater (at the hike's 5.4-mile mark).

The hike's remaining 2.2 miles mostly retrace the route back to the trail-head, but includes some new-to-you stretches. Just after getting back on the Bushey Point Trail, turn right at the fork onto one such stretch. At the following junction, turn left onto a gravel path. At the one after that, turn right to rejoin the main trail. Then work your way back to the railroad trestle and ravine to reach a junction. There, turn right onto the new-to-you eastern part of the Powell's Creek Trail. At the next junction, turn right to do the final short leg back to the trail-head. Follow the signs, and don't be led astray by the fire roads.

NEARBY/RELATED ACTIVITIES

Visit the visitor center (summer only) to see its absorbing history and science exhibits. Attend the annual Leesylvania Natural Heritage Day, held in May (contact the park for details).

Sample the nearby Julie J. Metz Mitigation Bank, a 200-acre expanse of wetlands along Neabsco Creek. It has both trails and a convenient parking lot (on Neabsco Road, 1 mile west of the park). Eventually, it will be connected to the park by a segment of the evolving Potomac Heritage National Scenic Trail (see Hike 29, page 143) that will pass through an undeveloped 34.4-acre park section donated by a developer in late 2005.

For an après-hike treat, visit Tim's Rivershore Restaurant & Crabhouse, (703) 441-1375. Located at the end of Cherry Hill Road on the Potomac River south of the park, in what feels like the middle of nowhere, it's a great place to get good food and impressive river views—and discuss the probably inevitable development of the Cherry Hill area.

WILDCAT MOUNTAIN NATURAL AREA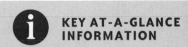

IN BRIEF

Tucked away in the peaceful farmlands of Virginia's Fauquier County near Warrenton lies a private nature preserve that provides a rich habitat for flora, a haven for fauna, and a secluded and little-visited hiking venue for humans who appreciate both natural and human history.

DESCRIPTION

Located on the western flanks of the Blue Ridge foothills between about 500 and 1,200 feet above sea level, the Wildcat Mountain Natural Area is a small gem of a sanctuary that owes its existence and splendor to nature, a generous family, happenstance, and the Nature Conservancy (TNC). Back in the 18th and 19th centuries, much of the 655-acre area was cleared as hardwood forests gave way to subsistence farmlands and woodlots. But that trend was gradually reversed as the surrounding region endured first the Civil War and then the Great Depression. Farming and logging ended in the 1940s, and, as humans left, plants and animals slowly reclaimed the land. In the 1960s, the Arundel family donated the land to

KEY AT-A-GLANCE INFORMATION

LENGTH: 5.4 miles (with shorter option)

CONFIGURATION: Modified loop

DIFFICULTY: Easy–moderate

SCENERY: Hilly woodlands, with some farmland views in winter

EXPOSURE: Mostly shady; less so in winter

TRAFFIC: Usually very light

TRAIL SURFACE: Mostly dirt or dirt-and-gravel; some grass; rocky, rooty, muddy in places

HIKING TIME: 3–4 hours

SEASON: Year-round, but best in spring and especially in leafless late fall and winter

ACCESS: Open daily, dawn–dusk

MAPS: USGS Marshall; free contour map of preserve (available at trailhead and also on Web site)

FACILITIES: None

FOR MORE INFORMATION: Visit Nature Conservancy's Web site, www.nature.org; call its Virginia chapter, in Charlottesville, (804) 295-6106

Directions

From Capital Beltway (Interstate 495) in Merrifield, Virginia, take Exit 49 to get onto I-66 heading west. Proceed for 35.4 miles to Marshall, and then leave I-66 at Exit 28. At end of 0.2-mile exit ramp, turn left onto VA 17 and proceed for 0.25 miles. Then turn right onto VA 691 (Carters Run Road) and proceed for 5.1 miles, and turn left onto England Mountain Road. Continue for 0.2 miles on road that's initially paved but becomes gravel (note yellow "WMNA" signs), and pull into small parking area on right near information board.

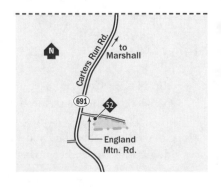

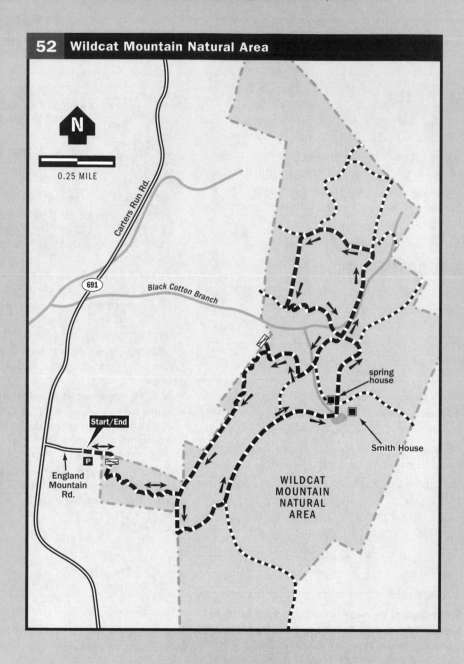

52 Wildcat Mountain Natural Area

N

0.25 MILE

Carters Run Rd.

691

Black Cotton Branch

spring house

Start/End

P

England Mountain Rd.

Smith House

WILDCAT MOUNTAIN NATURAL AREA

the Nature Conservancy, and the young organization used it to establish its first preserve in Virginia. And the rest is natural history.

The preserve is now covered mostly by stands of oak and hickory interspersed with beeches and other hardwoods, as well as some conifers. Redbuds, dogwoods, and other flowering trees brighten the spring landscape, as do a modest variety of wildflowers (including certain species, such as fame-flower, wild pink, and curlyhead, that grow on greenstone outcrops). The area is also home to deer, foxes, bobcats (for which it seems to be named), and smaller mammals, and bears. Some 200 species of birds are known to have visitation rights. The preserve is scenic year-round, but I prefer to trade off springtime floral color for leafless late-fall or winter vistas. Trail traffic is never a problem; I have yet to encounter any hikers there other than my companions.

A modest network of hiking trails crisscrosses the preserve, with access consisting of a steep trail from the trailhead. The network is a mix of fire roads, old farm roads, and dirt trails. They are all unnamed and well maintained, and mostly unsignposted (there are a few posted rondelles, or small round three-inch signs, bearing the conservancy's name and an oak leaf). I have used the network to devise a wiggly loop that covers 5.4 miles, with about 2,000 feet of elevation change (almost half of which is accounted for by the access trail). Along the route, you'll see an old farmhouse and mortarless stone walls.

The loop includes lots of turns, so I encourage you to carefully follow my directions and map. Also, stay on the designated trails (except, perhaps, for the ten-yard bushwhack I include), in that some plant habitats are fragile, some side trails lead onto private property without notice, and the native species include poison ivy. There are several streams to cross, but they are all narrow or naturally equipped with stepping-stones.

To get started, continue on foot uphill on the gravel road for 200 yards until you reach a T-junction. There, turn right onto an old unpaved farm road and follow it gently uphill for another 200 yards and past a chain gate. At a green "Trail" sign, turn left and head uphill on a dirt trail that zigzags for almost half a mile up to the ridge. The trail is faint in places, so watch for TNC rondelles on the trees. Also watch your step, in that the trail is steep in some places and rocky in others (note the distinctive outcrops of greenstone). Pause, too, not only to catch your breath but also to take in the distant ridge and farmland views to the west (behind you).

As the trail levels off, you'll reach and pass through a break in an old stone wall. Note the spot because it'll be a key junction later in the hike. Turn right and get on the trail that goes gently uphill next to the wall. As you go, peer over the beautifully built wall for more views to the west. After some 300 yards of wall walking, follow the trail as it turns left and takes a level and gently downhill route for about 0.25 miles to reach an old fire road. Turn left there, and follow the road gently downhill for about 0.75 miles, ignoring the side trail on the left en route.

After passing an old farm pond on the right, you'll reach a grassy clearing that's the site of a boarded-up old homestead called the Smith House. Built in about 1910 by a local businessman and Baptist preacher named Enoch Smith, the house remained occupied at least through the 1940s. Walk around the house and note its lapped-wood walls, tin roof, and generous supply of brick chimneys. Take a brief side trip to the nearby spring house.

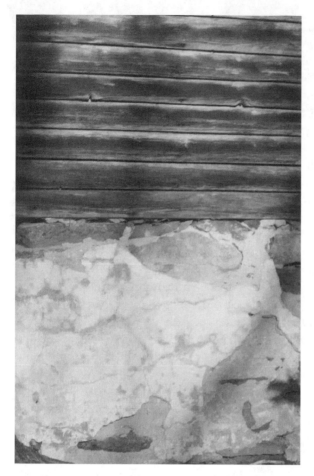

When at the Smith House, see if you think this white wall area looks like the U.S. map (note the Gulf, Florida, and East Coast).

From the front of the Smith House, get on the fire road ahead of you that's fairly level (ignore the uphill trail to the right). After 0.25 miles, you'll cross a small stream and reach a T-junction. There, turn left and head downhill for about 200 yards next to the just-crossed stream, and past a lone but comforting TNC rondelle. Arriving at a skewed four-way intersection (to which you'll return), turn right and proceed uphill on a fire road for about 0.5 miles though a somewhat open woodland area to get to a five-way intersection. There, swing left and go slightly downhill (shun the two ascending trails on the right, as well as the stump of a downhill trail on the far left). Over the next 0.25 miles, the road ascends gently, as you should, and passes a grand stand of pines on the left before leveling off and reaching a fork. There, go straight and downhill on a dirt trail for about 200 yards to a T-junction, marked by a large rock on the corner.

Turn left at the rock and continue downhill. In winter, it's worth pausing after about 150 yards to bushwhack carefully to the right for just ten yards to get lovely glimpses of Shenandoah National Park to the west. About 0.25 miles beyond the rock, swing left at a fork (where there are fine wintertime views off to the right) and follow the undulating trail for 0.25 miles back to the skewed four-way intersection. Along the way, you'll be on a grassy trail in a scenic open area and cross a stream called Black Cotton Branch. At the intersection, bear right and cross and recross a small stream to get onto another 0.25-mile dirt trail that leads to a fork. There, turn right and follow a 200-yard trail downhill, across two small streams, and then uphill to a T-junction.

Turn right and thereby get started on what I consider to be the hike's loveliest part—a 1.3-mile twisting and undulating ridgetop trail that leads scenically back to the break-in-the-stone-wall junction. After crossing another pair of streams (oddly, the preserve's streams seem to come in pairs), go uphill on an old road for 60 yards. Then turn left and uphill onto a faint dirt trail that may still be marked with pink flagging, and beyond which is a reassuring TNC rondelle (if you miss that turn, you'll wind up at a locked gate—in which case, return and try again). Keep going in a generally southwestward direction, passing more rondelles and perhaps more flagging, and take in the gorgeous leafless views off to your right. On reaching an eight-foot-high cone-shaped rock, turn right and then left to stay on the trail. When you get to the stone-wall junction, turn right and head back down to the trailhead, taking in the views ahead but also keeping an eye on your footing.

To shorten this short hike to 3 miles, on leaving the Smith House, take the trail to the left of the fire road, turn left at the next T-junction and right at the one after that, and then continue with what I call above the hike's loveliest part.

NEARBY/RELATED ACTIVITIES

See if you can spend a little time in the company of preserve steward Marvin Mitchell, who is knowledgeable and affable, and who lives nearby. Try calling him at (540) 347-7026.

53 SKY MEADOWS STATE PARK

KEY AT-A-GLANCE INFORMATION

LENGTH: 7.9 miles (with shorter options)

CONFIGURATION: Loop

DIFFICULTY: Moderate

SCENERY: Vista-rich upland meadows; woodlands

EXPOSURE: Mostly shady; less so in winter

TRAFFIC: Mostly very light–light; heavier on warm-weather weekends, holidays

TRAIL SURFACE: Mostly dirt; some gravel, grass; rocky, rooty in some places

HIKING TIME: 4.5–6.5 hours (including overlook looking)

SEASON: Year-round

ACCESS: Open daily, 8 a.m.–dusk; entrance fee

MAPS: USGS Upperville, Ashby Gap; PATC Map 8; sketch map in free park pamphlet

FACILITIES: Toilets, water, phone at trailhead; toilet near contact station

FOR MORE INFORMATION: Contact park, (540) 592-3556 or www.dcr.state.va.us/parks/sky meado.htm; look for knowledgeable ranger Bruce Baraniak at park; contact Appalachian Trail Conservancy, (304) 535-6331 or www.appalachiantrail.org

IN BRIEF

Sky Meadows State Park, in Virginia's portion of the Blue Ridge, lives up to its name. Up there, too, hikers can enjoy woodlands, wildlife, exercise, and an Appalachian Trail segment.

DESCRIPTION

Sky Meadows State Park, some 60 miles west of Washington, is a wonderfully tilted place. Suspended from the Appalachian Trail (AT), it spreads across the Blue Ridge's eastern flanks down to the Piedmont. It consists of almost nothing but slopes. Some support broad meadows reminiscent of the Alps, with vistas unsurpassed in the metro area. Others carry woodlands harboring a wealth of flora and fauna. Throughout the park are canted trails conducive to the release of human endorphins and sweat.

The 1,842-acre park lies within an extraordinary area of unspoiled, saved, and protected countryside along the border between Fauquier and Loudoun counties. The landscape is one of woodlands and fields dotted with an occasional pond or farm building and crossed by a few ribbons of country road. It seems ageless, tranquil, and inviting. In addition to the park, the larger area includes active

Directions

From Capital Beltway (Interstate 495) in Merrifield, Virginia, take Exit 49 to get on I-66 heading west. Proceed for about 40 miles, and take Exit 23 onto US 17 north. Proceed for 7.3 miles, and turn left into park on Edmonds Lane. Drive 0.7 miles to contact station, and then 0.6 miles to parking lot at visitor center.

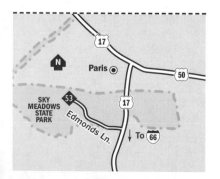

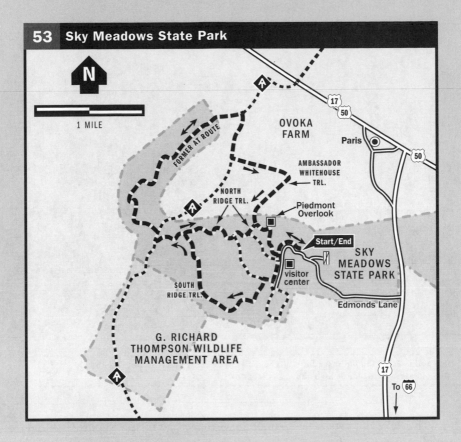

farms, the 4,000-acre Thompson Wildlife Management Area (WMA) (see Hike 54, page 261), and saved-from-development 1,500-acre Ovoka Farm, acquired jointly in 2003 by the National Park Service (NPS) and Piedmont Environmental Council (with support from the Appalachian Trail Conservancy).

As farmland, the park's core area has a heritage dating back three centuries. A series of families raised crops, livestock, and children there. Their cumulative history is preserved in the restored main building—called Mount Bleak—and other structures near the current parking lot. Sky Meadows's beginnings as a park date back to the mid-1960s, when philanthropist and local resident Paul Mellon (son of Andrew, who gave us the National Gallery of Art and other treasures) saved the area from becoming an upscale subdivision. He donated the property to the state of Virginia in 1975. After the park was opened in 1983, the state added additional acreage to protectively encase a stretch of the AT. Later, the park grew to its present size when Mellon donated a 462-acre area just across US 17 for the use of horses and their riders.

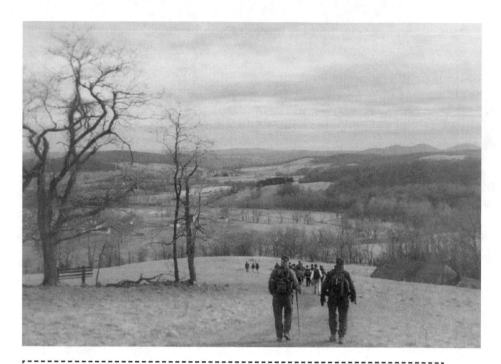

Opened in 2005, the Ambassador Whitehouse Trail enables hikers to traverse the old
Ovoka Farm grazing lands high above Sky Meadows.

This hike consists of a 7.9-mile loop that accumulates about 2,100 feet of elevation change (only a few of which are steep) and ranges across the meadows and woodlands of both the park and Ovoka Farm. It's a rewarding hike, with the landscape and seasons providing a continuum of change, some breathtaking views, and an occasional surprise (my best so far: seeing a bluebird in the snow, and, separately and mysteriously, a common loon on a high ridge). Oddly, though, the park lacks the botanical richness and diversity of the adjoining Thompson WMA (Ranger Baraniak thinks the difference may be the park's high density of safe-from-hunters deer). The trails are named, color coded, well marked, generally well maintained, and well mapped. Be sure to stay on them when in the woods, where poison ivy lurks. When in the meadows, steer clear of long grass (tick-tick-tick) and cow pies. Although animals are protected in the park, adjoining areas are open to hunters, so wear orange in the fall, especially on the AT.

To get started from the parking-lot trailhead, head for the nearby "Hiking Trails Campground" sign. Follow the dirt path for about 140 yards and then turn left onto a country lane. Follow the lane gently downhill, and then turn right to get onto the Gap Run Trail (0.5 miles into the hike). Go about 100 yards, and turn left onto the yellow-blazed South Ridge Trail. Keep going for about 1.6 miles on what was an old farm road, detouring en route to catch your breath at a vista-equipped bench on the right. After the trail levels out somewhat and slides into the woods, you'll reach its literally bench-marked T-junction with the blue-blazed North Ridge Trail. Turn left and continue uphill on the narrow rocky trail for about 0.5 miles to where it tops out and meets the white-blazed AT.

There, turn right and go about 200 yards to a significant T-junction. There, look straight ahead to see a new segment of the AT—but turn left to follow a 1.9-mile long former segment, now blazed purple (or is that mauve?). It's a woodland trail that goes downhill, turns right onto an old fire road, turns left (just before a gate across the road), and then winds and undulates through the trees. Watch for a couple of tricky turns. The first is where the trail leaves what seems to be the main trail to swing left at a blaze and acquire a rocky tread. The second occurs after the trail turns sharp left and goes downhill as an old narrow road; at the bottom, be sure to turn sharp right to get onto a dirt trail.

Continue until you find yourself at the signposted and white-blazed AT. Turn right to experience the relocated AT as it climbs gently out of the woods and out onto a high plateau on what were once Ovoka Farm pasturelands. Note the bird banding box on the left (if it's still there when you arrive). And after about 0.6 miles on the new AT (out of 1.3 miles total), turn left onto the signposted, light-blue–blazed, and new Ambassador Whitehouse Trail. It's 1.1 winding miles long and is a mowed-grass trail that offers panoramic views mostly to the south before dipping into the woods as a dirt trail to enter the park and end at the North Ridge Trail. There, turn left and follow the familiar blue blazes for about 200 yards, and turn left again onto the red-blazed and 0.7-mile long Piedmont Overlook Trail, which initially is somewhat rocky and goes uphill.

The trail levels off, crosses a stile, and emerges from the woods as a grassy trail where a couple of benches mark the magnificent Piedmont Overlook. Depending on the season and weather, you'll have views across the Piedmont to the east and south. Linger a while, and then head downhill through the meadow for over half a mile, following a line of trail markers and a seasonally mowed path. When cattle are present, the area resembles Europe's alpine pastures in several biological respects, so watch your step if cows are not your passion. But be grateful that their appetites and teeth help keep the meadows from reverting to woodland. Near the bottom, swing to the right, pass an old shed, turn left, cross a stile, turn left again onto the old country lane, and return to the trailhead. On leaving the park, watch along the entrance road for evidence that the park has one of Virginia's largest populations of redheaded woodpeckers.

Shorter hikes at Sky Meadows are worthwhile only if they include an overlook. One 3.6-mile option is to take the South Ridge Trail up and then the North Ridge Trail and Piedmont Overlook Trail back. Or for a vista-rich, 1.5-mile outing, just go up and down the overlook trail—which I sometimes do as an aerobic group-hike postscript to my elevation-free Virginia Arboretum outing (Hike 55, page 265).

NEARBY/RELATED ACTIVITIES

During the warm-weather months, tour Mount Bleak and sample the park's events and programs. Among them are the two-day Delaplane Strawberry Festival (late May), full-moon walks on the Piedmont Overlook Trail, and astronomy programs featuring telescopes, experts, and the dark night sky; contact the park for details.

After leaving the park, take a 6-mile detour on a beguiling country road that winds through woodlands and farmlands from US 17 to south of I-66. Start by heading south on US 17 for 0.5 miles and turning right onto VA 688 (Leeds Manor Road). Year-round, along that road, you'll find much scenery, a winery, and access to the Thompson Wildlife Management Area (see following hike profile). And from June to October, you'll find five family-run pick-your-own orchards offering cherries, berries, peaches, apples, and pumpkins (for details, visit **www.pickyourown/VAnorthern.htm**). In July and August, in fact, VA 688 becomes the county's "Peach Way," and in particular I favor the remarkably flavorful Beekman variety grown at Hollins Farms (**www.hollinfarms.com**). In the fall, you'll find about 20 varieties of apple (plus fresh cider) at the Hartland-Troy Orchard (**www.hartlandorchard.com**). Stock up and then head back east on I-66.

THOMPSON WILDLIFE MANAGEMENT AREA

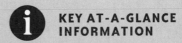

IN BRIEF

The Thompson Wildlife Management Area, in Virginia's Fauquier County, is richly supplied with trees, wildflowers, and wildlife, and enough trails to make it a rewarding hiking venue.

DESCRIPTION

The G. Richard Thompson Wildlife Management Area (WMA) covers almost 4,000 acres on the eastern slopes of the Blue Ridge. Lying about 10 miles east of Front Royal and 60 plus miles west of Washington, the state-owned, well-wooded WMA is managed chiefly to provide habitat for deer, black bears, and other creatures. For hikers, the habitat itself is the major draw, especially in spring, when trilliums are in bloom. The WMA is graced with what is probably North America's largest trillium stand (up to 30 million). It's also one of Virginia's richest botanical areas, and myriad other wildflower blooms carpet the woods from late spring to late fall. And resident and migrating birds, and butterflies, add both color and movement. Fall is also the main hunting season, when it's best to hike elsewhere (check with the state game department or Appalachian Trail Conservancy on dates). Even so, Sunday is officially a no-hunting day throughout Virginia.

Directions

From Capital Beltway (I-495) in Merrifield, Virginia, take Exit 49 and get on I-66 heading west. Proceed for about 50 miles to Linden. There, leave I-66 at Exit 13, take first left, go under I-66, and take first left to get onto US 55 heading east. Proceed for 1.3 miles and turn left onto VA 638. Drive 3.8 miles, and pull into Upper Ted Lake parking area on right.

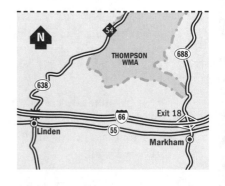

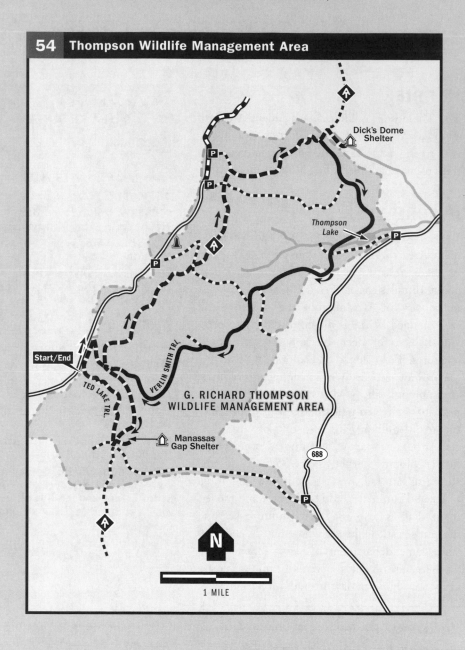

The hike described here consists of a 10.3-mile clockwise loop that includes an Appalachian Trail (AT) segment and approximately 3,200 feet of elevation change. As signposts and blazes are not abundant, use the following directions well.

To get started from the parking-area trailhead, take the old dirt road at the back and follow it downhill for 70 yards, and turn left onto a narrow dirt trail. After about 200 yards, turn right onto another old road (the Verlin Smith Trail) and follow it downhill for 200 yards to its junction with the northbound AT (the southbound AT is 100 yards farther down the road). Turn left onto the white-blazed and undulating AT and keep going northward for 3.6 miles close to the Blue Ridge crest line to your left. En route, in late April and May, watch for large-flowered trilliums, with their three broad leaves and three large white or pink petals. In trillium areas, stay on the trail. The plants grow slowly, taking up to eight years to produce their first flowers. They're easily killed by a heavy foot or grasping hand.

After passing the second and larger of two big rocks on the right and easing downhill for about half a mile, you'll reach a three-way junction. There, turn left to stay on the AT. After about 200 yards, leave the AT and turn right onto a blue-blazed path. Follow it and a small stream (Whiskey Hollow Creek) downhill. On reaching Dick's Dome Shelter, a stopover for AT through-hikers, be sure to peruse the logbook (trail register) for information and amusement.

From there, retrace your steps to the AT and then back to the three-way junction. This time, turn left, onto an unblazed trail that wanders generally south and downhill. After almost half a mile, you'll reach another junction—and be about halfway through the hike. There, bear left onto a seasonally overgrown road for another half mile to get to Thompson Lake. Follow the trail around the ten-acre lake's western shore. In high summer, watch especially for butterflies.

At the next intersection, go straight and ascend a steep hill. At a junction marked by a converted red barn, turn right to follow the WMA boundary gently uphill. At the next junction, turn right to begin a long woodland ascent. After a third of a mile, reach a pair of trail junctions. Turn right at the first one, and then left at the second one, next to a ruined metal shack. After going uphill on a dirt path, you'll reach a stream (Wildcat Hollow Creek) and discover that, for about 50 yards, the stream and trail vie for the same space.

After that, you'll be on the lower end of the Verlin Smith Trail. Swing sharply right, stop climbing, and again have trilliums for company. At the next junction, turn left onto the AT to start the hike's last leg by going uphill·and then gently downhill for almost a mile. Then, at a signposted T-junction, detour 120 yards to your left on a blue-blazed trail to experience the Manassas Gap Shelter and its thru-hiker logbook entries. Return to the T-junction, turn left, go 100 yards on the AT to another T-junction, and turn right and uphill onto the blue-blazed Ted Lake Trail. Keep going on the old road for about three-quarters of a mile to reach the trailhead and your car.

For a trillium-rich, 2-mile sampler loop, go south instead of north on the AT when you're first on the Verlin Smith Trail (see the map). To do the full hike (and a bit more) and end with an easy downhill leg, start at the parking area along VA 688 (Leeds Manor Road) near the lake (see the map and also Hike 53, page 256, for directions).

NEARBY/RELATED ACTIVITIES

Visit the family-run Apple House, (540) 635-2118, at I-66 Exit 13 in Linden. It's an eccentric mix of restaurant, gift shop, general store, and apple stand, plus bathrooms. Try its Alpenglow, a nonalcoholic fizzy cider invented by the family. If you like fresh apples, visit the pick-your-own Stribling Orchard (www.striblingorchard.com), in nearby Markham, on VA 688 (Leeds Manor Road) just south of both VA 55 and I-66 at Exit 18. Family-owned for six generations (so far), the orchard also offers eight peach varieties and is the southernmost of the five orchards along VA 688 that cause the road to sprout colorful "Peach Way" signs in summer (also see Hike 53, page 256).

VIRGINIA STATE ARBORETUM 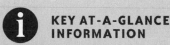 55

IN BRIEF

The Virginia State Arboretum lies amid the farmlands of northwestern Virginia. As a year-round hiking venue, it is novel, uncrowded, and picturesque.

DESCRIPTION

The Virginia State Arboretum covers 172 acres of gently rolling Clarke County countryside just west of the Shenandoah River and roughly 60 crow miles west of Washington, D.C. Officially, it's the Orland E. White Arboretum and part of a 700-acre agricultural research station operated by the University of Virginia. Although hiking there is physically unchallenging, it offers superlative aesthetic pleasures. The core setting consists of open woods and broad meadows. The woods range from dense research plots to spacious groupings of native trees, shrubs, and associated non-native species. The meadows furnish serene vistas all year and erupt in vivid wildflower color in the warm-weather months. This core area is surrounded by the research station's other lands, which in turn are encircled by commercial farms. Consequently, an arboretum hike feels like a journey through a countryside stretching to the horizon.

KEY AT-A-GLANCE INFORMATION

LENGTH: 5.3 miles (with shorter options—and a longer one)

CONFIGURATION: Modified loop

DIFFICULTY: Easy

SCENERY: Gentle hills, meadows, open woods, farmlands, ephemeral ponds

EXPOSURE: Mostly open

TRAFFIC: Very light; heavier on warm-weather weekends, holidays near trailhead

TRAIL SURFACE: Mostly grass; some dirt, gravel, pavement

HIKING TIME: 3–4 hours (scenery-gazing and label-reading included)

SEASON: Year-round, but usually loveliest in spring and fall

ACCESS: Open daily, dawn–dusk

MAPS: USGS Boyce; sketch maps in free facility pamphlets (accuracy is iffy)

FACILITIES: All near trailhead: toilets, water, emergency pay phone at Quarters; water at picnic area

FOR MORE INFORMATION: Contact Blandy Experimental Farm, (540) 837-1758 or www.virginia.edu/~blandy

---

Directions

From Capital Beltway (Interstate 495) in Merrifield, Virginia, take Exit 49 and get on I-66 heading west. Proceed for about 40 miles, and take Exit 23 onto US 17 north. Go 8 miles, and turn left onto US 50 west (also US 17 north). Continue for 7.9 miles to brown "Arboretum" sign on right. Get in left lane immediately and 0.2 miles later, turn left into arboretum on Blandy Farm Road. Drive 0.5 miles to main parking lot.

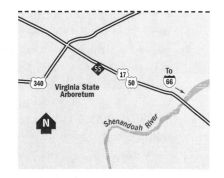

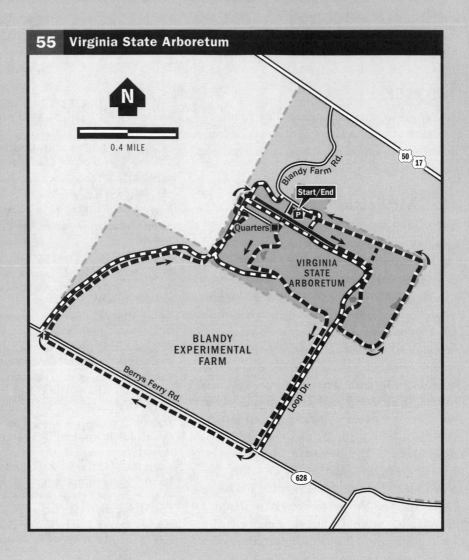

The arboretum also can be wonderful beyond the colorful attractions of spring and fall. In summer, you can freely roam the colorful meadows on broad mowed pathways (but beware the beating sun). In winter, crossing the withered grasslands under a slate sky can evoke starkly beautiful images of Western plains or Brontean moors. In good weather at any season, try ending your outing by walking across the meadows and into the sunset when the evening seems spread out against the sky. Yet another year-round pleasure is that the arboretum offers solitude and tranquility. Visitors are mostly researchers, gardening enthusiasts, and a few tourists, nearly all of whom stay close to the Quarters.

This easy, 5.3-mile hike covers most of the arboretum and a bit of the research station. In using the following description, keep in mind that distances are short, many trees are labeled, and the bluebird nesting boxes are numerous—as are both the species and numbers of birds, so take along field glasses. You'll also see gnarled trees, stone walls, old roads, a large old mansion beyond the fence, and other signs that the area is rich in history.

The mansion dates from the 1830s, when Joseph Tuly had it built on his plantation and named it Tuleyries (possibly a playful variant on the name of the famous French palace). Eventually, a stockbroker named Graham Blandy acquired the property. When he died in 1926, he left most of his 900 acres to the University of Virginia with the mansion and remaining acreage remaining in private hands. The following year, Orland E. White joined the university faculty as a professor of agricultural biology and director of the new Blandy Experimental Farm. Gradually, he transformed the property into a renowned research institution. After he retired in the mid-1950s, the arboretum was named in his honor. It became Virginia's state arboretum in 1986.

Get started by leaving the parking lot, browsing at the nearby information kiosk, and then taking the paved path leading to a two-story brick building. Known as the Quarters, it houses offices, a laboratory, a library, and researchers' living quarters. It's actually two buildings separated by a century. The left-hand wing was part of the plantation's slave quarters. The other wing and the linking portion were added in the 1940s. Walk through the link's arched passageway and then across the flower-rimmed courtyard lawn on a short paved path. At the path's end, first swing right to admire the large Korean dogwood planted in 1976 in memory of Graham Bland. Then swing left across a broad, grassy, and tree-lined avenue to reach the signposted Conifer Trail, which is actually just a series of numbered posts bordering a strip of conifers. Note number 5, a weeping Norway spruce that's worth admiring. At number 7, turn right and return to the avenue.

There, turn left and walk across the weathered, cacti-dotted bedrock that seems to have heaved up through the grass. Then pass ephemeral Lake Georgette on your left and head for a small green cinderblock structure, just beyond a ruined stone wall. Swing left in front of the wall and proceed gently uphill on an old road. On the left is a regal line of Sawara cypresses (native to Japan); on the right, though, next to the ruined wall, is a forlorn line of cypress stumps. After the ground levels off and the road disappears, keep going across the grass and through a grove of black walnut trees. Then, turn left onto a gravel side road. For the next half mile, you'll be close to the arboretum's southern property line, which is shrouded in a tangle of shrubbery.

After the road ends in roughly 200 yards, continue across the grass, edging right to pass through a stone wall. This area is filled with magnolias, dominated by a huge cucumber tree, or cucumber magnolia. From there, traverse a tree-flanked meadow, staying to the right of center. Watch for numbered posts that mark the

Broadleaf Trail. My route uses only a few of them, and out of sequence at that. After passing number 11 and number 4, veer right and around an unmowed area and proceed through wooded areas devoted to the rose family and pea family, then pass posts number 5, 9, and 8.

When you get to a gravel road (it's the one-day Loop Drive), turn right and follow it out of the arboretum, into the open, and into the farming part of Blandy Experimental Farm. Be alert for occasional vehicles approaching from behind. Cultivated fields and a few farm buildings surround you, with the Blue Ridge crest line as a hazy backdrop. Also note a distinctive horse-head trail sign on the right and opposite a fenced paddock on your left. That's the trailhead for Blandy's new, 5.3-mile-long Bridle Trail (the farm's only named trail), which coincides with parts of my hike route but ventures deep into Blandy's meadows to the east and scrubland to the west as a simple mowed-grass pathway (but is not shown on the map).

Turn right onto paved VA 628, which marks the farm's southern limit. It's lightly traveled, but you should cross and walk on the shoulder. Note the private cattle farm on your left. After about 0.8 miles, recross the road and turn right onto a gravel-surfaced lane that's part of the Loop Drive and winds through an overgrown research woodlot.

Then mark the hike's halfway point by veering left off the lane to detour through a glorious grove of more than 300 ginkgo trees. Walk under a canopy of yellow flowers in spring, fan-shaped green leaves in summer, and bright yellow leaves in the fall. Beyond the native-to-China gingkos, at all seasons, the Tuleyries remains visible.

Back on the road, march down a handsome row of cedars of Lebanon (a nonnative species that's very rare in the metro area). At the side road after the one signposted "Parking," and especially if it's spring, take another short detour. Turn right onto the side road, climb a grassy slope, and circle through a scenic area of pines and azaleas. Then return to the Loop Drive.

Next, turn right onto Dogwood Lane. Lined with restored field-limestone walls and dazzling-in-spring dogwoods, it will take you past an amphitheater and the Quarters to the front end of the Loop Drive. Staying alert for cars, follow the drive as it traces an L-shaped course across wildflower-laced meadows for almost half a mile. Along the way, semicircle to the left to visit an ephemeral pond (Lake Arnold) and several huge and wonderful willows. Just before the Loop Drive leaves the arboretum, turn left to follow the fence line. Remain close to it for almost 2 miles, moving across gently rolling terrain and mowed-in-season terrain, and pass through several groves.

The first grove consists of maples that nicely slow down a fall hike. As you reach a corner of the arboretum, turn left and head down a gentle grassy slope toward a large woodpile. Beyond the pile, cut through a band of woods and veer to the right around a small pond. Then proceed gently uphill until you reach a second arboretum corner. Turn left there and continue across the tree-dotted grassland and along the fence line. Depending on what creatures may be lurking in the grass, watch for hawks overhead (twice I've seen six little feet dangling beneath powerful wings). Pressing on, head for a gravel road (it's the Loop Drive again). Swing right and follow the road about 100 yards back to the trailhead.

Use the map to devise a shorter hike for yourself, such as cutting out the Loop Drive segment around the Blandy fields. Or lengthen the hike by incorporating parts of the Bridle Trail (see the map).

NEARBY/RELATED ACTIVITIES

Plan your arboretum visit to coincide with a scheduled program or event, such as the Garden Fair on Mother's Day Weekend in May, summer concerts in the amphitheater, or Arborfest in October. Call for details, (540) 837-1758. Visit the historic Burwell-Morgan Mill in nearby Millwood, (540) 837-1799.

56 SHENANDOAH RIVER STATE PARK

KEY AT-A-GLANCE INFORMATION

LENGTH: 11 miles (with shorter options plus hike and paddle option)

CONFIGURATION: Modified loop

DIFFICULTY: Hard

SCENERY: River views in variety and abundance, woodlands, grassy floodplain, forested mountain slopes in distance

EXPOSURE: About 60% open; more so in winter

TRAFFIC: Usually very light; relatively heavier in trailhead vicinity

TRAIL SURFACE: Chiefly dirt, with stretches of pavement, gravel, grass, wood chips; rooty, rocky, muddy in places

HIKING TIME: 5.5–7 hours

SEASON: Year-round, but can be too sunny and hot in summer

ACCESS: Open daily, 8 a.m.–dusk ("weather permitting"); entrance fee

MAPS: USGS Bentonville; sketch map in free park brochure, posted near trailhead and at Web site below

FACILITIES: Toilets, water, phones at trailhead; toilet at stables; toilets off-trail at outfitters at Bentonville Landing

FOR MORE INFORMATION: Contact park, (540) 622-6840 or www.dcr .state.va.us/parks/andygues.htm

IN BRIEF

Hidden in northwestern Virginia's Warren County lies a splendid state park where hikers can find a plethora of trails, scenery, flora, fauna, aerobic opportunity, and solitude.

DESCRIPTION

Opened in 1999, Shenandoah River State Park is definitely one of Virginia's newest state parks—and probably still one of its best-kept secrets. I surmise that it suffers from being overshadowed as a recreational destination by Shenandoah National Park and as a conspicuous tract of public land by Massanutten Mountain. Even so, I rank it as one of the metro area's most overlooked, most scenically varied, most underhiked, and loveliest hiking venues. As corroborating evidence, I offer you this hike, which I have devised jointly with Mike Darzi.

The park lies near Bentonville, about 8 miles southwest of Front Royal and 60-plus miles west of the Capital Beltway. Officially named the Raymond "Andy" Guest Jr.

Directions ⟶

From Capital Beltway (Interstate 495) in Merrifield, Virginia, take Exit 49 and get on I-66 heading west. Proceed for about 50 miles to Linden. There, leave I-66 at Exit 13, take first left, go under I-66, and take first right to get onto US 55 heading west. Proceed for 5.3 miles to Front Royal, turn left onto US 340, and drive south for 8.1 miles toward Bentonville; then turn right onto Shenandoah River State Park's entrance road. Proceed for 0.4 miles to contact station. Then continue for about 1.5 miles and downhill to T-junction, turn left, and go 0.25 miles to far end of large parking area, near shelter number 1.

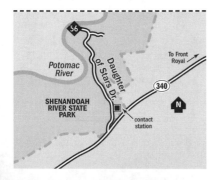

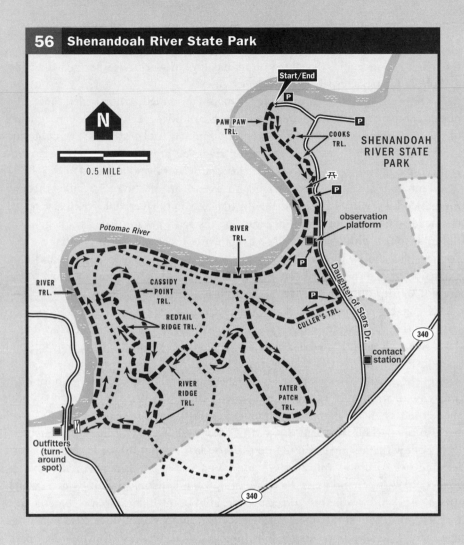

56 Shenandoah River State Park

Start/End

PAW PAW TRL.

COOKS TRL.

SHENANDOAH RIVER STATE PARK

N

0.5 MILE

observation platform

Potomac River

RIVER TRL.

RIVER TRL.

CASSIDY POINT TRL.

REDTAIL RIDGE TRL.

Daughter of Stars Dr.

CULLER'S TRL.

340

contact station

RIVER RIDGE TRL.

TATER PATCH TRL.

Outfitters (turn-around spot)

340

Shenandoah River State Park (for a state assemblyman from Front Royal), it extends 6 miles along the scenic (but, alas, complexly and mysteriously polluted) North Fork of the Shenandoah River and encompasses 1,604 acres of chiefly rugged and wooded hills, plus a grassy floodplain and some pastures and former farm fields.

The locale is rich in flora, including such deciduous trees as oaks, hickories, beeches, tulip trees, sycamores, dogwoods, black walnuts, and fruit-bearing paw-paws, along with some stands of pines. There's also a rich understory of wild-flowers and bushes (including lots of raspberry, blackberry, and blueberry bushes—and yes, you're allowed to pluck the fruit), plus poison ivy along the river (but, oddly, not inland). The park's animal life includes myriad birds and also bears, deer, foxes, and other, smaller creatures. You'll also encounter horses, but they're domestic and there because equestrians are attracted to the park's trails and riding stable. (Speaking of animal life, in warm weather guard against and check for ticks, especially tiny deer ticks.)

The trails are all well maintained, mapped, named, color coded, and sign-posted. Some of them are blazed, but others are not—perhaps as a consequence of the park being a work in slow progress. Human trail traffic is very light, and most visitors seem to be attracted to the riverside areas, where there are picnic and camping amenities and access for boaters, waders, and anglers.

Our hike consists of a loopy inland excursion of about 7.5 miles through the park's hilly woodlands, and then a flat, 3.5-mile riverbank trek back to the trailhead—but with the option of returning instead by water (see next page). The full hike comes with about 3,000 feet of elevation change, all in the first part, so you can also choose to stay on the level the whole way by doing an out-and-back excursion on the riverbank. You can also use the trail description and map to fig-ure out shorter options.

I suggest starting the hike with a stretch-your-legs 0.75-mile mini-loop between the trailhead (nominally shelter 1) and the riverbank at Fish Trap Rapid. To do that, head for shelter 3 and cut diagonally across the tidy, mowed, and tree-dotted picnic area to take a 30-yard-long gravel ramp leading to the river. There, check out the view, raspberry bushes, and walnut trees, and then look for a narrow dirt trail that follows the wooded riverbank upstream. At an open area that's used as a canoe launch, turn left and follow a gravel path and paved road back to the parking area and the start of the Paw Paw Trail (blazed black).

Follow the mostly dirt trail into the woods for about 30 yards, and then turn left and steeply uphill onto the 0.2-mile Clean Sweep Trail (purple). Continue as that trail levels off and joins the undulating 0.5-mile Cook's Trail (white), which offers vista glimpses before traversing the Highpoint Picnic Area to emerge at a parking area. Out in the open, turn right onto the park entrance road and surge uphill for 1.2 miles, including a short detour to the Cullers Overlook, an obser-vation platform with fine views of Massanutten Mountain and the river, and a plaque about the pre-park owners.

Then, at the next side road, turn right to proceed for 0.7 miles through a parking lot, into the woods, along a gravel road, and onto the Culler's Trail (orange). Continue past the paved side road to Indian Hollow Stables on the left, and proceed downhill on a broad trail that goes past an unnamed side trail on the left, over a small bridge, and into a level open area. There, turn left at a sign-post, go roughly 70 yards on a gravel road, and turn left again to get onto the signposted Tater Patch Trail (light blue). Proceed, initially uphill, on that mostly broad trail (partly an old farm road), which forms a 1.3-mile up-and-down par-tial loop that ends at the Sawmill Hollow Trail (gray). There, turn left, go about 0.2 miles uphill, turn left onto the River Ridge Trail (teal) at a T-junction, and proceed uphill for 0.4 miles.

Then, at an asymmetric intersection marked by a picnic table, turn right onto the Cassidy Point Trail (light green)—and note the nearby Redtail Ridge you'll be on later. Follow the light-green blazes for 0.7 miles on a broad and mostly level trail that threads through open woods and then dips steeply downhill to reach a gravel road at a signpost near a boarded-up tin-roofed cabin. Turn left, walk a few yards to another signpost, and turn left to head uphill and back into the woods on the 0.5-mile-long Redtail Ridge Trail (red). You'll follow a streambed, cross a small gully, and, within about 200 yards, reach a T-junction and a red-blazed tree bearing a promising one-word sign ("view").

Turn right to ascend 50 yards on a rough trail leading to a tree-shaded spot just past a cedar that has a lower trunk resembling the bulgy head of a grouper. There you'll find some fine sitting rocks and backrest trees, plus panoramic views of the dark and hulking Massanutten, the sparkling and burbling Shenandoah (you'll hear it, too), and the overarching sky. Ah, what a great lunch and siesta spot!

Then, refreshed, return to the main trail and keep going on what is an oddly overblazed trail that stays close to the ridgeline (and provides nice winter views), crosses several gullies, and takes you to a familiar, table-equipped intersection. There, turn right to do the remainder of the River Ridge Trail (almost a mile). Then, after making a sharp right, turn at a bench next to an officially closed trail, and start heading downhill on a trail that gets quite steep and rocky and crosses crumbly shale outcrops before leveling off and crossing 100 yards of grassy floodplain to reach the gravel road. There, turn left to follow the road for 0.3 miles through a gate, out of the park, down a paved road, and across Rocky Hollow Road to the hike's turnaround spot, where you should decide whether to return the 3.5 miles to the trailhead by river or riverbank.

That decision spot is the location of Shenandoah River Trips, (800) 727-4371 or www.shenandoah.cc (see Hike 58, page 280, for details). The river journey takes about one to two hours and is both scenic and safe (even for beginners). You'll have a choice of canoe, kayak, raft, or tube, which you'll just leave at the state park for the outfitter to retrieve. The take-out point is at the park's canoe launch, near the trailhead (although tubers have to land almost a mile upstream from there and walk down to the trailhead).

To do the riverbank hike to the trailhead from the outfitter's, return to the junction of the gravel road and the River Ridge Trail. From there, bushwhack 50 yards across the grass to the left to reach and cross a small bridge to get onto the River Trail (green). The trail is easy to follow (when in doubt, stay to the left) and has a surface that is variously dirt, gravel, and grass. You'll be out in the open for roughly a mile and a half, with hayfields and horse-dotted pastures rising to low wooded bluffs on your right. And on the left, on the river's far bank, you'll see little more than a few small trailers and canvas "porches"—private summer camps—against a backdrop of forested slopes.

As you go around a well-kept cabin—the Brown Cabin—nestled in a bend of the river, mourn the sad fact that it's not available as a park rental cottage but is reserved for summer work crews and other official guests. Watch on your right for the tin-roofed cabin you passed earlier; note the stovepipe chimney and porch, and try to connect what you see with the fact that almost a century ago, the building was the railroad-ticket office in Bentonville. Then, after passing the tube take-out and a picnic table, you'll be on the broad, mile-long, and shaded Paw Paw Trail (black) leading to the trailhead.

NEARBY/RELATED ACTIVITIES

Sample the park's programs, which include kayaking, a night float, "River Rocks/ White Socks" (for snorkelers), campfires, and a riverbank night hike; contact the park for details. Arrange to sample the trails on horseback starting at Indian Hollow Stables, (540) 636-4756. Do historic Front Royal's self-guided walking tour; get the free guide at the visitor center, (800) 338-2576 or **www.ci.front-royal.va.us.**

OVERALL RUN AND HEISKELL HOLLOW

IN BRIEF

Definition of dream hiking venue: a secluded, protected, and accessible area of rugged, forested, and stream-laced mountains; abundant flora and fauna; well-marked but very lightly used trails; vista-rich overlooks; and rock pools that welcome a hiker's body and spirit—in other words, Overall Run and Heiskell Hollow.

DESCRIPTION

The northern section of Shenandoah National Park straddles the Blue Ridge in northwestern Virginia somewhat more than 60 miles west of the Capital Beltway. Tucked away on the section's western flanks, about 10 miles southwest of Front Royal, lies an isolated and rugged area of side ridges and hollows that, for me, form one of the park's very best hiking venues.

My hike in this area (as previewed in the June 2006 issue of *Sierra* magazine) consists of a strenuous modified-loop trek of 12 miles, with 5,500 feet of elevation change. Also included here is a slightly easier 10-mile version with 4,500 feet of elevation change. Both

KEY AT-A-GLANCE INFORMATION

LENGTH: 12 miles (with shorter options)

CONFIGURATION: Modified loop

DIFFICULTY: Extremely hard

SCENERY: Forested mountain slopes and valleys, cliff-top overlooks, sun-dappled streams with hiker-usable rock pools

EXPOSURE: Partially shady; much less so in winter

TRAFFIC: Usually very light

TRAIL SURFACE: Mostly dirt or grass, with much slippery-when-wet rockiness; some mud and rock-hop stream crossings after heavy rain

HIKING TIME: 6–7 hours

SEASON: Year-round, but best in high summer (the pools!) and winter (the leafless views!)

ACCESS: No restrictions

MAPS: USGS Bentonville; PATC Map 9

FACILITIES: None

FOR MORE INFORMATION: Visit park's Web site, www.nps.gov/shen; call park (540) 999-3500 (recording); consult *Potomac Appalachian Trail Club, Appalachian Trail Guide to Shenandoah National Park with Side Trails*

Directions ⟶

From Capital Beltway (I-495) in Merrifield, Virginia, take Exit 49 and get on I-66 heading west. Proceed for about 50 miles to Linden. There, leave I-66 at Exit 13, take first left, go under I-66, and take first right to get onto US 55 heading west. Proceed for 5.3 miles to Front Royal, turn left onto US 340, and drive south for 9.3 miles to Bentonville. There, just before post office, turn left onto VA 613 (Bentonville–Browntown Road), go 0.75 miles, turn right onto VA 630 (Thompson Hollow Road), and then proceed for about 2 miles, almost to road's end, and pull over into small parking area on right.

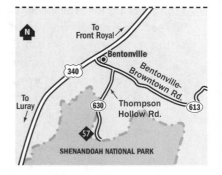

57 Overall Run and Heiskell Hollow

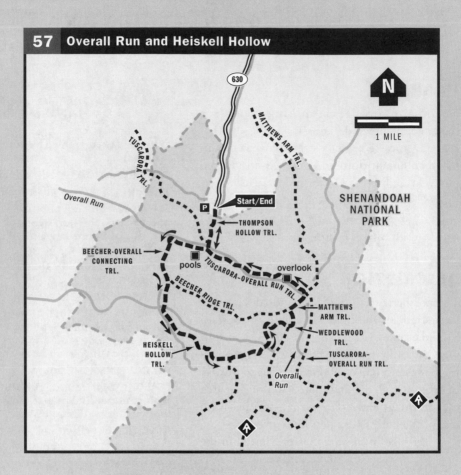

versions make fine use of Overall Run, a rocky, tree-lined stream dotted with cascades, waterfalls, and rock pools. The stream's lower course includes a wonderful cluster of pools that, in warm weather, invite hiker indulgence. That's why I often refer to this outing simply as "the pools hike."

The trails are named and blazed, and junctions are marked by concrete signposts. Some trail names, such as Heiskell Hollow Trail, invoke the area's prepark history, when such broad trails were dirt roads linking mountain communities. This section of the park contains few other reminders of the impoverished families that were displaced, starting in the 1920s, to make way for the national park—essentially a long-term experiment in returning exhausted land to wilderness. Eight decades later, the land carries heavy stands of oaks, hickories, and other hardwoods, with a healthy understory of bushes and wildflowers. And, from what I've seen, it is home to such creatures as bears, foxes, deer, bobcats, and rattlesnakes.

To get started from the trailhead, continue on foot to the end of the road, go around a chain gate, and head downhill on an unpaved driveway. At the bottom, turn right onto a narrow dirt trail—the Thompson Hollow Trail—and follow it past a boundary marker and into the park. You'll be on it for about a mile, heading uphill and then downhill through tangled and scrubby woods, and some fire-swept areas. En route, you will pass through a T-junction, and thereby also be on the blue-blazed Tuscarora Trail. At the next T-junction, take note of where you are, because you'll be returning there later in the hike using the trail that goes off to your left. This time, turn right to get onto the rather rocky Overall Run Trail and follow it gently downhill alongside its namesake stream.

About 200 yards down the blue-blazed Overall Run Trail, watch for an unmarked side trail on the left and use it to take a 100-yard detour for a preview of the pools area. Then continue down the main trail for 0.5 miles until it ends. There, turn left to get into the Beecher-Overall Connecting Trail and pick your way across lower Overall Run's several channels (rock-hop if the water level is high). On the far side, the dirt trail pitches quite steeply uphill for about 0.75 miles through an area of blueberry bushes. Pause as you climb, especially in summer (yes, you're allowed to collect fruit, nuts, and seeds in the park).

As the trail levels out, you'll reach a T-junction in a clearing, which provides the hike's first distant views (thanks to wildfires). There, turn right to stay on the connecting trail for another 0.75 miles as it curves mostly downhill into lower Heiskell Hollow. (Alternatively, to do the shorter, 10-mile version of the hike, go straight through the junction to get onto the yellow-blazed Beecher Ridge Trail, and follow it for 2.3 miles uphill.) After crossing a rock-strewn area and a stream, clamber up the bank to reach and turn left onto the blue-blazed Heiskell Hollow Trail.

At that point, be prepared for a long but mostly steady climb of about 1,500 feet over the course 3.1 miles. The first 1.8 miles and most of the elevation gain are on the broad, dirt-and-grass-surfaced Heiskell Hollow Trail. Turn left at the next trail junction to get onto and continue uphill on the narrow, somewhat rocky, and yellow-blazed Weddlewood Trail. Finally, after going straight through the next signposted T-junction, you'll reach the Weddlewood's junction with the yellow-blazed Mathews Arm Trail. Pause there to take a break, drink, and credit for having covered 7 of the hike's 12 miles and all but about 300 of its 2,500 feet of elevation gain.

Turn left onto the broad and mostly open Mathews Arm Trail (another old road) and gradually descend more than 0.5 miles to a T-junction, where you'll pass the uphill terminus of the Beecher Ridge Trail on your left (in case you're doing the shorter hike). Continuing on the level for 0.6 miles, you'll cross upper Overall Run (a stepping-stone challenge when the stream is full), and then swing left onto a rocky stretch of trail. At the next T-junction, turn left to stay on the Mathews Arm Trail, which stays twinned with the Tuscarora–Overall Run Trail for 200 yards. Watch on the left for a tree-shaded 30-foot cascade that's worth a look. At the next T-junction, turn left to leave the Mathews Arm Trail and to stay

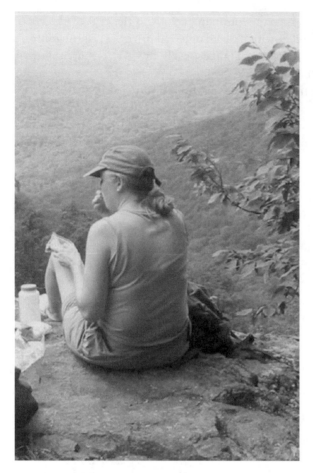

on the Tuscarora–Overall Run Trail.

The next segment of the trail has a narrow, rocky, and twisty character that should make you pay attention to your feet as it drops 1,400 feet over 2 miles. Halfway down, when the trailside landscape on the left disappears, raise your eyes to see that, 8.6 miles into the hike, you're on a cliff top dotted with several overlooks that work well as lunch stops. I recommend the overlook marked by a small tree with a crooked lower trunk. On a clear day, the view is to the west, where the great dark wall of Massanutten Mountain rises to the sky, and yonderer (as Carl Sandburg would say) loom the majestic Alleghenies. There's no direct sign of human activity anywhere in sight, and the feeling of wilderness is often enhanced by the wheeling presence of hawks and vultures, and the coarse cawing of ravens. Nearby, when water is plentiful, Overall Run continues downhill as a 93-foot plume—and the park's highest waterfall. Continuing, take your time in making your safe way downhill on what is the hike's steepest and rockiest part. Although the trail flattens out when it rejoins Overall Run, it doesn't give up its rockiness until it gets close to the T-junction with the combined Thompson Hollow–Tuscarora Trail, 1.8 miles from the overlook.

Proceed through the junction and down the trail for 200 yards to the turnoff for the pools. First, you'll find a dark pool deep enough for diving. Below that, the stream gently sluices across a smooth rocky surface with shallow depressions that nicely fit the recumbent human body. Then the stream feeds a little pool that's just right for standing and is bounded by a rock rim that serves as an armrest. Then it plunges down to a broad and shallow pool where one can swim short laps. Indulge yourself as you choose, and accept as a strange but welcome bonus that the insects in the pools area neither bite nor sting. Then retrace your steps the 1.4 miles back to the trailhead, using the Thompson Hollow Trail.

NEARBY/RELATED ACTIVITIES

Enhance your pool stay by secreting a well-stocked cooler there early in the hike. Return at another time to do a leisurely 3-mile round-trip hike to the pools with children and the cooler. On the posthike drive back, stay on two-lane and scenic US 55 to Delaplane before getting back onto I-66. En route, stop at the astonishing Apple House (in Linden near I-66 Exit 13) and pick apples at Stribling Orchard (in Markham, on VA 688 just south of US 55 and near I-66 Exit 18); for more information on these places, see page 264).

58 MASSANUTTEN MOUNTAIN AND SHENANDOAH RIVER

KEY AT-A-GLANCE INFORMATION

LENGTH: About 12 miles each on trail, river (with a lesser option)

CONFIGURATION: Out by trail, back by river

DIFFICULTY: Hard–extremely hard

SCENERY: Upland woods, Shenandoah Valley vistas and peeks, river views, Shenandoah hippos

EXPOSURE: Mostly shady on trail; shadeless on river

TRAFFIC: Very light on trail; light–moderate on river (rafting and tubing parties can make a difference)

TRAIL SURFACE: Mostly dirt, with much rock, gravel; moving water, with rapids, rocks

HIKING TIME: 4.5–5 hours at above-average pace; plus 3–5 hours on river (see text)

SEASON: Best from June–September (see text)

ACCESS: No restrictions on trail; outfitter's rules on river

MAPS: USGS Bentonville, Rileyville; PATC Map G

FACILITIES: Toilets, water, phone, camp store at outfitter's; grungy toilet at Seekford Landing

FOR MORE INFORMATION: See end of Description

IN BRIEF

Well west of Washington, D.C., lie scenic Massanutten Mountain and the Shenandoah River's lovely South Fork. They're so well arranged that a hike on one can be paired with a canoe trip on the other.

DESCRIPTION

This outing is an out-and-back excursion in the form of a 12-mile trek along a vista-equipped rocky mountain ridge, followed by a 12-mile canoe ride on a beautiful, rapids-dotted river. The ridge is a lofty one atop Massanutten Mountain, a massive, free-standing range in the Shenandoah Valley some 65 crow-miles west of Washington. The river is the Shenandoah River's exceptionally scenic (but, alas, polluted) South Fork, which meanders northward along the eastern foot of the range. The transfer point is Seekford Landing, where, by arrangement, the trekkers ford the river to switch to canoes (or kayaks) delivered by a trailhead outfitter.

Devised by veteran hiker and adventurer Cliff Noyes, this hike-and-paddle combo is a long day's journey into delight, especially

----

Directions

From Capital Beltway (Interstate 495) in Merrifield, Virginia, take Exit 49 and get onto I-66 heading west. Proceed for about 50 miles to Linden. There, leave I-66 at Exit 13, take first left, go under I-66, and take first right to get onto VA 55 heading west. Proceed for 5.3 miles to Front Royal. There, turn left and south onto US 340 and drive 9.3 miles to Bentonville. There, just past post office (on left), turn right onto VA 613 (Indian Hollow Road) and drive 0.8 miles to riverfront parking lot of either of two outfitters at Bentonville Landing.

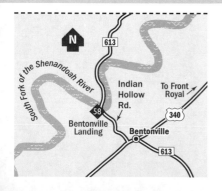

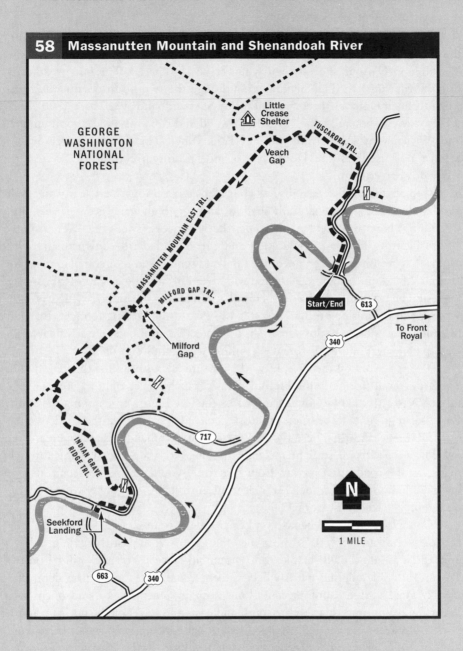

when it's organized as a group activity. It provides a strenuous and satisfying workout for both the upper and lower body, as well as for the senses. And it's best suited for people who can hike fairly fast for close to five hours while enduring about 4,100 feet of elevation change—and then paddle for three to five hours.

Plan on doing the outing when the weather is warm, the river level is right, the outfitters are open, hunters are absent (the Massanutten is part of George Washington National Forest), and you are well prepared. The best weather is usually from June through September, although the two outfitters operate from April through October. I recommend using Shenandoah River Trips, (800) 727-4371 or **www.shenandoah.cc,** which is owned and run with grace, good humor, and efficiency by Edith Appleton and Trace Noel. The other outfitter, which I have not used, is the Downriver Canoe Company, (800) 338-1963 or **www.downriver.com.**

Contact the outfitters to discuss your plans and options. Very low water isn't good because the river is naturally shallow, and very high water is dangerous. But, says Cliff, "Ninety percent of the time, the water level's just fine." That's why you're likely to have an exhilarating and current-aided ride downstream, over rapids that even novices can negotiate safely. I recommend that you plan to arrive around 7:30 a.m. to sign in, get fitted with a paddle and life jacket, obtain a river map, and be briefed by Trace; to be on the trail by 8 a.m.; to be on the water by 1 p.m.; and to finish by 6 p.m. Also plan to take along wading footgear (or plan to canoe in wet boots), plus sunscreen or protective clothing; to put valuables in waterproof bags; and to tie down everything when you're in the boat.

To get started on the hike, leave the outfitter's and head for the blue-blazed Tuscarora Trail (formerly the Big Blue Trail), which passes right by a gravel-surfaced VA 613 (Indian Hollow Road). Cross the low causeway spanning the South Fork. Keep going, and bear left at a fork about 50 yards down the road. Walk a third of a mile and then bear right at a fork onto Panhandle Road (which takes over as VA 613). Go straight through the junction after that. Passing through fields, as the road curves away from the river, you'll begin to ascend and be hemmed in by scrubby woods. At a clearing, turn left—or roughly west—to stay on the blue-blazed Tuscarora Trail.

Coming up next will be a second clearing, a "Road Closed" sign, and a gate across the trail (roughly 1.75 miles into the hike). Walk past the gate and head up a dirt trail amid oaks, maples, and mountain laurels. You will still be on the Tuscarora Trail, but the path will get steeper, the pines more prevalent, and the sky more visible. Continue on a long, straight, steep, rocky, and open trail. Savor the panoramic views to the south and east, and look for the curlicue South Fork 1,000 feet below and Shenandoah National Park spread across the horizon. Look more closely and try to discern your trailhead, some 2 crow-miles away. And search the sky for hawks, turkey vultures, ravens, and crows.

Trekking upward, you'll finally slide into a shady area and a trail junction. There, say good-bye to the Tuscarora Trail and turn left onto the orange-blazed Massanutten Mountain East Trail. At that point, you'll be done with the hike's most arduous uphill and over half of its elevation gain, and be almost a third of the way to the boats. Staying on or close to the crest of a long ridge, the trail extends south for almost 5 miles as one of the finest and wildest stretches of mountain trail in this book, if not the metro area. It has beguiling scenery that's more rockscape than landscape and offers some splemdid vistas. The trail bumps up and down and the surface ranges from rocky to very rocky, but you won't face any stiff climbs. Just be sure to stay left at each trail fork.

Be especially attentive at four places along the ridge trail. First, at a trail fork about 2 miles down the trail, swing left, as the blazes do. This rocky, below-the-crest trail has gorgeous views to the left. After that, emerge onto the crest and look left through the trees for glimpses of the Massanutten's western ridges. Second, thread your way carefully through the intersection at Milford Gap, the hike's 7-mile mark. There, the ridge trail crosses an old road that was once part of a stagecoach route across the Massanutten. That road—now the Milford Gap Trail—slides downhill at the intersection. But you should follow the orange blazes uphill and south. Third, heading downhill out in the open, stop at a huge rock and take in what I think is one of the ridge trail's best vistas. Finally, after negotiating the hike's rockiest stretch, watch for a signpost and a small oak daubed with orange and purple blazes. There, turn left onto the purple-blazed Indian Grave Ridge Trail to follow the hike's last segment.

The 2.5-mile-long trail follows a wooded side ridge that pushes east between two loops of the river (as is visible on a map, but not on the trail). The reputed burial mound is said to be somewhere in the woods and well plundered. Initially, the trail is steep and rocky. But the pitch slackens as the trail traverses a wet, muddy, and ferny area near the head of a small stream. It then veers to the right, away from the stream, and proceeds along a rocky hillside, where it's reassuring to see purple blazes again. After going steeply downhill again, the trail becomes flatter, wider, and less rocky. It then passes through an unattractive, disheveled area and reaches a gate and "Road Closed" sign. Walk around the gate and across a clearing. Proceed for about 40 yards on an old unpaved road, and then turn right onto a newer, gravel road. That's VA 717, which leads slightly downhill and around several curves for just over a mile.

As the road curves south and west, the high ridge bearing the ridge trail south of the colorful oak will loom directly ahead. At the end of an open field, and after passing a couple of telephone poles, turn left onto an unpaved side road—the first you'll encounter on VA 717. Walk a few hundred yards on the level and shady road. Where it curves to the left, watch for a dirt trail going right for about 15 yards to Seekford Landing.

Next, ford the rocky-bottomed, 200-yard-wide river. Aim for a small sand-bar slightly upstream on the far side, which is where canoes are typically left. Wear appropriate footgear and with empty pants pockets, cross the river as a group (if you have one). Once across, get going on your 12-mile cruise to the trailhead, paying close attention to the outfitter's river map.

For a less rigorous outing, do an out-and-back hike to the Tuscarora Trail's junction with the ridgetop trail for an aerobic outing of 7.4 miles, about 2,600 feet in elevation change, and lovely views; then have the outfitter launch you 3 miles or 7.5 miles upriver so that you can also spend time on the water.

For more information on Massanutten Mountain, contact the U.S. Forest Service's Lee District headquarters in Edinburg, (540) 984-4101; for more information on the trails, contact the Potomac Appalachian Trail Club, (703) 242-0693 or www.patc.net.

NEARBY/RELATED ACTIVITIES

Make the most of canoeing down a gorgeous river. I recommend pulling out for a picnic and a swim just below Compton Rapid. If you get to the outfitter's to find that you can't get on the river, do the Overall Run and Heiskell Hollow hike instead (Hike 57, page 275).

Also, to train for this arduous outing on the mountains and river, do my Shenandoah River State Park hike and its canoeing option see Hike 56, page 270).

APPALACHIAN TRAIL:
Blue Ridge Center to Weverton | 59

IN BRIEF

On this eclectic trek, hikers visit three states, cross two famous rivers, traverse a much-fought-over town, and sample two great trails, a rocky ridge, and a private preserve.

DESCRIPTION

Some 60 miles northwest of Washington, D.C., the AT leaves the Blue Ridge to span the Shenandoah River, pass through history-soaked Harpers Ferry, and then cross the Potomac River to head downstream between that river and the ruins of the storied C&O Canal. My aim here is to encourage you to do exactly the same thing—and get to know the Blue Ridge Center (BRC).

- -

Directions ────────────────▶

Car shuttle is required, so first drive to car drop-off and then convoy to trailhead. From junction of Beltway (Interstate 495) and I-270 spur in Maryland, drive northwest for 31 miles on I-270 to Frederick. At Exit 32, swing right to get onto I-70. Proceed for 0.4 miles and, at next fork, stay to left to get onto I-70 heading west. Proceed for 0.9 miles and then turn right at next fork (I-70 exit 52) to get onto US 340 heading west. Proceed for about 14.5 miles. Then turn right onto MD 67, go 0.1 mile, turn right onto Weverton Road, and go 0.2 miles to gravel parking area on right. Park there, at car drop-off. Next, get back on US 340 heading toward Harpers Ferry. Go 1.8 miles, crossing Potomac River, and turn left at first traffic light onto Harpers Ferry Road (VA 671). Go south for 2 miles to Neersville and watch on right for small "Blue Ridge Center for Environmental Stewardship" sign. There, turn right and take gravel entrance road for 0.3 miles to parking area near barnlike main building.

KEY AT-A-GLANCE INFORMATION

LENGTH: 10.7 miles

CONFIGURATION: One-way

DIFFICULTY: Hard

SCENERY: Mountain woodlands, valley peeks, townscapes, river views

EXPOSURE: About half shady; less so in winter

TRAFFIC: Usually very light; heavier in Harpers Ferry, especially in lower town on warm-weather weekends, holidays

TRAIL SURFACE: Chiefly dirt and grass at Blue Ridge Center; rocks and dirt on AT; pavement and stone in town; dirt on towpath

HIKING TIME: 6–7 hours

SEASON: Year-round, but town itself mostly closed in tourist off-season

ACCESS: No AT or in-town restrictions; Blue Ridge Center, towpath open daily, dawn–dusk

MAPS: USGS Harpers Ferry, Charles Town; PATC Map 7; local sketch maps

FACILITIES: None at car drop-off; toilets at trailhead; toilets, water, phones in town

FOR MORE INFORMATION: Contact or visit Appalachian Trail Conservancy (in town), Harpers Ferry National Historical Park visitor center, Blue Ridge Center; for details, see text

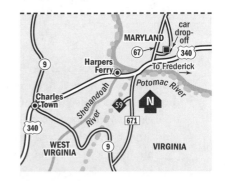

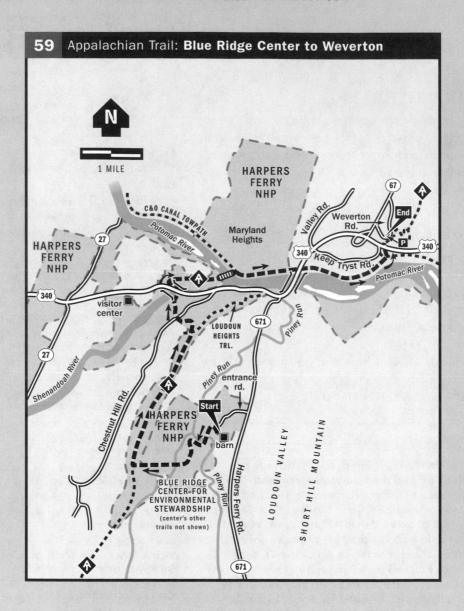

The Georgia-to-Maine AT was conceived in the 1920s by a forester, planner, and visionary named Benton MacKaye. A primitive version was in place by 1937, but it took decades to refine the route, secure public ownership, and arrange permanent maintenance. Now officially called the Appalachian National Scenic Trail and under National Park Service administration, the 2,168-mile trail is managed by the Appalachian Trail Conservancy (ATC) and maintained by local organizations and their volunteers. The Potomac Appalachian Trail Club (PATC), for example, takes care of the AT and its side trails throughout the mid-Atlantic states.

Harpers Ferry lies on a promontory bounded by the Potomac and its chief tributary, the Shenandoah, just upstream from where the Potomac punches through the Blue Ridge. A federal arsenal was built there in the 1790s. The arrival of the railroad and C&O Canal early in the 19th century spurred the town's growth as an industrial center and transportation hub. In October 1859, abolitionist John Brown led a raid on the arsenal to initiate his campaign to free Virginia's slaves. The raid fizzled, but helped ignite the Civil War less than two years later. During that conflict, Harpers Ferry was taken and retaken by both sides enough times to leave much of it in ruins. In the following decades, it was battered by a series of floods. Eventually, Congress stepped in and designated much of it as a national monument in the 1940s and then as a national historical park in 1963. Harpers Ferry National Historical Park now covers more than 2,500 acres in three states, and the town itself is West Virginia's most visited tourist attraction. Its restored and replicated buildings form a quaint and industry-free mini-version of the grimy antebellum community.

This hike can be rewarding year-round. Late spring is colorful on the out-of-town trail segments, thanks to trees, wildflowers, and migrating birds. Summer is colorful in town, thanks to bedecked tourists. Fall paints pretty pictures on the upland trail segments—and you should wear something orange because the protected AT right-of-way is narrow (but all three states do have a no-hunting-anywhere-on-Sunday rule). Winter is more monochromatic, but offers solitude, silence, and leaf-free views.

This 10.7-mile one-way hike (with 3,000 feet of elevation change), starts at what is officially the Blue Ridge Center for Environmental Stewardship. Rich in wildflowers, wildlife, and butterflies, the 900-acre former farm was bought by the Robert and Dee Leggett Foundation to both help buffer the AT lands and serve as an open-to-the-public preserve involved in conservation, organic farm- ing, education, recreation, and research (for details, visit **www.blueridgecenter .org**). Opened in 2004, it has 12 miles of mostly signposted and well-mapped trails (free sketch maps are available at BRC).

From the parking-area trailhead (BRC map in hand), walk back down the entrance road for about 60 yards, and turn sharply left onto an old road. After passing a pond, stay left at a fork and proceed through several intersections as the road gives way to dirt trails. At a Little Turtle Trail signpost, turn left and care- fully rock-hop across Piney Run, swing left along the stream, and continue. Next, you'll turn right onto the Arnold Trail, pass a campsite (on the left), cross Sweet Run, and turn left onto the Wood Thrush Trail. At a power-line right-of-way, turn right onto Butterfly Alley (not named on the BRC map), and follow the pylons steeply uphill to turn right onto the AT, 2.6 miles into the hike.

For the next 2.4 miles, you'll mostly ease uphill on a rocky trail that wigwags between Virginia and West Virginia and is shaded by oaks, hickories, beeches, and maples. Then, on reaching a fork marked by a large brown trail sign, turn left and plunge downhill for about a mile. (To the right is the blue-blazed Loudoun Heights Trail, which was part of the AT until the AT was re-routed through Harpers Ferry in the mid-1980s.) Halfway down, be careful crossing Chestnut Hill Road. And in July, turn right to walk along the road for 50 yards to a right-of-way where, says hiker-forager David Bailey, you'll find wineberries galore (they're now-wild raspberries native to Asia).

You'll finally reach level ground, where US 340 crosses the Shenandoah River, at the hike's 5-mile mark. There, take an underpass beneath the heavily traveled highway and then a bridge walkway across the river. Walk along US 340 for about 100 yards, cross Shenandoah Street, and follow the white blazes of the undulating AT eastward through the town on what's initially a dirt trail and then a paved one. En route, watch for a signpost marking a side trail to the headquarters of the ATC—also reachable at (304) 535–6331 or www.appalachiantrail.org.

Turn left when you reach a white-blazed brown sign. Then continue to follow the white blazes so that you swing right at a fork and go straight through a four-way intersection. Proceeding downhill, veer right to visit flat-topped Jefferson Rock. The view impressed pre-presidential Thomas Jefferson in 1783: "The passage of the Potowmac through the Blue ridge is perhaps one of the most stupendous scenes in nature." The Potomac is no longer clearly visible, and the rock itself is probably not the one Jefferson knew. But the view of the Shenandoah remains splendid.

Back on the main trail, continue downhill. Take a flight of steps hewn in a sloping slab of rock, passing Harper House on the left. Completed around 1780, it's now the town's oldest existing house and open to the public (take a peek). Owner Robert Harper ran a flour mill nearby, provided ferry service for his farmer customers, and is commemorated in various local names in addition to the town's (those rock steps, for instance, are carved in Harper phyllite). At the bottom of the steps, turn right onto High Street. On reaching Shenandoah Street at the bottom of the hill, turn right to get to the park's visitor center, in the exhibit-filled Master Armorer's House. Nearby are small museums, souvenir shops, and eateries.

Then walk back along Shenandoah Street, reach the restored and relocated federal armory, and turn right under an old trestle to reach a spacious overlook. There, you'll get panoramic views of the river junction and the forested slopes rising on all sides. Note the obelisk marking where Colonel Robert E. Lee captured John Brown. Then head for a bulletin board on the Potomac side of the overlook area and get on a brick walkway that leads to a footbridge across the river.

On the far and Maryland side, you'll find the C&O Canal towpath, the ruined canal, and rarely more than a few tourists. Turn right onto the towpath, which, for the next 3 miles, stays close to the river and doubles as a weirdly flat stretch of the AT. Note Loudoun Heights off to the right, and what Jefferson called "the terrible precipice hanging in fragments over you"—meaning Maryland Heights—to the left.

In Weverton, turn left at a bulletin board and AT signpost pointing left to start the hike's final half mile. Use the grade crossing—over an active railroad line—to get to a road that turns sharply left. Walk across a grassy triangle to pick up the AT, which heads uphill and under US 340. At the next intersection, go left and follow the customary white blazes. Leave the AT where it passes close to your waiting car.

NEARBY/RELATED ACTIVITIES

Further explore the lower town, using free maps and other guides from the visitor center, (304) 535-6029, and from the park's Web site, **www.nps.gov/hafe.** Take the Virginius Island Trail for a fascinating look at the town's industrial heritage and ingenious use of waterpower. Ask about the park's many ranger-led tours and other events. Return to hike up Maryland Heights. And be sure to sample more of BRC's delightful trail system.

60 ROLLING RIDGE FOUNDATION LANDS AND APPALACHIAN TRAIL

KEY AT-A-GLANCE INFORMATION

LENGTH: 8.9 miles (with shorter options)

CONFIGURATION: Modified loop

DIFFICULTY: Moderate–hard

SCENERY: Hilly woodlands, with great views from AT overlook

EXPOSURE: Mostly shady; less in winter

TRAFFIC: Usually very light

TRAIL SURFACE: Mostly dirt or dirt and gravel; some rocky upland stretches; some grassy stretches also prone to muddiness

HIKING TIME: 5–6.5 hours

SEASON: Year-round, but best in spring and when leaves are down

ACCESS: No restrictions, but contact resident manager before visiting

MAPS: USGS Round Hill; PATC Map 7; free sketch map of property (available from resident manager)

FACILITIES: Toilet on lower end of Friends Trail

FOR MORE INFORMATION: Contact resident manager Sheila Bach, (304) 728-8743 or snbach@earthlink.net; visit Friends Wilderness Center (www.friendswilderness.org); visit Rolling Ridge Study Retreat Community (www.rollingridge.net), for information on property's history

IN BRIEF

In West Virginia's Jefferson County, some 20 miles south of Harpers Ferry and 13 miles east of Charles Town, lies a remarkable private nature sanctuary that is dedicated to the preservation of the area's native plants and animals, open to the public with permission, and (as the owner foundation suggests) "ideal for meditative retreats, hiking, bird watching, and nature study."

DESCRIPTION

The nonprofit Rolling Ridge Foundation owns about 1,400 acres of land on the heavily hardwooded western slopes of the Blue Ridge just

---

Directions

From Capital Beltway (Interstate 495) in McLean, Virginia, take Exit 45 to get onto Dulles Toll Road heading west. Proceed for 12.2 miles (going past Dulles airport) to toll plaza for Greenway. Continue on westbound Greenway for 12.4 miles to outskirts of Leesburg. Stay in left lane (Exit 1A), which curves left and merges into westbound VA 7. Proceed on VA 7 for 4.1 miles, and then turn right onto 0.2-mile-long exit ramp to reach westbound VA 9. Stay on VA 9 (which becomes WVA 9) for 15.7 miles, passing through Hillsboro and Mannings. Just beyond Mannings, turn left onto Mission Road and proceed southward for 6.3 miles. Then, at Rolling Ridge sign, turn left onto unpaved road (actually Mission Road continued) and bear in mind that next 1.6 miles are on rough, narrow, twisty, and rocky-in-places country roads, as follows: Go 0.8 miles and turn right at four-way intersection; go 0.4 miles and turn left at "Niles Cabin Retreat" sign at next intersection; go 0.4 miles, following "Niles Cabin Retreat" signs (ignore "Retreat House" sign) and taking two right turns to reach cabin; park on gravel if possible.

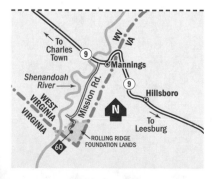

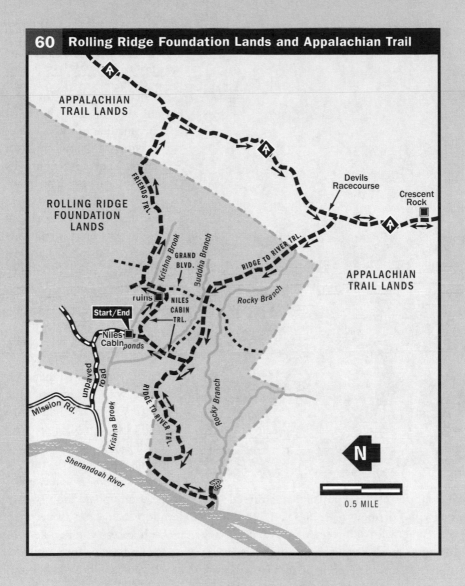

60 Rolling Ridge Foundation Lands and Appalachian Trail

APPALACHIAN
TRAIL LANDS

ROLLING RIDGE
FOUNDATION
LANDS

FRIENDS TRL.

Krishna Brook

GRAND
BLVD.

Buddha Branch

Devils
Racecourse

Crescent
Rock

RIDGE TO RIVER TRL.

APPALACHIAN
TRAIL LANDS

Rocky Branch

ruins

NILES
CABIN
TRL.

Start/End

Niles
Cabin ponds

Rocky Branch

RIDGE TO RIVER TRL.

unpaved road

Mission Rd.

Krishna Brook

Shenandoah River

N

0.5 MILE

east of the Shenandoah River. Rich in flora and fauna, the preserve is the legacy of Henry and Mary Cushing Niles, a Quaker couple who established the foundation in 1974 to preserve the land in perpetuity, as well as to provide for the use of the property "to minister to the needs of people for the strengthening of spirit, mind, and body." Accordingly, three nonprofit organizations lease small areas on the property for educational or humanitarian purposes. One of them is the Friends Wilderness Center (FWC), a Quaker organization that maintains the Niles Cabin Retreat (a 40-year-old building on the site of the original farmhouse,

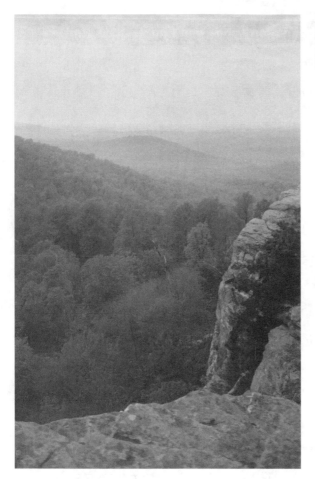

This photo only hints at why, when I take hikers to the open cliff top at Crescent Rock, I have such a hard time getting them to leave.

which was lost to fire) and an outdoor area intended for meditation and other activities in harmony with nature. The center and its effervescent resident manager welcome both Quakers and non-Quakers to attend its events and programs and to hike on a network of trails.

The principal trail is the Ridge to River Trail, which was constructed in cooperation with the National Park Service. I have incorporated that trail, along with a segment of the nearby Appalachian Trail (AT), into an 8.9-mile hike with 2,600 feet of elevation change that covers much of the preserve. If you want to do a shorter hike, use my map and directions to do either an upland loop (with a great vista) of about 6.4 miles and 2,000 feet of elevation change, or a river loop of 3 miles with 600 feet of elevation change. In both cases, you're likely to encounter much flora, some fauna (deer and maybe even a bear or fox), and few or no other people (except at an AT overlook). (*Note:* If you're interested in hunting, ask Rolling Ridge resident manager Sheila Bach, page 290, where and when it is allowed on the property in fall and winter.)

The hike's first mile consists of several short trail segments that zig and zag and go a little uphill to the meditation area. Starting from the Niles Cabin, head for the nearby pond, and follow the grassy bank counterclockwise past a bench and around the pond to a signposted intersection. There, go straight and gently uphill on a dirt trail. Then turn right onto a broad grassy trail and keep going. Pause, though, to veer left to walk around some old house foundations and a large restored chimney. Then swing left at what looks like an intersection but isn't, and proceed. Turn left at the next signposted T-junction onto an old gravel road, which is grandly called Grand Boulevard. Follow it across a tiny stream and then uphill. At the next T-junction, also signposted, turn right to stay on the briefly combined and generally level Grand Boulevard and Friends Trail. At the T-junction after that, turn right again to proceed on the Friends Trail.

From that point on, the trail is initially broad and level but then becomes narrow, rocky, somewhat eroded, and upwardly inclined. After a few hundred yards, after passing a "Quiet" sign, you'll reach a picnic table and fire circle in a small woodland clearing on the left. That's the FWC's meditation area, which also includes a roofed tree house, a yurt, and a toilet. Pause to explore or perhaps use the area, and then step around a large fallen tree and continue uphill for 1.1 miles on what was once a steep wagon road. As you go, pause to catch your breath. Also, watch on the right for a few spindly American chestnut trees, which are remarkable for simply being alive (a blight wiped out the U.S. chestnut forests during the first half of the 20th century).

Continuing, you'll cross the unmarked boundary between the Rolling Ridge property and the federally owned AT lands and be on a trail that becomes progressively fainter. On reaching a fork on level ground, ignore the trail to the right that curves downhill. Instead, swing left and take the trail that goes gently uphill, and pick your way past the small fallen trees that crisscross the trail. When the trail seems to disappear, keep going for about a hundred yards or so and look to your right for rock outcrops and a gently rising wooded slope. Pick your way uphill for about 20 yards and you'll suddenly find the AT beneath your feet (at the hike's 2-mile mark). It's just a narrow, rock-bordered dirt trail in the woods with not a trail sign in sight. Turn right and head south. You'll be on the white-blazed trail for 1.6 miles, going mostly downhill on a rocky treadway in thick woods.

On the last 200 yards, just after crossing a power-line right-of-way, you'll be walking downhill alongside a dramatic boulder field known as the Devils Racecourse. At the bottom, where the AT joins the signposted Ridge to River Trail (3.6 miles into hike), turn left to scramble across the boulder field and stay on the AT for a 1.2-mile out-and-back side trip to Crescent Rock. You'll climb quite steeply for 0.3 miles and then reach a fork, where you should stay on the AT by staying to the right and continuing for another 0.3 miles gently downhill to Crescent Rock, on the right. There, you'll be on an open cliff top with superb views of the Shenandoah Valley to the west and northwest, and on clear days, you'll see the sunlight glinting on the Shenandoah River.

Then leave the overlook and return to the AT's junction with the Ridge to River Trail (4.8 miles into the hike). From there, do as that trail's name suggests and hike the 2.5 mostly downhill miles to the river. You'll be on old farm roads for much of the way, but be careful to follow the blue blazes. So, just after passing the southern end of Grand Boulevard on the right, leave the road and swing left onto a blue-blazed woodland trail. While on that trail, take note of—but ignore for now—a T-junction where a purple-blazed trail goes off to the right. At the end of the trail, turn right onto an old road, follow the blue blazes for 150 yards, and then turn left past a gate to continue on another old road. Eventually, you'll be on the well-wooded floodplain and an often-muddy road leading to the Shenandoah River (7.3 miles into the hike).

Rest a while there, or even take a dip. Then start retracing your steps uphill. Soon after leaving the river, watch on the right for Rocky Branch, a small stream that's about to join the river. Follow a narrow and steep dirt trail up that stream bank for about a hundred yards to see a small waterfall and also the six stone viewing chairs left there long ago by the Niles family. Then resume your return journey. When you get back to the purple-blazed trail (the Niles Cabin Trail), turn left and follow it as it crosses an old road and then, as an undulating grassy trail, crosses a small stream and takes you uphill to the trailhead area (8.9 miles into the hike).

NEARBY/RELATED ACTIVITIES

I recommend doing the hike as an AT loop and a river loop with a prepared lunch at the Niles Cabin in between (by arrangement with Sheila Bach), thereby adding about 0.5 miles to the hike's total distance. Also consider reserving space for an overnight stay at the cabin; it has two comfortable bedrooms, a screened porch, lots of nature-related reference books, modest rates, and an accommodating live-in chef. In summer, staying over fits nicely with a late-afternoon dip in the river or the pond closest to the cabin, as well as with stargazing on a clear night. And check with Sheila (see page 290) about upcoming events at Friends Wilderness Center and about the long and long-planned Perimeter Trail.

60 HIKES
WITHIN 60 MILES

WASHINGTON, D.C.
INCLUDING
SUBURBAN AND OUTLYING AREAS OF
MARYLAND AND VIRGINIA

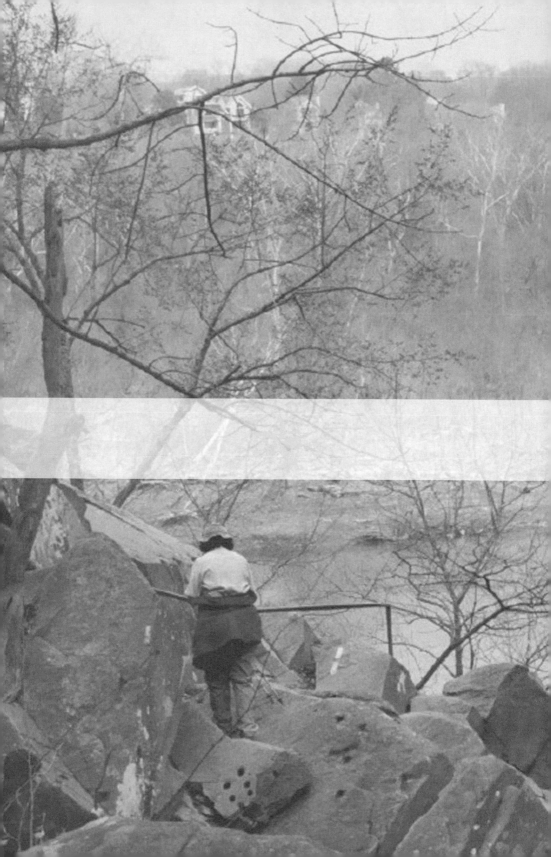

APPENDIXES AND INDEX

APPENDIX A:
HIKING CLUBS AND OTHER INFORMATION

All of the following regional or local organizations offer group day hikes year-round. Some of them also organize backpacking trips, bike rides, canoe outings, trail maintenance and other kinds of service trips, and social events. All of them post outings schedules on their Web sites, and some also provide printed versions.

Aleph Outdoors
groups.yahoo.com/group/aleph-outdoors

Appalachian Mountain Club,
Washington, DC, Chapter
www.amc-dc.org
www.outdoors.org
(AMC's national Web site)

C&O Canal Association
www.candocanal.org

Capital Hiking Club
www.capitalhikingclub.org

Center Hiking Club
www.centerhikingclub.org

Chesapeake Hiking and Outdoor Society
www.chaoshikers.org

Maryland Outdoor Club
www.marylandoutdoorclub.org

Mosaic Outdoor Mountain Club of Maryland
www.mosaics.org/maryland

Mountain Club of Maryland
www.mcomd.org

Northern Virginia Hiking Club
(703) 440-1805
www.nvhc.com

Potomac Appalachian Trail Club
(703) 242-0963 *(call for activities tape)*
www.patc.net

Sierra Club, Maryland Chapter
maryland.sierraclub.org

Sierra Club, Maryland Chapter's
Howard County Group
maryland.sierraclub.org/hc

Sierra Club, Metropolitan Washington
Regional Outings Program
(Organizes outings for the club's Maryland, Virginia, and Washington, D.C., chapters)
(202) 547-2326
www.mwrop.org

Wanderbirds Hiking Club
www.wanderbirds.org

Washington Women Outdoors
www.washingtonwomenoutdoors.org

APPENDIX B:
PLACES TO BUY MAPS

ADC Map & Travel Center
www.adcmap.com
1636 I Street NW
Washington, DC
(202) 628-2608, (800) 544-2659

Eastern Mountain Sports
www.ems.com
2554 Solomon's Island Road
Annapolis, Maryland
(410) 573-1240

2800 Clarendon Boulevard
Arlington, Virginia
(703) 248-8310

Plus store in Timonium, Maryland

Hudson Trail Outfitters
www.hudsontrail.com
4530 Wisconsin Avenue
Washington, DC
(202) 363-9810

12085 Rockville Pike
Rockville, Maryla
(301) 881-4955

1101 South Joyce Street
Arlington, Virginia
(703) 415-4861

Plus stores in Annapolis, Gaithersburg, and Towson, Maryland; Fairfax and Springfield, Virginia

L. L. Bean
www.llbean.com
10300 Little Patuxent Parkway
Columbia, Maryland
(410) 715-7020

1961 Chain Bridge Road
McLean, Virginia
(703) 288-4466

Potomac Appalachian Trail Club
www.patc.net
(Produces and sells excellent topographic and trail maps)

118 Park Street SE
Vienna, Virginia
(703) 242-0693
7 p.m.–9 p.m., Monday–Thursday;
noon–2 p.m., Thursday and Friday

REI
www.rei.com
9801 Rhode Island Avenue
College Park, Maryland
(301) 982-9681

1701 Rockville Pike
Rockville, Maryland
(301) 230-7670

3509 Carlin Springs Road
Baileys Crossroads, Virginia
(703) 379-9400

11950 Grand Commons Avenue
Fairfax, Virginia
(703) 522-6568

Plus store in Timonium, Maryland

APPENDIX C:
HIKING STORES

Eastern Mountain Sports
2800 Clarendon Boulevard
Arlington, Virginia
(703) 248-8310
Plus two other metro-area stores

Fleet Feet
1841 Columbia Road NW
Washington, DC
(202) 387-3888

Galyan's
2 Grand Corner Avenue
Gaithersburg, Maryland
(301) 947-0200

12501 Fairfax Lakes Circle
Fairfax, Virginia
(703) 803-0300

Hudson Trail Outfitters
4530 Wisconsin Avenue
Washington, DC
(202) 363-9810

12085 Rockville Pike
Rockville, Maryland
(301) 881-495

1101 South Joyce Street
Arlington, Virginia
(703) 415-4861
Plus five other metro-area stores

L. L. Bean
10300 Little Patuxent Parkway
Columbia, Maryland
(410) 715-7020
Plus store in McLean, Virginia

Metro Run & Walk
1776 East Jefferson Street
Rockville, Maryland
(301) 984-2900

7516 Leesburg Pike
Falls Church, Virginia
(703) 790-3338
Plus store in Springfield, Virginia

Mountain Trails
212 East Cork Street
Winchester, Virginia
(540) 667-0030

Pacers
1301 King Street
Alexandria, Virginia
(703) 836-1463

3100 Clarendon Boulevard
Arlington, Virginia
(703) 248-6883

Patagonia
1048 Wisconsin Avenue NW
Washington, DC
(202) 333-1776

REI
9801 Rhode Island Avenue
College Park, Maryland
(301) 982-9681

1701 Rockville Pike
Rockville, Maryland
(301) 230-7670

APPENDIX C:
HIKING STORES (CONTINUED)

REI *(continued)*

3509 Carlin Springs Road
Baileys Crossroads, Virginia
(703) 379-9400

11950 Grand Commons Avenue
Fairfax, Virginia
(703) 522-6568

Plus store in Timonium, Maryland

The Sports Authority

110 Odendhal Avenue
Gaithersburg, Maryland
(301) 926-3445

3701 Jefferson Davis Highway
Alexandria, Virginia
(703) 684-3204

8355 Leesburg Pike
Vienna, Virginia
(703) 827-2206

Plus 11 other metro-area stores

DEAR CUSTOMERS AND FRIENDS,

SUPPORTING YOUR INTEREST IN OUTDOOR ADVENTURE, travel, and an active lifestyle is central to our operations, from the authors we choose to the locations we detail to the way we design our books. Menasha Ridge Press was incorporated in 1982 by a group of veteran outdoorsmen and professional outfitters. For 25 years now, we've specialized in creating books that benefit the outdoors enthusiast.

Almost immediately, Menasha Ridge Press earned a reputation for revolutionizing outdoors- and travel-guidebook publishing. For such activities as canoeing, kayaking, hiking, backpacking, and mountain biking, we established new standards of quality that transformed the whole genre, resulting in outdoor-recreation guides of great sophistication and solid content. Menasha Ridge continues to be outdoor publishing's greatest innovator.

The folks at Menasha Ridge Press are as at home on a white-water river or mountain trail as they are editing a manuscript. The books we build for you are the best they can be, because we're responding to your needs. Plus, we use and depend on them ourselves.

We look forward to seeing you on the river or the trail. If you'd like to contact us directly, join in at www.trekalong.com or visit us at www.menasharidge.com. We thank you for your interest in our books and the natural world around us all.

SAFE TRAVELS,

Bob Sehlinger

BOB SEHLINGER
PUBLISHER

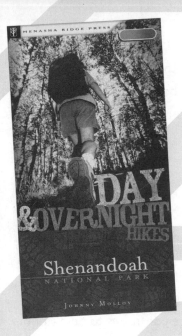
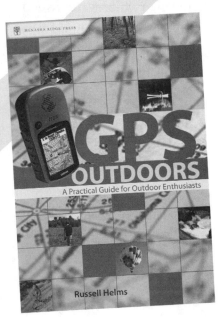